Introduction Surgical Nursing

3

Introduction to Surgical Nursing

Edited by

Penelope Simpson MSc, Dip Ed, Cert Ed, DN (Lond), RCNT, RN
Senior Lecturer, School of Health Studies, University of Portsmouth, UK

A member of the Hodder Headline Group
LONDON • SYDNEY • AUCKLAND

First published in Great Britain in 1998 by
Arnold, a member of the Hodder Headline Group
338 Euston Road, London NW1 3BH

British Library Cataloguing in Publication Data
A catalogue record for this book is available from the British Library

Library of Congress Cataloging-in-Publication Data
A catalog record for this book is available from the Library of Congress

ISBN 0 340 63176 7

Publisher: Clare Parker
Production Editor: James Rabson
Production Controller: Rose James
Cover design: Mouse Mat Design

Composition in $9\frac{1}{2}/11\frac{1}{2}$ Palatino by Photoprint, Torquay, Devon
Printed and bound in Great Britain by The Bath Press

Contents

List of contributors

Marva D.F. Brown
Senior Nurse Manager, Royal National Throat, Nose and Ear Hospital, London, UK.

Lysette G. Butler, RN, RNT, DipN, Cert Ed (FE)
Gynaecology Ward Manager, Southend Health Care Trust, Southend, UK.

Clare Carroll (née Beattie) RN, RCNT
Freelance nurse, London, UK.

Mark Collier BA(Hons), RN, ONC, RCNT, RNT
Nurse Consultant in Tissue viability/kinetic therapy, KCI Medical Ltd, Witney, Oxon, UK.

Helen Fawcett-Adamson BSc(Hons), RN, Cert M
Product Manager, Fresenuis Ltd, UK.

Vivienne Mathews RN, RNT, Cert Ed
Senior Lecturer, University of Portsmouth, Portsmouth, UK.

Dominic Mawdsley BA(Hons), (UEA), BA(Hons) (Manchester), RN
Senior Lecturer, Department of Health and Continuing Professional Studies, De Montfort University, Leicester, UK.

Anne Murray RN, RCNT, DipEd, BSc(Hons)
Nurse Tutor, Nottingham University School of Nursing, Nottingham, UK.

Helen Neary
Sister, Cardiothoracic Intensive Care Unit, Southampton General Hospital, Southampton, UK.

Somduth Parboteeah MSc, DipNurs, RCNT, RNT, RN
Senior Lecturer, School of Health Studies, University of Portsmouth, Portsmouth, UK.

Barbara Richards RN, Dip. in Otolaryngology
Clinical Nurse Manager, Royal National Throat, Nose and Ear Hosptial, London, UK.

Penelope Simpson MSc, DipEd, CertEd, DN(Lond), RCNT, RN
Senior Lecturer, University of Portsmouth School of Health Studies, Portsmouth, UK.

Jennifer S. Wesson RN, ENB100 & 998
Sister, Cardiothoracic Intensive Care Unit, Southampton General Hospital, Southampton, UK.

Preface

Introduction to Surgical Nursing is designed for nurses working in surgical settings, be they students, qualified nurses in a new specialty, returners to nursing or enrolled nurses converting to first level.

The book's purpose is to back up the precise and focused care of the patient undergoing a variety of commonly performed surgical procedures. It thus cannot be a comprehensive guide to every type of surgery. It need not be used in isolation, nor read from cover to cover: it is an 'enquire within', to be dipped into when needed.

The first thing asked of readers is that they be familiar with the relevant anatomy and physiology, and individual specialist chapters may suggest texts for this.

The first part of the book covers general principles of care for the patient undergoing surgery.

The specialist chapters that follow identify the specifics of care for a range of problems. Principles of care are offered, as policies and practice will vary in detail from place to place.

Throughout, references to research and publications are made to support the material, and further readings are offered.

Technical language is used, as it has very precise meanings, so use of a nurses' dictionary may be advisable. A glossary can be found at the end of the book. Where possible, we have quoted from the patients' own experiences.

On the whole, we have referred to the patient by one sex or another for the sake of a more comfortable flow of language. The first section uses the feminine gender.

Penelope Simpson

PART ONE

Introduction to surgical nursing

1

Penelope Simpson

Introduction

The special function of the surgical nurse is to support patients through this major event in their lives. To the team, much of what nurses do becomes routine and obvious, but it is alien to the patient, so a constant 'drip-feed' of information and explanation is essential.

The whole process of becoming a patient can be disorientating, debilitating and dysfunctional. There is, first, the condition for which the surgery is required, second, the surgery itself, and, third, the anaesthetic to contend with, physically, emotionally and socially. The surgical nurse has to take account of where the patient was admitted from and is returning to in order to offer appropriate individual levels of care, support and information. The more detailed knowledge that the nurse is able to provide, the more likely is her

care to be effective. This implies an awareness not only of the patient's physical state, but also of her levels of psychological and social well-being, as these markedly influence her recovery.

Orem's self-care nursing model has relevance to surgical nursing, with its trend towards ever-shorter stays. The nurse can act for or do for the patient, guide and support the patient, provide an environment that promotes personal development and teach the patient (Behi, 1986).

Holistic care offered as part of a health service (rather than a sickness service with a 'repair shop' mentality) suggests that we function as health promoters in our everyday work, enabling our patients to make healthier choices as a result of our interventions. There is, in the section on leaving hospital, below, a checklist of areas to consider when planning for discharge, which starts as soon as the patient is admitted. Using convalescence creatively can be enormously helpful to patients, some of whom respond very well to a 'nursing prescription' after discussions of what is relevant to them. The subtle use of a nursing history is likely to highlight lifestyle areas that might respond to guidance. Taken to its logical conclusion, this may well save some patients from readmission. As all projections predict that surgical nurses will become busier, this would appear to be a cost-effective way of working.

What is surgery?

Surgery is usually an invasive procedure, involving cutting through normal structures in order to correct deformity, improve function or remove diseased tissue, leaving an external or internal wound or scar. Some surgery is exploratory, investigative or diagnostic. Some form of anaesthesia is always available (see p. 21).

One significant feature of surgical nursing is that a rapid change can occur in the patient's condition. A seemingly healthy, independent patient can be temporarily rendered acutely ill and totally dependent by the combination of the operation and the anaesthetic. Other patients arrive in very poor condition and are much improved by surgery. For some, surgery is only palliative, i.e. it does not cure the basic problem, but provides much-needed relief from symptoms in order to improve quality of life.

The routes by which patients present for surgical nursing care include:

- planned admission from the waiting list;
- emergency admission from Accident and Emergency department (A&E), outpatient department (OPD), another ward or hospital, or via the GP;
- transfer from the OPD, another ward or a different hospital.

Introduction

The purpose of surgical nursing is to support the patient safely through pre-operative preparation, anaesthetic, operation, recovery, the post-operative phase, convalescence and follow-up. Giving information is an essential part of the surgical nurse's role.

Communication, or information flow

Since a general anaesthetic may render a patient incapable of identifying herself or securing her own safety, the accurate flow of information to, from and about patients is vital to prevent errors, from simple misunderstandings to performing the wrong operation. How the written documentation is organized varies from unit to unit. Most of the suggestions in this section relate to the person who is undergoing planned surgery, with additional material about surgical emergencies and day cases.

Providing information can reduce the incidence of post-operative complications, including infection (Boore, 1978; Bysshe, 1988; Bond and Barton 1994).

Pre-admission

Once a patient knows her admission date, the following information is needed:

- patient handbook – what to bring; a drug form for the GP to complete;

- A briefing sheet on the operation – what is involved, length of stay;
- A telephone number for further information.

This information should be available in other languages, large print and audiotape and video-tape versions. Many people are unaware, for example, that driving after a general anaesthetic is illegal for 5–10 days because of slowed reaction times.

Patient comments

'I wish the handbook had suggested ear-plugs.'

'I needed to ask someone about the nitty gritty of the operation.'

Someone who is admitted as an emergency will have had no such preparation time. Neither the patient nor family will have had a chance to adjust to the realization that surgery is needed. The physical and mental preparation of the patient may be limited to the absolute essentials, which may increase the risks of the surgery and anaesthetic.

DAY SURGERY

Patients may be considered suitable for day case surgery, in which case information needs to be precise and unambiguous. The benefits of such surgery include increased comfort and conveni-ence for the patient, less stress and disruption for the family, less time off work and the psycho-logical benefit of no overnight stay. Patients unsuitable for day case surgery are those who:

- have a chronic illness such as heart disease, insulin-dependent diabetes, severe psychiatric disorder or obesity;
- have no adult to take them home and to support them there for the first 24 hours after surgery;
- do not have access to a telephone;
- live more than a 30-minute car journey from the hospital.

Markanday and Platzer (1994) and Bond and Barton (1994) make a case for nursing pre-assessment of day case patients to ensure that they are checked, carefully selected, and well prepared. Information in various formats must be available for patients to take away and digest. Overnight beds must be available for the 1 in 50 patients who do not feel up to going home at the end of the day.

Patient comment

'It was so much more comfortable to recover in my own bed.'

Other advantages include reduced risks of cross-infection and the comfort of being at home and able to move freely to promote circulation, thus reducing the risk of deep venous thrombo-sis.

MINIMAL ACCESS SURGERY

The massive increase in the use of 'keyhole' sur-gery will have major implications. The surgeon operates using a miniature camera at the end of a telescopic tube, inserted into the body through a minute incision. Further tiny incisions are made for long-handled instruments, guided via a tele-vision monitor. It is likely that a high percentage of surgery as we know it can be undertaken either as day case procedures or within a minimal-access surgery facility, with specially trained staff and adjacent hotel facilities for pre-discharge patients (Cushieri, 1994). The advant-ages to the patients include:

- reduced waiting-list times;
- fewer last-minute cancellations;
- shorter hospital stays;
- reduced trauma;
- less post-operative pain;
- faster recovery rates;
- fewer respiratory and wound complications.

The whole team will need training in the skills needed to support patients undergoing these procedures.

Admission

Next will be admission to the unit itself. The ward is likely to have a printed list of planned admissions, with outline information on the prob-able surgery for each person, so that the staff know whom to expect. It helps information flow and improves the welcome if beds are already allocated for patients before they arrive. Wound infection rates can be higher in open wards with a bed occupancy of 25 or more (Bibby *et al.* 1986), which may influence choice. If documents are also assembled ready for completion, it is apparent to all staff, although not yet to the patient, which member of the team will be caring for her. Some similar form of preparation is necessary for those arriving as emergencies, providing there is sufficient warning, and for those having day surgery.

On arrival at the ward, the patient should be welcomed and taken to her bed without delay. This is where an effective ward clerk can add immeasurably to the smooth functioning of the team. The nurse needs to introduce herself and outline the likely sequence of events and what the patient is expected to do. An information sheet in every locker, plastic coated and in large print, can back up verbal details. These may include a map of the ward and a description of the nursing team, even of which uniform means which level of nurse. It is necessary for the patient to identify 'her' named nurse as soon as possible, thus starting to reduce unpleasant disorientation.

Patient comments

'Nothing reinforces the feeling of being the lowest form of life more than staff busily hurrying about, and ignoring you.'

'It was so helpful to see things in print and to reread them several times'.

The admission process is used to:

- show the patient around;
- meet the team;
- identify the word routines;
- observe the patient;
- get to know her;
- identify her worries, fears and strengths;
- take a nursing history (see p. 7);
- generate a care plan with the patient to prepare her for surgery, anaesthetic and convalescence.

Patient comments

'I felt such a fool, wandering around, looking for my nurse, not realizing that I was allowed to ring.'

'I didn't want to bother the busy nurses to ask the way to the bathroom.'

At some stage, the patient will also be seen by the surgical house officer or registrar and 'clerked'. This involves checking information gained in the OPD and any pre-admission tests and investigations, reviewing the state of the main body systems and arranging for further checks to ensure fitness of the patient for anaesthetic and surgery. These may include a chest X-ray and full blood screen. Some units now perform these at a pre-admission clerking clinic to cut down the time in hospital waiting for the results. This system is ideal for patients having day surgery. The consequent reduction in the patient's hospital stay, thus avoiding colonization of the patient's skin by hospital bacteria (Spencer and Bale, 1990), is a cost-effective move. The concept of a nursing assessment and medical work-up 10–14 days before admission to hospital is supported by Bond and Barton (1994) and Haines and Viellion (1990), the latter believing it inappropriate to expect an anxious patient to learn new information the evening before surgery.

For clerking and examination, the inpatient may need to wear nightclothes. Check what access is needed. Many of the questions are relevant to how the patient is to be nursed. Consider delaying taking the full nursing history until you have seen the post-clerking, completed medical notes. Another advantage of the nursing history following the medical history is that the nurse may require more details from the patient about a particular area in order to plan effective nursing intervention. Also, the patient herself may require clarification on some points previously made.

Patient comment

'Don't these people talk to each other? I have answered that question before.'

Once all inpatients have been visited, the surgical house officer or registrar generates an operation list from which the whole team works, in order to co-ordinate their efforts and to make sure that things go as smoothly as possible.

Identification

Formal identification of the patient using a plastic wrist-band must be handled tactfully. It can make the patient feel depersonalized if combined with an inappropriate use of nightclothes. The information on the band should include name, age or date of birth, hospital identification number and ward name. This should preclude a problem should there be another patient of the same name in the hospital at the same time. It enables identification of patients at all times, particularly when they are unable to answer for themselves, such as during general anaesthesia.

Pre-operative visits

The anaesthetist visits the patient pre-operatively and needs access to the medical notes, results of relevant tests and significant nursing information in order to assess the patient's fitness for anaesthetic. At this stage, premedication, post-operative pain relief and anti-emetic therapy will be prescribed. The patient should be encouraged to discuss any anaesthetic concerns with the anaesthetist. It is a good idea for patients to jot down their questions in order to make the most of the interaction.

Pre-operative visits by theatre nurses occur in some units, enhancing the patient's level of preparedness and ensuring an individualized approach to patient care. This may be seen as part of the implementation of primary nursing in theatre or as a practice designed to improve information flow and hence patient care (Wicker, 1990). Patients can find it immensely reassuring that they are 'known' to someone in the strange environment of the operating theatre. This has the potential to increase the level of effective communication between ward and theatre nurses, and lessen the patient's anxiety (Martin, 1996). The potential problems that can be detected by this pre-operative assessment visit may include, for example:

- specific anxieties about the anaesthetic – patients can be better informed by the theatre

nurse, who can in turn ensure that the anaesthetist is informed;
- generalized worries about the operation, which may be allayed by more precise information;
- mobility difficulties that affect positioning on the table – a specific per-operative care plan will be generated for that patient;
- sensory deficits, such as hearing or visual impairment, requiring additional communication support.

Selected patients will be visited pre-operatively by a physiotherapist who will teach them exercises to perform immediately post-operatively. The physiotherapist will need access to the medical and nursing records. In some units, the physiotherapist is able to write a plan on the patient's nursing documents which are kept at the bedside, so that the whole team is informed and can maintain the regimen.

Patients may need the services of a dietitian, cancer care counsellor, social worker, stoma nurse or other clinical nurse specialist for their particular needs, as determined at assessment.

Pre-operative preparation

The objective of pre-operative nursing care is to render the patient in the best possible condition for surgery and convalescence. Thus, she must be carefully assessed, including taking a nursing history. In some cases, such as unconsciousness or confusion, the history may have to be obtained from a carer.

Nursing history and patient assessment

The patient needs time to settle into the ward before she can identify what she needs to know. The process is really an exchange of information: for the team to best prepare her, and so that she herself can feel well-prepared.

Most units work to some sort of nursing model, such as those of Roper, Logan and Tierney, or Orem (Aggleton and Chalmers, 1986) in order to assess their patients systematically to agreed criteria. Within this, it is likely that each nurse will develop her own eclectic model based on what has been found to be effective.

The areas that need to be assessed depend to some extent on the magnitude of the proposed surgery and the degree of urgency.

A system-by-system approach may benefit some, while others work better with broader guidelines. Some suggestions are offered here on areas that may need to be covered by the nursing history and assessment:

BREATHING

The respiratory system will have been examined by the house surgeon. The team needs to identify any problems in order to minimize the respiratory complications of the anaesthetic. Some indications will be given by the patient's colour and her ability to complete a long sentence without pausing for breath. Another way is to find out how far she can walk, and how fast, before becoming breathless. An exercise tolerance test such as stairclimbing may be indicated. Anxiety may well be making the patient breathe more quickly than normal, and pain may cause shallow breathing. The patient may be asthmatic, so check whether she has brought her inhaler with her.

Smoking not only increases anaesthetic risk and the incidence of post-operative respiratory complications, but is also associated with chronic cardiovascular and respiratory pathology (Wilson-Barnett and Fordham, 1982). Explain to the patient the need to reduce smoking to the absolute minimum prior to surgery. It may be helpful to find less destructive ways in which the patient

can deal with her anxiety, such as visualization, relaxation and/or distraction.

CARDIOVASCULAR SYSTEM

The state of the heart and blood vessels is relevant to the physical response to the anaesthetic and operation. The findings enable the nursing team to monitor the patient's condition, using the blood pressure and pulse as a reference point. To take these readings very shortly after admission for planned surgery is illogical, as the anxiety associated with becoming a patient is likely to distort the findings. A more realistic set of measurements will be achieved when the patient has been put more at ease. They can then be relied on as a baseline, to identify when the post-operative patient is returning to her normal levels.

For the emergency admission patient, a series of recordings is needed to determine the progress and condition of an already sick person. None of these readings can be truly regarded as baseline, but only as a detection of trends.

CLEANSING/DRESSING/MAINTAINING BODY TEMPERATURE

The patient's ability to achieve a reasonable degree of personal hygiene needs to be assessed. Any help she requires can be found out by tactful questioning and by offering the level of support she might find helpful. A plan can then be written to minimize her having to explain to each member of the team what is required.

The patient's clothes are a form of non-verbal communication, indicating something about her mental state, ethnic origin, economic status and self-care abilities. The extent to which she can dress and undress herself must be determined in order to plan for any necessary assistance. By noticing the fit of her clothes, some impression of weight loss or gain can be acquired.

At some stage after admission, the patient's temperature is taken to use as a baseline. A raised temperature may indicate an infection, which may preclude surgery. This needs to be reported. The temperature is usually also taken on the day of surgery for the same reason.

DYING/SENSE OF LOSS/PLANS FOR THE FUTURE

The varying emphases needed in these areas of assessment will emerge from the questions the patient chooses to ask, or more significantly, not to ask. Some people have a real fear of dying under anaesthetic, and if the team do not elicit such fears and help to alleviate them, there are implications for patient safety. The possibility of death or disability may be highlighted by the proximity of other sick people or by the patient's diagnosis. Ask her what she thinks is wrong with her and what this means to her. This can highlight misconceptions and areas of ignorance that can then be tackled. The care plan can then be based upon what the patient knows or fears.

For most people, an operation is a major event. It may make them question their values, habits and beliefs. Many feel the need for spiritual comfort at this time, even if this does not feature much in their everyday lives. It is thus worth asking the patient about her religious observances in order to be able to offer the services of the relevant minister. It also ensures that the team do not unknowingly violate religious prohibitions.

Loss of autonomy can be part of becoming a patient; she may feel no longer in control of her life but at the mercy of others. Some fear the loss of control they feel is part of being unconscious during the operation. They worry, for example, about loss of continence or about saying something embarrassing.

Patient comment

'I was terrified that I would blurt out some dark secret.'

The nurse needs to assure her that these events are highly unlikely, and that privacy will be secured.

As surgery usually involves the removal of some body tissue, there may be a sense of loss related to a change in body image. This may be no longer feeling whole and healthy or may be a major mental reorganization in coming to terms with what is perceived as a mutilation. The nurse needs to use all her counselling skills to determine the patient's postion and help her to cope. Many units can call on a range of nurse specialists, such as breast care counsellors and stoma nurse specialists, to help in this.

The patient may have been so preoccupied with her impending surgery that she may not have thought beyond it. Part of assessing the patient's needs includes identifying what she thinks will happen to her after the operation. As a result, short- and long-term plans can begin to be made, from estimating her length of stay in hospital, through the immediate convalescent phase to plans for further into the future.

EATING

Taking an effective dietary history can be vital to the patient's well-being during and after surgery, providing significant findings are acted upon. Unacceptably high levels of malnutrition have been consistently reported in surgical patients (Lennard-Jones, 1992). It has been found that malnourished patients heal better when their nutritional status is improved before surgery than when it is only improved post-operatively (Stotts, 1992). Scanlon et al. (1994) have developed a tool with a scoring system, and an action plan, based on the Waterlow system. A diary/recall system, which seems to be useful and accurate, involves the patient writing down what she remembers eating and drinking the previous day, then the day before that, and so on, as far back as she can recall. Once she has done this, it needs to be established whether this is her typical diet or whether it has recently changed. If there has been recent change, for example owing to diarrhoea and/or vomiting, it may be possible to discount this: what counts is what the patient *usually* eats. One way of looking at such a system and checking crudely for balance is to use the 'tilted plate' method. It can be a helpful health-promotion tool if the analysis is carried out with the patient. For this, each food consumed is assigned to one of six main groups:

- vegetables and fruit;
- carbohydrates;
- proteins;
- dairy products;
- sugars and alcohol;
- fats and oils.

The amount consumed in each group is then assessed by weight. The best pattern for food balance is:

- vegetables and fruit: raw, cooked, frozen, dried and juice – 33%;
- complex carbohydrate foods – 33%;
- proteins, including nuts, eggs and pulses – 12%;
- dairy (low fat) – 14%;
- oils, fats, sugars and alcohol – keep to 8%.

STUDENT ACTIVITY

Recall your food intake over the past 24–48 hours.
  Record the amounts in the relevant sections and estimate the relative weights.

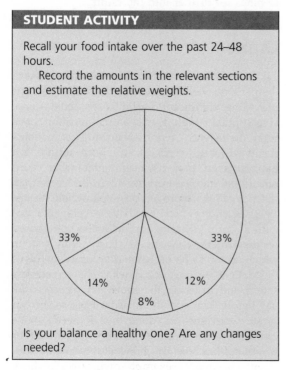

Is your balance a healthy one? Are any changes needed?

If an unhealthy pattern is noted, the nurse could work with the patient on how to adapt her diet during convalescence to promote good healing. Verbal advice will need to be backed up in writing. The aim is to tap into the patient's motivation to return to normal. A dietary change lasting for about 3 months can become a habit and less likely to revert.

Deficiencies of energy, protein, vitamins or minerals may affect drug metabolism, altering drug toxicity. The toxicity of the drug is generally increased when it exerts a direct action on tissue and decreased if metabolism must take place before the drug can act (Holmes, 1986).

After elective surgery, the patient's energy expenditure increases by 24%. This increase in nutritional requirement results from the stress of the operation increasing the patient's blood cortisone level and thus raising metabolic rate. Malnutrition is of concern because it has been associated with impaired immune response, prolonged recovery and an increase in the risks of the surgery itself (Moynihan, 1994).

ELIMINATION

Questions about the patient's usual elimination patterns and any recent changes are best treated in a matter-of-fact approach to a potentially embarassing area. The purpose is to establish the current pattern. Every patient thinks her pattern is normal, but some interesting variants can emerge.

Patient comment

'I get up to pass water about three times a night, just like everyone else.'

Early on in the admission process, a specimen of urine is tested to exclude renal problems. Some opportunistic diagnoses of diabetes mellitus are made by this route.

It may be appropriate to use this opportunity to teach the patient pelvic floor exercises:

1 The patient sits with her feet slightly apart, abdominal and buttock muscles relaxed.

2 She is asked to imagine that she is trying to stop herself passing wind from the bowel by squeezing the muscle around the anus.

3 This muscle needs to be squeezed and lifted so that the patient can feel it move. Her buttocks and legs should not move at all.

4 She is then asked to imagine that she is bursting to pass urine, and to tighten the ring of muscles to prevent a leak, holding it for 4 seconds. She must not push her legs together, and must let the contraction go slowly.

5 This movement needs to be repeated four times, and the whole sequence repeated as often as she remembers during the day, every day.

6 Persistence markedly reduces the risk of stress incontinence. It can be helpful to have a written prompt for the patient to work from.

Ensure that the patient has had an effective bowel action before she goes to theatre. If help is needed, laxatives, suppositories or an enema may be used. More rigorous preparation of the bowel will be dealt with in Chapter 8.

EXERCISE AND ACTIVITY

The amount of exercise taken by the patient needs to be established as part of her overall fitness assessment. How active a person is prior to surgery can affect her ability to 'bounce back'. If she starts from a reasonable baseline, even if she has not been able to achieve as much recently, she will still be in a better position than someone who tends to be inactive.

There is no reason why most patients should become sedentary on arrival in hospital. On a working day, it is likely that a person will be active for an average of 8.5 hours, which falls to 3.5 hours in hospital. The time in bed or a chair can increase from 15.5 to 21.5 hours (Wilson-Barnett and Fordham, 1982). Providing patients are available when members of the team need to see them, they should be positively encouraged to keep active while they can move freely without pain. This can help to reduce the risk of deep venous thrombosis.

Risk factors for thromboembolism (Caprini et al., 1988) include:

- Age over 40 years
- Prior major surgery
- Previous thromboembolism
- Immobilization
- Stasis – congestive cardiac failure, myocardial infarction, cardiomyopathy, constrictive pericarditis, leg oedema, venous stasis and varicose veins
- Cancer
- Sepsis
- Stroke
- Obesity
- Inflammatory bowel disease
- Pregnancy
- Oestrogen therapy
- Nephrotic syndrome
- Polycythaemia rubra vera
- Inherited risk factors

All those at risk should be fitted with anti-embolism stockings and scheduled for early ambulation and leg elevation. Those with two or more risk factors should be prescribed anticoagulant therapy such as heparin.

EXPRESSION OF SEXUALITY/TAKE-UP OF HEALTH SCREENING

There is great potential for the nurse to act as an effective health promoter in these areas while the patient may be more receptive to health suggestions.

How the patient expresses her sexuality is not necessarily the nurse's concern, but being a source of accurate information on contraception and/or safe sex is. A woman of childbearing age may be taking the contraceptive pill, for example, which tends to speed up blood clotting time, and hence increase the risk of deep venous thrombosis. It may be the nurse who finds out that the patient has failed to stop taking the pill in anticipation of surgery and must therefore inform the medical staff in case anticoagulant therapy is indicated.

The nurse can find out whether the patient attends health-screening activities appropriate to her age and sexual activity. If she does not, for example, attend for cervical smears, there may be a chance to discuss this and to explore any misconceptions. It could be an opportunity to teach breast or testicular self-examination. Leaflets on a range of topics can be made available to have most impact while patients are concentrating on their health.

Patient comment

'Having to have surgery did make me rethink some aspects of my sex life. It was very nice to be able to discuss it with someone knowledgeable.'

FLUID INTAKE, INCLUDING ALCOHOL

The fluid intake of the patient can also be established using a diary recall system. This results in a more accurate picture than do questions about 'typical' or 'usual' intake. The more neutral and non-judgemental the nurse's approach, the better. No comment needs to be made at this stage, except to encourage the patient to continue giving information. The nurse needs to determine whether the recalled intake has changed from what the patient perceives as 'normal'; again, what matters is the day-in, day-out intake. Assessment will include the level of caffeine intake from coffee, tea and cola drinks. No more than five a day of these are recommended, especially if they are taken full strength with no decaffeinated alternatives. The total volume needs to be estimated to confirm that the patient is drinking 30 ml/kg body weight per 24 hours, excluding alcohol, which is dehydrating. As the patient's fluid intake is likely to be restricted for the investigations and anaesthetic, she needs to be encouraged to drink the equivalent of one glass of water per hour while awake to ensure god hydration. Patients with renal or cardiovascular disease may have a more restricted intake.

When analysing the patient's alcohol intake, the nurse is looking for a healthy amount and pattern. A convenient way of estimating this is to use the unit system. A unit of alcohol is reckoned to be one glass of wine, one measure of spirits or half a pint of beer, these being pub measures, as home measures are inclined to be more generous. The safe limits are currently set at 21 units per week for men and 14 for women. A very light woman would not be safe at this level and would have to scale her intake down accordingly. The healthiest pattern is to avoid binging and to have two alcohol-free days per week. This is an area that cannot be ignored, as men with alcohol-related health problems now occupy one hospital bed in five, and women one in seven. Any person who is in the habit of drinking too much may not admit it but may manifest problems during their hospital stay. The actual pattern and amount may emerge over time once the patient trusts the nurse. 'Sanctioning' (Shanks, 1992) – permission from other people (the nurse) to recognize it as a problem and to seek help – may be needed.

HAIR AND NAILS

The state of the patient's hair may give clues to other areas of assessment. If the hair is poorly cared for, this may reflect loss of energy or motivation owing to the illness or to lack of mobility.

Dry, sparse hair may reflect an underlying condition such as hypothyroidism. Most patients need to be advised to wash their hair prior to surgery. Those who cannot will need help so that they enter the operating theatre in as clean a state as possible.

The patient's nails can be discreetly inspected when shaking hands, for example, or while observing them during the nursing interview. They may show the blue colour of cyanosis, indicating some deficit of oxygen intake, or the pallor of anaemia. The nails may be spoon-shaped from some long-standing cardiac problem. There may be flecks or horizontal ridges, showing general health problems, or the nails may be long and uncared-for, pointing towards a potential lack of self-care ability.

HEALTH/DRUGS HISTORY

These can be discerned from the medical notes, but the nurse needs to question the patient to clarify relevant issues. For example, some drugs may interact with food and have an impact on nutritional status (Holmes, 1986).

The patient may have brought in the prescribed drugs she is currently taking. The medical staff need to know about these, as decisions have to be made on which are to be continued. For example, it is probably important that short-acting beta-blockers are continued when the patient is fasted in the peri-operative period, in order to reduce the possibility of myocardial infarction or cerebral vascular accident resulting from rebound hypertension (Lloyd, 1989). The anaesthetist needs to know whether patients are taking monoamine oxidase inhibitors as these can interact with opiods such as pethidine, with fatal results (Bass and Kerwin, 1989; Coe and Laurent, 1989).

It is necessary to include questions about over-the-counter medicines, or recreational drugs that the patient may not view as drugs, which might interact unfavourably with other treatments. Equally, it is useful for the team to know about any current use of complementary therapy. A patient who misuses narcotic drugs may be aggressive, have communication difficulties and need very large doses of anaesthetics to achieve the desired effect. She will also be at high risk of HIV, be resistant to the effects of post-operative narcotic analgesics and be at high risk of their side-effects, including respiratory depression.

HOBBIES

These are relevant in showing the patient's life-style and can give pointers to physical, mental and social levels of activity. It is helpful to the patient to know that there will probably be a wait before surgery; some hobbies can be encouraged to fill the gap and relax the patient.

Patient comments

'If I had known that there would be all this hanging about, I would have brought in something to do.'

'I was so thankful that I had my own music with headphones. I was able to tune out the rest of the ward.'

Knowing the patient's hobbies can aid in offering precise, focused discharge advice.

HOUSING

The patient's living conditions, especially if the accommodation is in some way unsuitable for a convalescent patient, are relevant as discharge planning begins on arrival. She may need to arrange to stay with friends or family, or have someone to come in to help her. This is best organized while she is still relatively fit before surgery. It is useful to know whether she needs to be able to climb steps before she can be safely transferred home.

MENTAL STATE

Assessment is needed in order to tailor the flow of information to the patient's needs. Some clues will be gained during the initial interview and can subsequently be checked. The likelihood is that the anxiety of coming into hospital for surgery will to reduce most people's ability to concentrate and retain information. This state needs to be differentiated from:

- toxic states that can also temporarily affect short-term memory;
- more long-term mental health problems or learning difficulties.

Patients with a degree of pre-operative mental impairment may be vulnerable to the effects of anaesthesia (Carter, 1989), with a consequent impact upon their recovery time.

MOBILITY

This can be in part assessed by observation of how well and how much a patient can move, and will be backed up by thoughtful questioning about work, hobbies and any previous injuries. One way of determining limitations to movement is to ask the patient what she is unable to do for herself. This can be documented immediately as useful information for the nursing care plan. It may also be relevant to the position in which she will be placed during surgery. Referral to the physiotherapist may be needed.

MOUTH AND TEETH

The state of the patient's mouth and teeth needs to be established. Any loose teeth, crowns or caps must be documented, so that the anaesthetist is informed and can avoid vulnerable areas when passing tubes into the patient's mouth. Dentures must be removed before surgery. Ill-fitting dentures may be a cause of mouth ulceration or poor nutrition, and this needs to be rectified. It is helpful if dentures are labelled or at least if the patient has a marked container of water to place them in when not wearing them. This reduces the chances of their being mislaid while the patient is in theatre.

The tongue should be inspected and the mucosa checked for normal colour, freedom from ulcers, and so on. Any abnormalities must be reported as they may warrant further investigation, being indicative of other conditions. It can be useful to determine the patient's last visit to the dentist, with perhaps a suggestion that 6-monthly visits are best. If the patient's mouth is in a poorly cared-for state, some discussion might be indicated. In patients with black or oriental skins, the inside of the mouth or the eyelid will be where jaundice, cyanosis or pallor shows most clearly.

PAIN

A pain history can help to establish a diagnosis or achieve effective pain relief at an early stage of the patient's stay. Facts to elicit about the pain include its:

- intensity – how bad is it?
- duration – how long does it last/has it lasted?;
- location – where is it?;
- nature – what type of pain is it?, what words does the patient use to describe it?;
- triggers – what starts it off?;
- exacerbation – what makes it worse?;
- remission – what makes it better?

Observe the patient's hand gestures as she is likely to point to a sharp, localized pain. A more diffuse pain will be indicated by a circular hand movement over the offending area. Patients with communication difficulties may prefer to use a body outline chart to indicate the site of the pain. If a pen is used to mark the chart, the size of the area inked in has a bearing on the patient's perception of the pain. A 'serious' pain is often indicated by a large patch on the chart. This may mean either that it is very painful or that the patient is worried about it; facial expression will help to clarify this. A visual analogue scale in which 0 is no pain and 10 is the worst pain imaginable can be used. The patient marks on the line the level of her pain.

Anxiety and tension will tend to increase pain, so anything that will reduce the patient's anxiety is beneficial. It may be that simple relaxation exercises will enhance the patient's preparedness. If these are isometric (muscles are tensed and then relaxed in turn), they are unsuitable for those with hypertension. In such cases, the patient can be encouraged to focus her awareness on each area, rather than actually using the muscle, before consciously relaxing it. A quick relaxation technique suggested by McCaffery (1983) is:

breathe in deeply, clenching your fists
breathe out as far as you can and go limp all over
start yawning

This can repeated as often as necessary, keeping in sequence. A taped relaxation sequence can benefit many patients, enabling them to feel in control of their pain. One hospital radio broadcasted the tape at a specific time every evening, and patients were encouraged to tune in.

SKIN INTEGRITY

The condition of the patient's skin is assessed by questioning and observation, looking for potential or actual problems and noting bruises, rashes, ulcers, oedema, jaundice and soreness. For example, pimples in the area where the incision is to be made may be a reason to delay surgery until the infection has resolved. If the patient has many bruises but no recollection of trauma, she may have a clotting defect or a memory problem. The skin may show evidence of other problems that need addressing or resolving, such as allergies, recent body piercing (Langford, 1996) or intravenous drug use. A scoring system such as the Waterlow scale will assess the patient's risk of pressure sores. If the patient is in an 'at-risk' category, preventive measures can immediately be implemented. The assessment of the probable rate of healing will involve weighing up the 'plus' and 'minus' factors.

SLEEPING

Find out the patient's normal sleeping pattern and whether it has recently changed. Try to keep to the normal pattern in hospital. It is worth eliciting her normal bedtime routines and recommending that she try to keep to these as much as possible.

Patient comment

'It was very comforting to hear the tick of my usual bedside alarm clock every time I woke up, and to know what time it was without bothering the nurses.'

If the patient is used to sleeping with someone else, she may find it difficult to settle on her own. Having a small item of that person's clothing, with its familiar smell, will help to reduce the strangeness. Equally, if she usually sleeps alone, sharing a room with others, especially noisy ones,

PLUS factors that promote rapid healing:

- Young
- Good blood supply
- Fit
- Warm
- Well-nourished
- Mentally well-prepared patient
- Continent
- Relaxed
- Normal haemoglobin level
- Low anxiety
- Well oxygenated

MINUS factors that tend to delay healing:

- Advanced age
- Smoker
- Unfit
- Mentally unprepared patient
- Malignant disease
- Tense
- Steroid treatment
- Anxious
- Chemotherapy or radiotherapy
- Confused in time, place or person
- Poorly oxygenated
- Recurrent trauma
- Anaemic
- Oedema
- Malnourished (especially lack of protein, vitamin C, vitamin K and zinc)
- Excess exudate
- Diabetic
- Necrotic tissue
- Infected
- Foreign bodies
- Abdominal wound
- Renal failure
- Poor blood supply
- Jaundice
- Cold
- Inflammatory disease
- Obese

can be unsettling. Earplugs and sleepmasks may be helpful. Others may use a few drops of lavender essential oil on the pillowcase.

Identifying a sleep deficit has implications for nursing care. The patient will need support and encouragement to rest and may need a hypnotic drug to aid sleep before the operation. Lack of sleep is also likely to affect the patient's concentration and ability to retain new information. Post-operatively, adequate sleep will be necessary, because it enhances anabolism and reduces catabolism.

SMOKING

The smoking habits of the patient are relevant to her respiratory response to a general anaesthetic. The amount smoked needs to be elicited tactfully and non-judgementally. It is also useful to determine whether a non-smoker is exposed to others'

smoking, i.e. is a passive smoker. The more time the patient stays free of cigarette smoke, the less likely are respiratory complications after a general anaesthetic. This may be a good time to assess her motivation for reducing her consumption or giving up.

SPECIAL SENSES

Sight

Any impairment of sight must be established as early as possible so the patient can be treated appropriately. For further suggestions, see Chapter 4. Find out where the patient wears glasses or contact lenses, and try to ensure that these are worn as usual. In an emergency admission, always query and check for the presence of contact lenses before allowing the patient to go to theatre. If left in, even if they are of the extended-wear type, severe corneal abrasions can result. The patient may express a preference for wearing her glasses until she is anaesthetized. It is the responsibility of the ward nurse to take them away afterwards and make them available as soon as the patient needs them again.

Hearing

Early detection of hearing impairment improves communication between the patient and the health-care team. Assess whether the patient wears a hearing aid or relies on lip reading or sign language. The hearing aid may need to go to theatre with the patient to ensure she is informed of what is to happen and what is asked of her. In this case, it must be labelled, and reinserted in the recovery room to ease post-operative communication.

Smell

Hospitals do not just look, feel and sound strange to the patient: they also smell alien. The sense of smell is very primitive and can powerfully affect our emotions. Patients need encouragement to surround themselves with familiar smells to help them to settle in, for example a usual talcum powder or bedjacket.

SPEECH AND COMMUNICATION

Concentration is likely to be impaired by anxiety. It is useful to determine the patient's abilities, in case there are language or learning difficulties, or residual speech problems after a stroke. The initial interaction between the nurse and patient will provide information on problems and how these may be minimized or overcome. Eliciting specific anxieties from the patient about the type of operation, for example, can identify the main focus for information and reassurance.

If the patient does not speak English, a family member may be available to translate. Most units have a list of translators available via the switchboard.

SUPPORT SYSTEM

The patient's family and friends form part of the support system that is likely to be called upon while she is in hospital and when she goes home. Establish who is most significant in the patient's life and what the patient is likely to expect of them. Find out who is able to visit and who is looking after any dependents. The stress of impending surgery may highlight family tensions and difficulties. The nurse needs to know upon whom to rely and may suggest that one member of the immediate family or significant person (not necessarily the 'next of kin') should be nominated by the patient as the co-ordinator. This will save repeated telephone calls and nursing time.

WEIGHT AND HEIGHT

The patient's weight will help in estimating the correct dose of anaesthetic. Ask the patient what she thinks she weighs and note whether there has been any change. If there has been significant (for example 10%) weight loss, there are serious implications for operative morbidity and mortality. The medical staff need to be informed, as decisions must be made on whether to proceed with surgery or boost the patient nutritionally first. It may only be necessary to give the patient a liquid supplement to significantly shorten her stay (Mason, 1992). The dietary history will have highlighted whether there is a protein or calorie deficit.

The patient's height is determined in order to estimate the body mass index (BMI), calculated by dividing the patient's weight (kg) by the height (m) squared. The resulting figure provides a useful guideline on whether the patient is in a healthy or an unhealthy band:

- < 19 = underweight
- 20–24.9 = normal
- 25–29.9 = grade I obesity/plump
- 30–39.9 = grade II obesity
- 40+ = grade III obesity.

The BMI is not calculated if the patient is a child, oedematous, dehydrated, pregnant or an amputee.

The combination of known dietary and drinking habits and BMI may form the basis of health-promotion activities planned with and for the patient.

WORK

The patient's profession, or retirement or unemployment, has to be established so that planning for convalescence can begin early. Many patients may have little idea of how they are going to feel and for how long after surgery. Discussion of what is involved in their daily work and leisure means that advice can be precisely targeted to their circumstances.

> Nurses have a duty to ensure that patients and relatives understand what is being proposed and have an opportunity to talk over their hopes and fears for the outcome of an operation. There is also an obligation to give a nursing assessment of the patient's condition, documenting problems which may be unknown to or overlooked by surgical staff (*Nursing Times*, 1992).

Patient comment

'I was worried that I wouldn't come round after the operation.'

Following on from the nursing interview, nursing assessment continues throughout the patient's stay. Its purpose is to ensure that the whole team possesses relevant information in order to make the best decisions for the patient's care. This could, for example, avoid heroic surgery on unsuitable patients who might end up featuring in the *National Confidential Enquiry into Peri-operative Deaths* (Campling *et al.*, 1992). The process is two-way, as information passes to the patient throughout her stay, with the intention of reducing her anxiety to manageable levels. This has been shown to reduce the patient's perception of post-operative pain (Hayward, 1975).

A well-informed patient is more likely to retain her feelings of control over what is happening. A patient who is under stress and depressed requires more medication and anaesthesic, has lower immune functioning, is more likely to suffer complications and will take longer to heal (Dossey, 1991). One way of reducing stress is for the patient to use her inner resources to calm or energize herself. Guided imagery and relaxation techniques can be of positive benefit.

Investigations

Fear of the unknown in patients about to undergo a diagnostic test, and distress during the procedure, can be eased by valid descriptions of the physical sensations associated with the procedure (Clark and Gregor, 1988).

Patient comment

'It helped that the nurse was able to warn me about the "hot flush" feeling of the dye going in. I was then not so worried by it when it happened.'

Experienced nurses are able to call upon their knowledge, gleaned from many patients. Less experienced nurses can build up their knowledge by conscientiously asking every patient who has had an investigation to describe the physical sensations involved. The specialist chapters in Part Two outline specific investigations for relevant areas of surgery. Further details will be found in Booth's *Handbook of Investigations* (Booth, 1983).

At all stages of preparation for investigation and surgery, the patient must be encouraged to ask questions and express her concerns. Her consent cannot be taken for granted. It must be explicitly obtained for everything that happens to her in hospital. The duty to care includes respect-

ing patients' autonomy, even if they refuse the treatment offered (Robson, 1994).

The patient also needs to be prepared for the experience of premedication, induction of anaesthesia and the immediate post-operative phase. Any equipment used, strange locations encountered or sensations felt should be described, shown, visited or discussed. The use of videotapes, audiotapes and booklets, if carefully chosen and not used as a substitute for one-to-one explanations, can greatly enhance the patient's understanding and co-operation.

Consent

Consent to the anaesthetic and operation cannot be assumed by the fact that the patient has voluntarily come into hospital. Gaining informed consent is a serious matter, with ethical and legal implications. It is the doctor's responsibility to explain the advantages and risks of the proposed treatment and, if possible, give the patient thinking time before she signs a consent form. 'What is primarily needed is knowledge of the alternative courses of treatment and those risks and side-effects which have a bearing on the patient's life plans and values' (Strong, 1979). The nursing team can help the patient by reinforcing or translating what the patient has been told by the doctor and checking with the patient what she wants to happen. If necessary, refer back to the doctor.

Points to bear in mind for gaining valid consent to surgery include:

- information – what the reasonable doctor decides to tell (Alderson 1995);
- competence;
- voluntariness;
- lack of deceit.

A patient aged 16 or 17 has the right, under the 1969 Family Law Reform Act, to consent to or refuse treatment. In law, a child of almost any age can consent to treatment if deemed capable of understanding the implications. In practice, however, many units tend to gain the consent of a parent or guardian to any proposed treatment of a patient under 18 years of age. Dissent requires understanding of a higher order than does consent.

People with a learning disability should be seen as competent to make decisions until proved otherwise (Law Commission, 1991). With patients with dementia, nurses must try to be aware of and respect the person's capacity for making decisions for herself. If, however, treatment is necessary to safeguard life, health or well-being, health professionals are legally bound to give treatment without consent. If patients are unable to give consent because of continuing mental incapacity, the nurse must act in their best interests (Phair, 1996).

In a serious emergency, when the patient is unconscious or virtually unconscious on admission, it is possible for the surgeon to operate without formal consent from the patient or family, providing the treatment is administered without negligence and, in an emergency, in the best interests of the patient (Pinfold, 1991). A hospital manager can be asked to document the circumstances.

In the case of religious or other objections to treatment, such as a Jehovah's Witness refusing to consent to a blood transfusion, there is a valid restriction on the doctor's right to treat the patient: 'A conscious, rational patient is entitled to refuse any medical treatment and the doctor must comply, no matter how ill-advised he may believe that instruction to be' (Mr Justice Donnelly, cited by Pinfold, 1991).

An adult who is incompetent within the meaning of the Mental Health Act 1983 may have surgery if it is necessary in her best interests (Pinfold, 1991).

No-one else may consent to treatment on behalf of an adult. Doctors may consult with relatives or next of kin before surgery and may even gain their written or verbal consent. This is not valid consent or a legal obligation but good medical practice (Buchanan, 1995).

The minimum aim in gaining consent (Buchanan, 1995) is to:

- present the patient with understandable information;
- give patients time to think about their decisions;

- enable them to change their minds if they so choose.

Consent can be withdrawn at any time, and then even written consent is invalid.

Deep breathing and coughing exercises

Some patients are at high risk of developing post-operative pulmonary complications, such as atelectasis (collapse of a lung segment) and pneumonia. The negative factors include:

- being elderly;
- being a smoker;
- being obese;
- suffering from chronic lung disease;
- having an upper abdominal or thoracic incision.

These patients will need to be taught diaphragmatic breathing and coughing exercises for the early post-operative period. The best time to teach these is before pain and the anaesthetic decrease the ability to retain information.

Breathing exercises

The patient is asked to:

- sit up in bed
- with her back supported by pillows
- rest her hands just down from axillae
- take six deep breaths
- feel the chest expanding with each breath
- feel the abdomen rising with each breath, showing use of diaphragm
- cough, with the knees bent if necessary

If abdominal surgery is planned,

- place the hands either side of incision
- press to equalize pressure
- while coughing

Leg exercises

Flexing and extending the feet, rotating the feet and ankles, and extending the legs will be taught pre-operatively, so that the patient will be familiar with the movements post-operatively. They improve venous return, by exercising the muscle pump of the calf. In a patient on prolonged bedrest, or at high risk of deep venous thrombosis (30% of those aged over 40 according to Scurr *et al.*, 1988), exercise may be enhanced by simultaneously applying pressure to the sole of the foot, which increases venous return. This should be done ten times an hour. Other measures to combat deep venous thrombosis include:

- posture – any position that promotes venous stasis, such as sitting still for long periods, crossing the legs (Evans, 1991) or pressure on the calves from a pillow, should be avoided;
- deep breathing exercises to use the respiratory pump, as negative pressures within the pleural cavity exert a suction effect, improving venous return;
- avoidance of dehydration;
- early ambulation;
- subcutaneous heparin;
- graded compression stockings, except in those with arterial insufficiency of the legs.

Planning and action to prevent deep venous thrombosis start as soon as the risk is identified and continue throughout the patient's stay and into convalescence.

Fasting

The patient can usually eat and drink normally on the day before surgery, unless the bowel is to be operated on (*see* Chapter 8). For a safe induction of anaesthetic, the aim is to render the patient's stomach volume less than 25 ml and the pH less than 2.5 (Roberts and Shirley, 1974; cited by Chapman, 1996). This is usually achieved by giving no food for at least 4 hours pre-operatively and by restricting fluids for a shorter time. Anxiety will slow stomach emptying, so the time is often extended to 6 or more hours. Explain to the patient that the purpose of the fast is to prevent her from vomiting while under anaesthetic. This is, however, not a large cause of deaths associated with anaesthesia when compared with hypovolaemia (Thomas, 1987). The patient's understanding needs to be checked and her co-

operation gained. A 'nil by mouth' sign on the bed keeps the team informed.

The anaesthetist is likely to be more lenient than the nursing staff in permitting fluids (Thomas, 1987). Studies have shown that 150–240 ml of water, coffee and pulp-free orange juice administered 2–3 hours prior to surgery produces no significant increase in residual gastric volume or acidity, and, indeed, that 50–1000 ml of clear fluids ingested up to 3 hours before surgery results in no significant difference in residual volume or pH (Maltby *et al.*, 1986, 1988, 1991, cited in Chapman, 1996).

When a patient is admitted as an emergency, the time she last ate or drank must be established, as must any vomiting. If she has a serious condition, she may have to go to theatre with a full stomach and either have it emptied with a wide-bore tube or have Sellick's manoeuvre performed (*see* below) to protect her airway. If a delay can be tolerated, the patient may be monitored for a few hours to let the stomach empty safely.

Critical factors that render a patient at risk of perioperative aspiration of gastric contents are:

- a residual gastric volume greater than 25 ml
- a pH of less than 2.5

Skin preparation

As an intact epithelium is the body's chief defence against invading bacteria, each portal of entry for surgery, intravenous access or drains poses an increased risk of infection.

In order to minimize this risk, the patient's skin must be rendered as free from micro-organisms as possible by the time of operation. This is usually achieved by a bath or, better still, a shower with an antibacterial agent shortly beforehand. In an emergency, or if the patient is unable to get out of bed, a bedbath or assisted wash may be given.

All make-up, including nail polish, must be removed to ensure that the patient's true colour can be detected. Jewellery, hairgrips and prostheses must be removed for safety, as they can be lost or contribute to burns if they contain metal and diathermy is used in theatre. Some patients may have navel rings or other studs (Langford, 1996). If the patient does not wish to remove her wedding ring, it can be secured with adhesive tape.

The patient is given clean bedlinen and dressed in a special operation gown, usually opening down the back for ease of removal. Knickers may be left on if surgery is not on the immediate area. Because skin scales are shed continuously, along with normal skin flora such as *Staphylococcus epidermidis* and any organisms that have colonized the skin since hospitalization, for example *Staphylococcus aureus*, Pseudomonas or *Escherichia coli* (Spencer and Bale, 1990), regular changes of bedlinen must be part of surgical care in order to reduce the risk of wound infection.

For certain types of surgery (for example, those involving orthopaedic implants), a more energetic regimen is demanded, which may include the repeated application of antibacterial lotions to the skin, a series of showers with antibacterial lotion and/or the removal of body hair in the region of the operation.

Despite evidence to suggest that pre-operative shaving increases the risk of wound infection (Seropian and Reynolds, 1971, and Cruse and Foord, 1980, are two examples), many units continue this practice (Spencer and Bale, 1990). There may be many reasons for this, including the convenience of applying adhesive theatre drapes and dressings to hairless skin.

If body hair must be removed, a depilatory preparation can be used if there is no adverse reaction. If there is insufficient time to determine this, shaving is indicated. This is best done as late as possible before the surgery to reduce the risk of colonization of the broken skin surface. The best equipment is a sharp disposable razor, shaving foam, enough time and a good light. If possible, it is best for the patient to do this herself, as she can take time and trouble over the task. Shaving is more effective (i.e. closer) if it is against the growth of the hair shaft. Unless absolutely essential, removal of pubic hair is to be avoided as regrowth is very uncomfortable.

Patient comment

'The itching from the shaved area nearly drove me mad.'

In an emergency, shaving may have to be carried out in the anaesthetic room once the patient has been anaesthetized.

Infection rates are always lower when elective operations are performed, because there is time to ensure that the patient is properly nourished and hydrated and receiving prophylactic antibiotics (Gould, 1994). These are most effective when given within 2 hours of the first incision (Classen *et al.*, 1992), which is particularly relevant for a patient undergoing emergency surgery, when they may be included with the premedication.

Before premedication is given or the patient taken to theatre, some or all of the following points will be noted on a form of checklist:

- Allergies recorded
- Bladder emptied
- Consent form signed
- Contact lenses/ artificial eyes removed
- Crowns/caps/loose teeth noted
- Dentures/prostheses removed
- Head on canvas
- Hearing aid worn/ removed

- Identity bracelet
- Jewellery removed/ wedding ring taped
- Last food
- Last fluid
- Make-up/nail polish/ underwear removed
- Pacemaker reported
- Pressure sore risk score
- Psychological status
- Skin prepared
- Site marked

STUDENT ACTIVITY

Find the theatre checklist for your unit and compare it with the one above. Is anything missing from either of them? Do you consider this to be important?

Premedication

This consists of one or more drugs given before the patient goes to theatre to render her in an optimum state for induction of the anaesthetic. Premedication takes many forms, for example papaveretum, pethidine or morphine to initiate analgesia and reduce anxiety with their euphoric effect, coupled with an anti-emetic such as metoclopramide. Many anaesthetists prescribe a sedative–hypnotic benzodiazepine such as temazepam to allay anxiety, provide sedation and assist in the smooth induction of anaesthesia (Mirakhur, 1991).

The premedication may include an anticholinergic drug, such as atropine or hyoscine, to dry up secretions and protect against vagal overactivity. The patient will notice the effect of a dry mouth. The use of such drugs is declining (Mirakhur, 1991).

Premedication also includes other drugs that will act while the patient is in theatre, such as subcutaneous heparin for those at risk of deep venous thrombosis.

It is particularly important to administer oral premedication with a drink. It is safe to give 60 ml water with the tablet even in the patient starved for surgery since the stomach produces about 125 ml/hour of gastric juices anyway. (Channer, 1985)

In an emergency, there may be no time for a premedication to work, so the necessary drugs may be given intravenously in the anaesthetic room.

Patients undergoing day case surgery may not necessarily be given a premedication.

Anaesthetics

Anaesthesia denotes the state of being without physical sensation. **Analgesia** is the state of being without pain.

Anaesthesia can be achieved locally or generally.

Local anaesthesia

It is not always necessary to have the patient unconscious during operation. Local anaesthesia removes the pain and temperature sensations from the area to be operated upon, usually leaving sensations of pressure, movement and stretching. It can be achieved in a number of ways:

- topical/surface, using drops, sprays, lozenges, ointment or cream;
- infiltration by subcutaneous injection;
- field block, creating a zone of analgesia around the operative site;
- nerve block – a small amount of anaesthetic solution injected around a nerve will block impulses arising in that nerve's distribution;
- spinal and epidural anaesthesia – a nerve or group of nerves can be blocked near the spinal cord, either as the nerve roots traverse the cerebrospinal fluid (CSF) (spinal; Fig. 1.1) or after they have pierced the dura mater but are

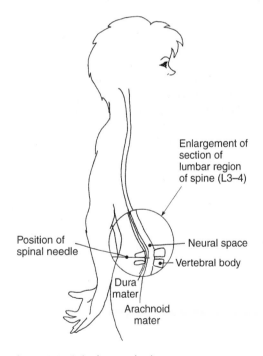

Figure 1.1 Spinal anaesthetic

still within the spinal column (epidural) (Strathern, 1996).

A nerve blocked in this way, so close to the spinal cord, will affect sensation from all nerve branches. The intensity and duration of the block depend upon the agent used and its concentration. The area rendered insensitive depends upon the site and volume of injection and the relative position of the spine.

An intravenous infusion for access is always set up before commencement of the spinal or epidural injection.

After the injection is complete, the anaesthetist supervises the careful positioning of the patient, explaining what is going on and what to expect. A successful block will produce warmth and tingling in the area to be operated on, followed by heaviness of the limb, reduced power and reduced sensation. The patient's blood pressure will be measured regularly throughout the operation.

Overdose or toxicity will be indicated by pallor, anxiety, nausea, falling blood pressure, failing slow pulse, twitching or convulsions, and cardio-respiratory collapse. Resuscitation will require oxygen, ventilation and anticonvulsant and hypertensive drugs (Wood, 1987a).

Intravenous block can be used to anaesthetize a limb. The limb is elevated and a tourniquet applied; then a precise dose of intravenous anaesthetic is injected through a previously sited cannula. The tourniquet can only be left inflated for 1 hour and is then deflated in stages to allow slow release of the local anaesthetic into the general circulation.

The possible complications following a nerve or intravenous block are severe hypotension, convulsions and respiratory or cardiac arrest. Thus oxygen must be available, an intravenous cannula in place, a blood pressure cuff in position, the patient placed on a tipping trolley and general anaesthetic equipment available.

General anaesthesia

INDUCTION

Drugs used for general anaesthesia comprise a triad of hypnotic, analgesic and relaxant (paralysing) agents. The first two are used to achieve a reversible loss of consciousness and pain relief; the third paralyses the patient's muscles. They can induce anaesthesia by two routes: intravenous or inhalational.

Intravenous induction

The agent is injected into a superficial vein, usually via an intravenous cannula in the back of the hand. The drug travels through the vein to the right side of the heart, the pulmonary circulation, the left side of the heart and thence to the brain. Most patients, except those with poor circulation, fall asleep within 30 seconds.

Patient comments

'I wish someone had told me what it felt like to be given the anaesthetic. It felt cold and I could feel it travel up my arm and then I went to sleep.'

'The drug gave me a buzzing sensation all over my skin, rather pleasant, then I suddenly blacked out.'

Inhalational induction

The patient breathes a mixture, usually of oxygen and nitrous oxide, and an anaesthetic vapour is slowly added to this, progressively deepening the anaesthesia. During this form of induction, the patient will exhibit the classical stages of anaesthesia:

- from full consciousness with diminished perception of pain (Milne, 1988);
- to the stage of excitement, during which she may move vigorously, cough, hold her breath or vomit (Wood, 1987a);
- gradually the anaesthetic deepens to stop the excitement (Wood, 1987a); and cause
- surgical anaesthesia to take its place.

As most anaesthetics are induced by rapid intravenous agents, these signs are usually masked (Wood, 1987a).

COMPLICATIONS OF GENERAL ANAESTHESIA

Cardiac arrest

Cardiac arrest is the most serious complication, occurring more frequently on induction or immediately after operation owing to myocardial depression caused by general anaesthesia (Milne, 1988). Thus all patients have electrocardiogram

(ECG) leads attached as a routine precaution, so that they can be monitored throughout surgery.

Vomiting

Vomiting during anaesthesia can and does lead to death. Active vomiting or passive regurgitation of stomach contents along the oesophagus to the pharynx may result in inhalation of acidic stomach contents and severely damage the lungs. Death can be caused immediately by acute airway obstruction or a few days later as a result of the lung damage. At-risk patients include those:

- who have eaten or drunk within the last 4 hours;
- who have eaten 6–8 hours earlier and then suffered a serious accident, which often halts digestion (sympathetic activity);
- with pyloric stenosis, leading to delayed emptying of the stomach;
- with large abdominal swellings, especially a pregnant uterus;
- with facial/pharyngeal injuries, who may have a large amount of blood in the stomach.

Precautions to prevent aspiration of stomach contents (Wood, 1987a; McGarvey, 1990) are:

- a rapid sequence of induction;
- emptying the stomach using drugs;
- the application of pressure to the cricoid, a ring of cartilage just below the larynx, which, when pressed backwards presses on and closes the oesophagus, which lies immediately behind it (Sellick's manoeuvre).

Respiratory depression

All anaesthetic agents depress respiration, some lasting beyond the end of anaesthesia (Milne, 1988).

Fall in core body temperature

Vasodilatation produced by anaesthesia causes a fall in body core temperature. Severe hypothermia may develop, especially if the operation involves exposing the viscera, causing a delayed return to consciousness, inadequate respiration and peripheral perfusion (Milne, 1988). Kurz *et al.* (1996) suggest that wound infection may be triggered by hypothermia.

MAINTENANCE OF GENERAL ANAESTHESIA

To keep the patient in a suitable state for safe and rapid surgery, the anaesthetist ensures that the patient:

- is asleep;
- is pain-free;
- does not make reflex movements;
- is paralysed if necessary.

This can be achieved by spontaneous or controlled ventilation, depending on the surgeon's requirements. In spontaneous ventilation, the patient is maintaining her own respiration automatically. In controlled ventilation, complete paralysis of all voluntary muscles is achieved by the injection of muscle relaxant. Cardiac and smooth muscle is unaffected, but respiration must be assisted as the respiratory muscles are paralysed. The patient will therefore have an endotracheal tube in place (intubation) (McGarvey, 1990) in order to maintain a clear airway. The surgical indications for this include:

- abdominal operations needing good muscle relaxation;
- thoracic operations needing controlled ventilation
- a patient position that may compromise spontaneous respiration, such as lying prone, head-down tilt or lithotomy (supine, with both legs up in stirrups);
- head and neck operations in which the anaesthetist's access may be limited or pressure will be applied, hindering respiration;
- intracranial operations.

Other reasons for controlled ventilation include recent food intake, shock, obesity, foreign material likely to compromise the airway (such as teeth, bone, pus or blood), a difficult airway and a lengthy operation (Wood, 1987a).

There is evidence for a degree of unconscious perception of auditory signals during general anaesthesia. The saying 'hearing is the last sense to go and the first to come back' may have to be revised in light of this. Some anaesthetists use this route to relay positive messages to the patient during the operation via headphones attached to a personal stereo (Holmboe and Williams, 1990).

This has been found to reduce mean post-operative stay and the incidence of pyrexia and gastrotintestinal problems (Evans and Richardson, 1988).

MONITORING DURING ANAESTHESIA

The patient is normally attached to a range of equipment to detect any abnormalities, including those of pulse, blood pressure and ECGS. Other monitors will be added as required by the patient's condition.

The patient's *pulse rate* is detected by digital palpation of an artery by the anaesthetist, by oximetry, by transducer in a finger cuff, by display on a dial or by display of the *heart rate* on the ECG monitor.

Finger plethysmography measures finger blood flow, providing information about heart *rhythm* and *rate* and a crude index of pump activity.

Blood pressure is detected by a oscillotonometer (a manually inflated cuff with the pressure read from needle movements across the dial), electronically (with automatic, intermittent cuff inflation and digital display) or by using an intra-arterial line connected to a pressure transducer via a saline catheter, continually displayed in a wave or digital form.

Central venous pressure is measured by introducing a saline-filled catheter into the large veins of the thorax via the veins of the neck, chest or arm. It is especially useful when large volumes of fluid are being lost and transfused.

The *electrocardiogram* (ECG) monitors the rate and rhythm of the heart by three or four leads on the chest, back or limbs, or a foil plate placed under the thorax. The trace is displayed on a screen.

Temperature is monitored electronically using a probe that may be placed in the oesophagus, ear or rectum to measure 'core' temperature. The readings are displayed on a dial or digital read-out. To compare the periphery with the core, toe or finger temperature can be measured.

Blood loss may be to some extent estimated by the amount of blood in the suction bottle and by weighing the swabs used.

Respiratory rate and *tidal volume* can be set and observed by the anaesthetist when the patient is artificially ventilated (Wood, 1987a).

Pulse oximetry determines the percentage of oxygenated haemoglobin, providing information about function of both the respiratory and the cardiovascular system.

Capnography, the measurement of end-tidal carbon dioxide levels, is performed for all operations.

A urinary catheter may be inserted into the bladder and *urine volume* measured hourly.

REVERSAL

The anaesthetic vapour and gases are switched off and the patient allowed to breathe room air and/or oxygen as her condition dictates. If muscle relaxants have been used, they are reversed with neostigmine, which slows the heart; glycopyrrolate or atropine is given to counteract this side-effect. Respiratory depression is a side-effect of the narcotic analgesic used. This is reversed, if present, using naloxone (Wood, 1987b).

Recovery glycopyrrolate from general anaesthesia

The patient is not left unattended until she is in full possession of her faculties. The anaesthetist hands the patient over to the recovery nurse with information on the:

- type of operation;
- general physical status;
- pain relief;
- state of consciousness;
- fluid balance;
- special observations to be made (e.g. neurological or neurovascular);
- need for oxygen.

Some patients exhibit post-operative tremors, thought to be a response to the pre-operative fall in body temperature or to the anaesthetic wearing off in the spine sooner than in the brain (Sessler, 1988). The patient will need warming up with an infra-red lamp or other heat source, as it appears to be cold skin rather than low core temperature than triggers the tremors. Shivering can increase oxygen consumption by 100–400%, may increase metabolic demand by as much as

300–400%, can cause distress to patients and can strain surgical repairs (Hind, 1994).

Patient comment

'It was very odd. I had the shakes quite violently, but I didn't feel cold.'

The recovery room exists mostly to deal with short-stay post anaesthetic patients who need continuous adequate supervision in an environment where all the necessary treatment facilities (oxygen, suction, drugs, defibrillator, tracheostomy set, etc.) are immediately available. The direction of nursing care in the recovery room is particularly focused towards the following.

AIRWAY

The patency of the upper air passages is secured, sometimes using a Guedel airway, so that the patient can breathe easily. This is frequently checked by feeling air coming out of the patient's nose or mouth onto the palm of the nurse's hand. In a straightforward uncomplicated recovery, the patient will wake up and either pull or spit the airway out. Oxygen is frequently prescribed by the anaesthetist. The nurse also observes the colour of the patient's skin.

VOMITING

Vomiting or regurgitation of gastric contents may occur after emergency surgery but is relatively unusual owing to the use of antiemetics. Suction is available to deal with this problem, and nasogastric tubes are left on free drainage at this stage.

RESTLESSNESS

Restlessness is a normal, transient feature of recovery from anaesthesia and may also be caused by such factors as pain, a full bladder, mental confusion, fear, lack of oxygen or discomfort from tight splints or bandages. A high staff-to-patient ratio means that the cause is likely to be detected before it becomes a problem. The patient is often placed on her bed, with the safety rails in position, so that she is unlikely to come to harm; restraint is rarely necessary.

CIRCULATION

The circulation is likely to be unstable owing to the premedication and anaesthetic drugs. The blood pressure, for example, is likely to be lower than normal and easily reduced further by movement, pain, anoxia, analgesics or vomiting. Pulse and blood pressure are measured frequently, and the patient is not usually returned to the ward unless the systolic pressure is above 100 mmHg and the pulse below 100 beats per minute.

Other specific observations may include temperature, urine output, neurovascular (colour, warmth and sensation) or neurological observations, and checking for bleeding or pain.

Once the patient has reached a satisfactory level of recovery, the anaesthetist is informed and the patient released into the care of the ward nurse. The latter will do a top-to-toe assessment of her patient, including:

- the general physical condition (last recorded observations, pink, warm and dry, pale/cyanosed, cold and clammy);
- the exact surgery that was performed and any unexpected findings or events;
- the presence and care of drains, catheters and infusions;
- the state of the wound dressing;
- the current state of pain relief, antiemesis and fluid replacement and their prescription for at least the next few hours;
- the patient's mental state.

Recovery from spinal anaesthesia

Until the spinal anaesthetic has worn off, there is a risk of hypotension if the patient sits up. She must therefore lie down on 2–3 pillows for approximately 6 hours on return to the ward. Once her blood pressure and other observations are satisfactory and the block has worn off, i.e. feeling has returned to the area, she should be able gradually to sit up. A slow intravenous infusion should be maintained for the first 6 hours in case fluids are needed to treat hypo-tension. If the infusion is not needed for other reasons, it may be removed once a satisfactory blood pressure is achieved. There is a low risk of headache following spinal anaesthetic owing to leakage of CSF, and lying flat will not prevent its development (usually at 2–4 days post-spinal). It occurs on standing or sitting up and is relieved by lying down. Simple analgesics and ensuring that the patient is well hydrated are also helpful. If the headache is troublesome, the anaesthetist

should produce a blood patch. Caffeine may also be used intravenously.

Epidural blood patch

To seal the hole that is leaking CSF:

- 10–15 ml of the patient's blood is taken
- This is injected into the epidural space
- A clot forms, covering the hole and preventing further loss

Post-operative care

Monitoring on the ward

Once the patient has been returned to the ward, she will be monitored regularly to detect trends in her condition. The most likely pattern will be half-hourly recording of respiration, pulse rate and blood pressure, with less frequent tem-perature measurements. If these stabilize as anticipated, the time between observations will gradually be lengthened to 4-hourly. At each observation point, the nurse will look, listen and feel, using the recovery room baseline, and real-istic anticipation of any likely complications (*see* below).

The patient can usually gradually sit up as her condition stabilizes and she is able to sustain a reasonable blood pressure. She may need several reminders that her operation is over and she is back in the ward. Any messages from family and friends can be relayed as her consciousness improves. It is not usually beneficial to have visitors at this point (as it uses up too much energy), except one significant person for a short while, as the patient needs to sleep the anaes-thetic off. She is likely to be disorientated in time and place, so cues such as a clock are helpful.

Complications

These may include the following:

SHOCK

Shock is a response of the body to peripheral circulatory failure. In this case, it is likely to be oligaemic/hypovolaemic (insufficient blood). It is manifested by pale, cold, clammy skin, accel-erated heart rate, reduced systolic pressure, low-ered pulse pressure, a weak thready pulse, subnormal temperature and lip cyanosis. The main objective is to restore the circulating blood volume, so immediate measures include arresting haemorrhage, increasing the speed of the intra-venous infusion and lying the patient down with her head on one pillow, her trunk horizontal and her legs elevated (except after gynaecological sur-gery; *see* Chapter 9).

BASAL CONSOLIDATION LEADING TO CHEST INFECTION

The risk of this is increased in smokers, de-hydrated patients, those with high abdominal and thoracic incisions, and those receiving nar-cotic analgesia. The patient will have a raised temperature, rapid, shallow respiration, decreased chest expansion, chest pain and a productive cough with mucopurulent sputum. Treatment will include chest physiotherapy, antibiotic ther-apy, incentive spirometry (Hall *et al.*, 1996), an increase in fluid intake, early ambulation and symptom relief.

RENAL FAILURE

Acute renal failure can occur during surgery owing to hypovolaemia and/or hypotension. It is shown by anuria (a urinary output below 100 mL/day) or oliguria (one of below 400 mL/day). It must be distinguished from *acute retention of urine*, which may afflict the post-operative patient, sometimes after pethidine has been administered. In renal failure, the patient is acutely ill, needing immediate, energetic treatment; in retention the distended bladder is the main cause of discomfort.

Measures to deal with retention include sitting the patient up to micturate, providing privacy, running water within earshot, dangling the patient's hands or feet in a bowl of water, placing her in a warm bath or, as a last resort, inserting a urinary catheter.

It is usually expected that the well-hydrated patient will pass urine within 24 hours of surgery; this must be documented.

DEEP VEIN THROMBOSIS

The veins most frequently affected are in the calf. Peak incidence is on day 5 after surgery, although vulnerability may persist for up to 12 weeks post-operatively (Voelker, 1996). Thrombosis is caused by a combination of dehydration, venous stasis, reduced venous return to the lower abdomen, trauma to the venous walls and increased co-agulability of the blood. The patient complains of pain or cramp in the calf and raised temperature; oedema and pallor in the leg will be noted, with warmth and redness over the affected vein and a positive Homan's sign (pain in the calf on dorsi-flexion of the foot). The immediate treatment is bedrest, elevation of the affected limb, anticoagulant therapy and elastic stockings. The aim is to prevent extension of the thombus, or dislodging of the clot leading to a pulmonary embolism.

PULMONARY EMBOLISM

The patient complains of sharp, stabbing pains in the chest, is anxious, dyspnoeic and cyanosed, perspires profusely, may show pupillary dilatation and has a rapid and irregular pulse, which rapidly becomes imperceptible as the patient dies from blockage of the pulmonary artery. Sometimes the first sign of a massive, lethal pulmonary embolism is a sudden urge to defaecate, followed by collapse. A smaller embolism may manifest itself in a more modest way, perhaps being mistaken for a chest infection until haemoptysis is noted. The immediate treatment is to sit the patient upright, administer oxygen and summon medical assistance.

NAUSEA AND VOMITING

These may be a reaction to opiate, anaesthetic, analgesic or other drugs, abdominal distension, pain or electrolyte imbalance.

The following factors increase the risk of post-operative nausea and vomiting (PONV) (Rowbotham, 1995):

- Age under 3 or over 70 years
- Puberty
- Post-pubertal females, particularly in the second half of the menstrual cycle
- Obesity
- Starvation or excessive pre-operative fluid restriction
- A history of motion sickness
- A previous history of PONV
- High anxiety
- Unpleasant sights, sounds and smells
- Pregnancy
- Laparoscopic procedures
- Cardiothoracic, gastrointestinal, gynaecological and orthopaedic surgery
- Opioid analgesics

PONV is treated by:

- determining and removing the cause, if known;
- positive intra-operative suggestions (Williams *et al.*, 1994);
- side-lying to prevent aspiration, which causes severe or fatal lung damage (Rowbotham, 1995);
- ensuring the availability of suction;
- withholding food or fluids until PONV subsides;
- giving sips of fluid (ice or ginger ale) and dry solid food (plain biscuits) once it subsides;

- performing frequent oral care;
- administering anti-emetic therapy, for example metoclopramide/ginger root (Bone *et al.*, 1990);
- applying wrist bands with buttons to press continuously on the acupressure meridians of both wrists.

DECUBITUS ULCERS

The patient at risk of pressure sores will have been identified pre-operatively using a scoring system. In theatre, a pressure-reduction device will have been placed beneath the patient and the bed equipped with one. Despite this, the patient will need rigorous attention to changes of position, monitoring of areas at risk, prompt attention to any broken skin and adequate oxygenation and nutritional support.

HAEMORRHAGE

Haemorrhage may be internal or detected by visible blood loss in drains, through dressings or from orifices. Primary haemorrhage occurs at the time of operation, reactionary haemorrhage within a few hours of surgery in response to increasing blood pressure, and secondary haemorrhage some days later as a result of infection. The patient will be apprehensive, restless and thirsty, with cold, pale, sweaty skin. The pulse will increase and 'air hunger' (deep rapid respiration) will be noted. Venous and arterial blood pressure will both rapidly decrease.

Treatment will be as for shock. Measures will be instituted to arrest bleeding. Plasma expanders will be administered until cross-matched blood is available. The patient may have to return to theatre for ligation of the bleeding vessel.

INFECTION

Infection can be acquired as a result of coming into hospital (nosocomial). The patient may acquire a wound, chest or urinary tract infection, especially if she is immunocompromised. Nursing measures of which scrupulous and timely handwashing is the most important, aim to minimize this possibility.

CONSTIPATION

This may go relatively unnoticed by the patient, who reasons that, with no food going in, no output is likely. However, the entire gut lining is still being shed as usual. Peristalsis will be decreased for at least 24 hours in patents undergoing pelvic or abdominal surgery. Constipation may be caused by dehydration, immobility and opiate analgesia; if these are present, bowel actions must be recorded.

ACUTE CONFUSION

Acute confusion may affect an elderly patient with no previous history of dementia. The key features are:

- a sudden onset, with clouding of consciousness over 24 hours and inappropriate or incoherent responses;
- impaired attention;
- apathy, purposeless movement or hyperactivity;
- thought, perception and short-term memory impairment;
- cognition and mood fluctuation, especially at night;
- impaired information-processing;
- disorientation in time, place and person;
- emotional lability;
- disturbed sleeping/waking pattern;
- hallucinations and delusions.

It tends to last less than a month, does not cause permanent brain damage and is usually followed by full recovery (Holden, 1995). For prevention and management, *see* Chapter 2.

The role of the nurse is to identify those at risk of such complications and try to prevent them, including monitoring for early signs. Griffiths *et al.* (1989) suggest that reduced grip strength in post-operative patients may be a useful predictor of complications. All patients after major vascular surgery had reduced grip on the first day. By the third day, grip had returned to normal in those who went on to have an uneventful recovery.

Pain

Most patients suffer pain after an operation, the function of which is to ensure that the injured part is rested. The aim of care for a patient in pain is to reduce its level sufficiently to enable her to avoid the hazards of immobility and other side-effects of pain but not to allow her to damage the healing process by excessive activity.

Patient comment

'The first thing that I was aware of was burning hot pain in my operated foot, and cool competent hands taking my blood pressure.'

Pain relief is prescribed by the anaesthetist, so it is helpful for the ward nurse to check that there is a written prescription before the patient returns to the ward. Opioids are frequently used in the first 48 hours following surgery, either intra-venously or intramuscularly. They have a range of side-effects that must be monitored closely:

- reduction in motility of the entire gastrointest-inal tract, resulting in delayed gastric empty-ing and constipation;
- nausea and vomiting, which are very common; an anti-emetic is usually prescribed;
- respiratory depression, which may be poten-tiated by other sedatives, such as alcohol and antipsychotic drugs; the respiratory rate is always carefully monitored in patients receiv-ing opiates;
- drowsiness, so levels of consciousness are checked regularly;
- postural hypotension, which may occur in fluid-depleted patients;
- interaction with monoamine oxidase inhibitors to produce hyperpyrexia, which can be fatal;

Systemic opioids must never be administered to patients receiving epidural narcotics (Strathern, 1996).

Fear of pain may be a major deterrent to per-forming deep breathing and coughing exercises or mobilizing adequately post-operatively: 'Suc-cess in giving patients the courage to be active is unlikely unless control of pain is adequate' (Wilson-Barnett and Fordham, 1982).

A pain management strategy should include the following:

DETAILED ASSESSMENT OF PAIN

This may involve use of a 'painometer', in which 0 = no pain and 10 = the worst possible pain the patient can imagine. By agreeing this scoring system pre-operatively, the patient can see that someone is going to take her pain seriously. A familiar idea will also be easier to implement with the drowsy patient. Scores can only be compared with previous ones from the same patient.

When scoring a patient's pain, it may be help-ful to score her wound, nasogastric tube and drain separately to gain an accurate picture of what is troubling her most. The pale, sweating, restless patient with raised respiratory and heart rates is showing all the physiological signs of acute pain.

PRESCRIBING AND DELIVERY OF ANALGESICS

The rise of continuous, intravenous pain relief via an infusion set or syringe driver is a welcome development, as is patient-controlled analgesia (PCA). This results in a more subtle and respon-sive form of pain relief.

OTHER TENSION-RELIEVING STRATEGIES

The patient can be encouraged to go limp in order to avoid increasing pain from muscle tension. The strategies described in the section on pre-operative pain can be useful here. Massage, well away from the area of the incision, may help, as may listening to pleasant music.

DYNAMIC EXERCISE

Dynamic exercise can itself relieve or avoid addi-tional muscle and joint aches induced by the awkward position and movement caused by pain.

Day case patients may have local analgesic blocks to treat their pain in hospital. By the time the

Patient-controlled analgesia

- Achieves
  - minimum effective blood analgesic concentration with
  - minimum side-effects
- Via
  - a syringe pump and
  - a timing system
- Is activated by the patient pressing a button
- Causing a small predetermined bolus dose of analgesic (e.g. 1 mg morphine) to be delivered into the venous circulation
- The epidural (Greenland, 1995; Strathern, 1996) and subcutaneous routes may also be used
- At the same time, a lock-out device is activated to ensure that another dose cannot be given until the first has exerted its full effect, usually in 5–10 minutes
- Most machines allow a continuous background infusion to be delivered independent of patient demand, so that sleeping patients are not woken by pain.

(Warwick, 1992; Thomas, 1995)

blocks wear off, they have probably returned home. An effective strategy, including written information, must be devised for ensuring that subsequent pain relief works (Firth, 1991).

Wound care

Woundcare is aimed at supporting a natural process. The theatre dressing is therefore usually left undisturbed for as long as possible.

Most uncontaminated surgical wounds heal by *primary intention*, in which all the layers are stitched closely together (approximated) to eliminate deadspace. This results in the minimum of granulation (the outgrowth of new young capillaries and connective tissue cells from the surface of an open wound) and therefore scar tissue once healing is complete (Tudor and Gupta, 1992). These scars usually fade with time.

Healing by *secondary intention* is necessary for wounds that cannot be sutured. They heal more slowly, filling the area in from the base, and have an increased chance of infection. Although considerable contraction takes place, the scarring tends to be more prominent than in a sutured wound.

Healing by *tertiary intention* is also known as delayed primary suturing; it is performed several days after wounding. The wound is more likely to be contaminated, so scarring will be greater (Long and Phipps, 1985).

Inflammation is the first phase of healing; the wound will be red, hot, swollen and painful, with loss of function of the affected part. The blood vessels cut during surgery will have bled, producing clots at the site of the injury to stop blood flow and provide a temporary glue at the wound edges. As fluid evaporates from the clot, it dries out to produce crusting – a 'scab' (Tudor and Gupta, 1992).

During the *destructive phase* of wound healing, non-viable tissue is removed and the wound site is supplied with granulocytes, phagocytes and immunoglobulins (Spencer and Bale, 1990).

Within 24 hours, epithelial cells from the edges of the wound start to migrate over the dermis, forming an epithelial layer under the deepest layer of the scab. The fibroblasts (collagen-producing cells) increase their activity over the next few days, reaching a maximum about 1 week post-surgery. At first disorganized, the collagen laid down later becomes a more organized network in response to the stresses on the wound and increases in tensile strength. This so-called *proliferative phase* may last for 3–4 weeks (Tudor and Gupta, 1992).

The *maturation phase* of wound healing may take 12–18 months from initial incision. The wound is remodelled many times, granulation tissue being replaced by an acellar fibrous mass. It is this phase that determines the final nature of the wound, including its maximum strength (Tudor and Gupta, 1992).

The best wound dressing provides a warm, moist, acidic environment at the wound surface, which excludes atmospheric oxygen and is impermeable to bacteria. Ideally, it is also non-adherent, non-toxic, non-allergenic and comfortable, provides protection and can be left in place for some time (Morison, 1992). Hydrocolloid dressings fulfil many of these criteria, and dressing changes must aim to maintain this optimum healing environment. The best cleansing solution is usually warmed normal saline, which is not dried off afterwards. If the wound is allowed to get cold, it can take 4 hours before cell division is back to its former level of activity. The wound should not be left exposed either, as it is best kept at a temperature of 37°C. The habit of taking dressings down for doctors' rounds is therefore counterproductive to healing (Glide, 1992).

The purpose of wound cleansing is to remove the debris and micro-organisms that might delay healing or cause infection. Wound exudate itself seems to be antibacterial so, unless the exudate is excessive and causing problems, it is best left undisturbed. If a wound is clean, there is little exudate and there are signs of healthy granulation (bright red, rough, like granulated sugar in appearance), repeated cleaning could do more harm than good. Unnecessary cleaning and dressing traumatize new, delicate tissues, cool the wound and remove the bactericidal exudate. They thus waste nursing time and delay wound healing (Glide, 1992).

It is rarely necessary to use antiseptic solutions on a healing wound as most are rapidly inactivated by body fluids. Many, such as Eusol, can adversely affect blood flow to the healing wound (Brennan et al., 1984). Used in sufficient strength to kill bacteria, they are likely to inactivate the quickly dividing cells needed for healing. The cleaning action of most antiseptics is largely mechanical and can be achieved more safely using normal physiological isotonic (0.9%) saline, preferably using an irrigation technique (Glide, 1992).

Items such as cotton wool balls, which shed fibres onto the wound surface, should be avoided, as the fibres become embedded in the granulation tissue. They may act as foci for infection or prolong the inflammatory phase of healing by activating the 'foreign body' response (Glide, 1992).

Wound exudate is usually haemoserous or serous. One indication for immediate dressing change is strike-through of exudate to the outside of the dressing. This provides a liquid pathway for bacteria to travel in both directions. Thus dressings with a reasonable degree of absorbency should be chosen. An assessment chart (e.g. Morison, 1992) can monitor progress.

When dressings are be changed, the main source of pain is often their adherence to the wound, so an effective non-adherent dressing material should be chosen, reducing the trauma to the delicate granulating tissue and thus promoting healing (Moody, 1992).

Sutures and clips

Suture removal is determined by the rate of tissue healing. The pre-operative assessment (see skin integrity) will give some idea of progress. Plans need to be flexible as there is a wide range of normal. The standard '7–10 days' offers a useful starting point.

Skin clips are used where there is little tension on the wound and a good blood supply. Thus they can be removed earlier than sutures, at approximately 4–5 days post-operatively. There is a removal instrument for each type of clip; all work by freeing the 'barbs' of the clips from the skin by distorting the clip. The action can be enhanced by rocking the clip remover gently before lifting the clip away.

Subcutaneous continuous sutures improve the cosmetic end-result and are fairly simple to remove. The retaining bead or button is cut next to the skin and the suture swiftly slid out. As it is removed, the patient usually complains of a sharp stinging sensation, which settles to an ache in a few minutes. It may make some patients nauseated.

Intermittent skin sutures are more complex to remove, and the patient may be reassured by the offer of analgesic cover. Because of the altered sensations of the wound, it is best for the nurse to be in a position where she can see the patient's face in order to determine which areas are very painful, which numb and which relatively normal. If possible, the patient should determine the rate of progress.

Patient comment

'It was like torture, this pain working its way steadily down my belly, and there was nothing I could do about it.'

Each knot is identified and lifted slightly, and the suture cut once, just below the knot, as close to the skin as possible. The objectives are to:

- prevent any part of the surface suture being pulled beneath the skin;
- remove the entire suture length;
- minimize trauma.

The suture is then pulled out across the wound to reduce traction on the skin edges.

If, after removal of sutures or clips, there is any doubt about the approximation of the skin edges, or any tendency to gape, self-adhesive skin closure strips are applied. They can remain in place for up to a week, and the patient can bathe or shower with them on. The end-result of good approximation is a narrower, more cosmetically pleasing scar.

In some areas, dissolvable sutures such as Dexon are used, which do not need removal but only trimming of the knots close to the skin before the patient goes home.

By the stage of suture removal, there is little physiological need for a dressing over the wound. The patient may, however, feel psychologically safer with such a barrier over the wound.

Drains

Wound drains are used to remove or divert body fluids, blood, bile and air from the operative area in order to promote healing.

Collections of fluid in the tissues can form a focus for infection. A tube is inserted into where the material is expected to collect and is led outside the body, usually via a puncture site separated from the main wound. The tube is stitched to the skin for safety. A sterile safety-pin may also be attached to the tube to prevent it slipping into the body cavity.

An open drain will be allowed to seep into dressing material. The current trend is to use closed drainage systems, which fall into two types – gravity and suction:

- Gravity drainage tubes are connected to drainage bags or bottles that hang lower than the patient. These are passive collectors.

- Suction drainage tubes are active collectors connected to:
  - a bottle that has been sucked out to create a vacuum. Indicators on the lid show whether the system is working or needs attention;
  - a bulb that is squeezed to create a vacuum before being connected to the tube. It slowly reinflates, collecting body fluid;
  - a bottle to collect the exudate, and an air outlet connected to a low-pressure suction pump, designed to exert steady, gentle suction as indicated on the dial;
  - underwater seal chest drains (see Chapter 7).

It is necessary, when caring for a patient with an open or closed wound drain, to use meticulous aseptic technique. Using wound drains has been found to increase infection rate, depending on the type of drain and how and where it is inserted. A closed suction drain through a separate stab wound poses the least risk (Cruse and Foord, 1980). Apart from infection, the complications associated with use of a drain (Nightingale, 1989) include:

- failure of the drain to function properly, because of incorrect positioning or too narrow a tube for the viscous fluid to pass through;
- an inflammatory reaction to the material of the drainage tube;
- damage to adjacent structures, caused by a rigid drain or too powerful a suction;
- accidental early removal if the drain is not properly secured with a suture, pin or tape.

Such complications can be a source of great pain and anxiety. Thus, if the use of a drain is anticipated, the patient must be informed beforehand and reminded why as often as necessary. If the drain is adequately secured, and the patient feels confident about this, she is less likely to limit her movements for fear of damaging it (Fig. 1.2).

Removal is largely determined by the decrease in amount of drainage. The patient may need analgesic cover as, even if pain is absent at the time, the disturbance to the tissues is likely to cause it. Aseptic technique is employed, the suture cut or safety pin removed and the drain carefully slid out, while the patient takes a series of deep breaths. The site is likely to seep for a

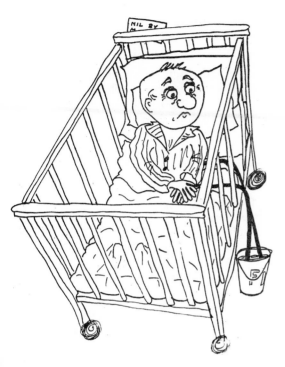

Figure 1.2 How does it feel to have a drain?

while, so an absorbent dressing needs to be applied.

Patient comments

'The tube itself came out all right, but it didn't half stir things up. I was left with a burning pain in the area for the rest of the day.'

'The nurse was thoughtful. He gave me a painkiller and gave it time to work. He also put me in charge of how quickly the tube came out. We agreed a system of signals to indicate stop or go, and he taught me deep breathing exercises to distract me from the pain.'

Nasogastric tubes

The patient may return from theatre with a nasogastric tube to manage gastric dilatation, paralytic ileus and vomiting after abdominal surgery. As the routine use of such tubes is associated with an increased incidence of post-operative

pulmonary infection, and as many as two-thirds of patients may have complications such as vomiting, nasopharyngeal soreness, cough and dysphagia, their use has to be clearly justified (Creagh, 1988).

STUDENT ACTIVITY

When you are hungry, use a stethoscope to listen to your own bowel sounds. Try again after a meal. How do they differ?

The criterion for nasogastric tube removal is the presence of normal bowel sounds. As nurses do not usually listen for these, nursing indicators will be absence of nausea, lack of abdominal distension and freely passed flatus. If the tube has been in position for some time, be aware that the end of the tube might become knotted, rendering the usual route of removal through the nose painful, traumatic or even impossible. Gaffney and Jones (1988) describe management in this event. Usually, however, tubes slide out relatively easily, to the relief of the patient.

Patient comment

'I was frightened that it was really going to hurt. The nurse let me pull it out myself, so I felt in control of what was going on. It was unpleasant, but nothing like I had imagined.'

Intravenous infusion

Many patients return to the ward with an intravenous infusion to replace fluid, restore electrolyte balance and provide access to the venous system for drug delivery. The most common fluid is 0.9% sodium chloride. Dextrose saline or dextrose (5% in water) may be used to provide a few calories. The longer an intravenous cannula site is in use, the more likely phlebitis is to develop (Hecker, 1988).

Patient comment

'The vein went hard, like a rope along my arm. It didn't go down for three months.'

Aseptic technique is essential when handling equipment; handwashing must be employed before dealing with intravenous equipment. Alcohol swabs should be used for any essential manipulation and disconnection. Each unit will have a written policy on care of an intravenous infusion, including recommendations on when to use filters and how often to change giving sets (usually between 48 and 72 hours). Using infusion pumps has reduced the amount of nursing time spent regulating infusions (Allan, 1988). The infusion will only remain until:

- the patient is tolerating oral fluids in sufficient quantities to render it unnecessary;
- the patient is no longer dehydrated, and it is anticipated that she will be able to gain sufficient calories orally. The giving set may then be removed, but the intravenous cannula is left in place if intravenous access might be needed for drug delivery.

The site needs to be regularly inspected for signs of phlebitis and extravasation, so a transparent sterile film dressing is advisable.

Patient comments

'The drip didn't hurt at all. I was hardly aware of it.'

'The place where the needle went in was painful, and my hand went red and swelled up. They had to take the needle out and put it in my other hand.'

Signs of extravasation (fluid delivery to tissues surrounding the vein, often called 'tissueing') are:

- swelling at the cannula site;
- discomfort, burning or pain at the cannula site;
- a feeling of tightness in the arm;
- blanching or coolness of the skin.

In the event of extravasation:

- the intravenous fluid should be turned off;
- the arm should be elevated to encourage venous absorption;
- medical attention should be sought;
- frequent checks should be made on the circulation and motor function (Lamb, 1995).

Signs of phlebitis (acute inflammation of the lining of the vein) include varying degrees of:

- painfulness at the cannula site;

- erythema (redness);
- swelling;
- a palpable venous cord

depending on how advanced it has become before detection and action. The cannula must be removed and a fresh one sited elsewhere. Parenteral intravenous therapy may be necessary to prevent generalized septicaemia (Lamb, 1995).

Circulatory overload may occur if an infusion is given too rapidly; it is manifested by (Lamb, 1995):

- increased pulse rate;
- hypertension;
- distended neck veins;
- dyspnoea (breathlessness);
- respiratory gurgles and wheezes;
- a generalized feeling of discomfort.

The infusion is stopped and symptomatic treatment that may include diuretics and chest physiotherapy started.

Blood transfusion

A transfusion may be necessary during or after surgery to restore circulating volume. If it was anticipated, this would have been explained to the patient prior to surgery. However, it can be a shock to a patient who is not expecting it.

Patient comment

'I was alarmed and revolted by the bag of blood hanging above my bed when I woke up. I thought it was only given to people who were dangerously ill.'

The blood will have been grouped and cross-matched, i.e. the patient's blood group identified and a check made that the donated blood is compatible with the recipient's. In some cases, autotransfusion is performed, achieved either by the patient donating blood for storage at a suitable point before surgery or by 'scavenging' shed blood during the operation, filtering it and returning it to the patient's circulation.

Each unit will have its own policies and procedures to ensure that the right blood gets to the right patient at the right time in the right condition.

Each patient will be monitored during transfusion by measuring, for example, temperature, pulse, blood pressure and respiration every half an hour. The patient will be observed for signs of an adverse reaction or any complication of blood transfusion, including:

- allergic reactions (*see* below);
- circulatory overload;
- disease transmission;
- a pyrogenic reaction;
- bacterial contamination;
- haemolytic reaction and incompatibility;
- hyperkalaemia (potassium excess);
- hypocalcaemia;
- air embolism.

If problems are detected, the first step will be to stop the transfusion and call for immediate assistance. Intravenous access will still be necessary, so the cannula must remain in place, kept open with normal saline, even if the transfusion set is disconnected.

Allergic reactions may occur soon after the transfusion has started or hours afterwards. These are potentially life-threatening and range from mild fever or rash, to shortness of breath, generalized oedema and possible cardiac arrest.

Mobilization

After minor surgery, the patient is encouraged to get out of bed the same day. After more major operations, this may be delayed until the next day or longer, depending on, for example, weightbearing restrictions. There must be good reasons for keeping patients in bed as 'the pathological physiology initiated by surgical trauma is one of stagnation involving blood, lymph, pulmonary gases and intestinal contents, and ... exercise, particularly walking, improves each' (Wilson-Barnett and Fordham, 1982).

All patients, as they come round from the anaesthetic, must be encouraged to do chest and leg exercises at regular intervals to minimize complications. As vital signs are regularly recorded, the presence of the nurse at this time can be a useful reminder.

It helps, while the patient is still sleepy from the anaesthetic, to place her in a position different from that of the operation, if this has not already been done in the recovery room. This contributes to relief of pressure and reduces the risk of pressure sores, many of which begin in theatre.

Major movement by the patient, as opposed to for the patient, can commence when she has a sustaining blood pressure, usually 2–4 hours after surgery, and has recovered from the anaesthetic.

Much of the strength of sutured wounds is present immediately after surgery, and only a small increase in wound strength results from healing over the following months (Wilson-Barnett and Fordham, 1932). The team can use this to encourage the, often reluctant, patient to greater mobilization in the immediate post-operative period. This will also help to reduce the risk of deep venous thrombosis, chest infection and other hazards of immobility.

Patient comment

'It really felt as if the wound would tear apart every time I moved. It was far worse when the nurses lifted me. What was best was for me to move myself an inch at a time, knowing when to stop, until I had got myself into the new position.'

Giving the patient time and control over the movement can be beneficial. Aids to enhance self-movement of the patient include:

- fitting a 'monkey pole' (trapeze) to the bed;
- showing her how to hold onto the bedframe under the mattress to steady herself and give her something to pull against – an infusion stand, if firmly attached to the bed, can be helpful for this;
- keeping the bed as low as possible to facilitate easy transfer to and from an armchair;
- a rope ladder attached to the foot of the bed for the patient to pull herself up hand over hand;
- rocking from hip to hip to move herself up the bed.

Ensuring that the patient's hygiene and elimination needs are met while she is recovering from the anaesthetic can contribute to the enhancement of her mobility. A few hours after returning from the recovery room, a face and hands wash may be appreciated. If it is appropriate, the patient's theatre gown should be removed and replaced with her own nightclothes. All this promotes a range of movement – avoiding stasis. Equally, when the patient needs to empty her bladder, a commode brought to the bedside or a short walk to the toilet is more natural than trying to use a bedpan.

Patient comment

'Trying to perch on a bedpan with a spinning head was almost impossible. It was such a relief to slump onto the commode.'

Sleep and rest

The first post-operative night is likely to be far from restful. Many patients seem to be 'slept-out' by the anaesthetic and do not sleep well, despite the fact that they feel tired.

Patient comment

'I seemed to wake every hour, needing a drink of water or a bedpan or something for the pain.'

The nurse needs to settle the patient as far as possible, with not only attention to pain relief, hydration, a clean mouth and an empty bladder, but also reassurance about events such as wakefulness and, vital signs monitoring. It is worth encouraging a rest in the afternoon for the first couple of post-operative days, balanced with gently increasing activity, as the patient's condition permits.

Eating and drinking

As soon as the patient can tolerate sips of water, the aim will be to make up for any dehydration incurred as a result of pre-, peri- and post-operative fasting and fluid loss, giving the equivalent of a glass of water per waking hour. It can be rendered more attractive by adding fruit squash.

The return of appetite may be delayed in the case of abdominal surgery or nausea and vomiting. No patient should be without food for more than 3 days because of the increased metabolic demands imposed by surgery. At this point, a decision has to be made, and documented, about what is to be done. This may be parenteral feeding if the gut is not working or is inaccessible, enteral feeding if the gut is functioning, by fine-bore nasogastric tube, gastrostomy or jejeunostomy, sip feeding with supplements, fortified diet or normal food. The aim is to establish a normal eating pattern as soon as possible to counteract the catabolism of major surgery. Small, frequent snacks are often more tolerable than 'great platefuls' at longer intervals. Tea, squash, clear soup and jellies are of no help as they fill the patient up without providing much by energy or many nutrients. Some units have a microwave and encourage family members to bring in favourite foods to tempt the patient's appetite. If necessary, a food and weight chart will record progress.

Planning for discharge starts as soon as the patient is admitted and preferably before. Written plans are helpful, each unit having its own version. Areas to consider are listed below in alphabetical order, no priority being intended:

Discharge advice

The following will be considered (in alphabetical order):

- bowels;
- complications;
- decisions;

- depression;
- dressing and bathing;
- driving;
- drugs;
- exercise;
- follow-up;

- food and fluids;
- hobbies;
- housework;
- probable progress through convalescence;
- rest and sleep;
- sexuality;
- specific recommendations or prohibitions;
- support system;
- weightlifting;
- work;
- wound care.

> **STUDENT ACTIVITY**
>
> Find a patient information leaflet designed for the patient to take home. Compare it with the checklist for advice on discharge. Are all the categories included?

Bowels

The patient may find that her bowel habit is altered when she returns home. There may be residual effects from the drugs taken in hospital, plus those taken home, be these constipating analgesics or diarrhoea-inducing antibiotics. Nausea will affect intake and hence bowel function; food and drink containing ginger can be a very effective anti-emetic. Certain operations have a specific impact on bowel habit, such as the tendency to diarrhoea after cholecystectomy (owing to the constant flow of dilute bile), which can take up to a year to settle. The patient must avoid straining at stool as it is likely to be very uncomfortable and should improve her soluble fibre (fruit, vegetables and oats) and fluid intake, plus her activity levels, to achieve a comfortable result.

Complications

The specialist chapters in Part Two outline possible complications to search for and inform the patient of. This is necessary realistically to involve the patient in her own care. Thoughtful advice reflecting reality can be given without

alarming the patient. For example, it would be irresponsible to ignore the likelihood of dehiscence (a 'burst abdomen') if someone has had a wound infection. Secondary haemorrhage owing to infection, for example, or deep venous thrombosis may occur once the patient has gone home.

Decisions

The slowed reaction time, tiredness, anxiety, insecurity, lack of concentration and pain suffered by many patients at home (Vaughan and Taylor, 1988) do not encourage good decision-making. Decisions should be deferred, if at all possible, until the patient is in a better frame of mind.

Depression

Post-anaesthetic depression may strike the unsuspecting patient between 7 and 10 days postoperatively, often when she has left hospital. She feels sad and weepy for no apparent reason. Lack of confidence may leave her feeling vulnerable and unable to cope. It is necessary to warn patients of this and that it will pass of its own accord in a few days.

Dressing and bathing

The main problem areas appear to be getting clothing on over the feet, and tightness and restriction over the wound (Vaughan and Taylor, 1988). Tracksuits or larger, looser than normal clothes can be more comfortable in the short term.

Whether or not to bathe and difficulties in getting in and out of the bath seem to concern patients once home (Vaughan and Taylor, 1988). While the stitches or clips are still in place, getting the wound wet is allowed, but a long soak is not recommended. Adding salt to the bath has no effect. It is suggested (Vaughan and Taylor, 1988) that a non-slip bath mat should be used, and a towel hooked around the taps can be helpful for the patient to pull herself up out of the bath. If the water is too hot, she may feel sick and faint on getting up. It can be reassuring to have someone else in the house while attempting the first bath. Showers are best as the patient does not 'stew in her own juice'. If difficulties with bathing are identified before the patient leaves hospital, a suitable bath aid can be suggested. Sources vary; aids may be available from occupational therapy or physiotherapy departments, a reputable chemist or the British Red Cross Society.

Driving

Anaesthetic drugs can take some considerable time to be metabolized. They tend to lodge in fatty tissues, from which they are reluctantly given up. This is especially relevant in females, who have a higher percentage of body fat than males. The result is slowed reaction times, which are most noticeable if the patient attempts to use machinery or drive. The recommendation is not to drive for 7–10 days after release from hospital, although the longer the period under anaesthetic, the longer the time the patient is affected. When the patient feels ready to resume driving, she must be capable of dealing with an emergency stop as well as normal driving. After some operations, there is a specific ban on driving for longer than 7–10 days (see the specialist chapters in Part Two).

Drugs

Written instructions are needed on the drugs that the patient is expected to take at home. If she is only briefed about them verbally at a late stage before leaving hospital, her ability to retain the information is likely to be limited, with consequent loss of compliance. The likelihood of drug–nutrient interaction (Holmes, 1985, 1986) must be taken into consideration, especially if the patient needs long-term treatment.

Exercise

Specific exercises are prescribed post-surgery to strengthen areas affected by the operation. These will be taught by the physiotherapist and must be performed adequately before the patient goes home. Patients are still at risk of deep venous thrombosis on returning home, so activity must be undertaken for up to 12 weeks post-operatively (Voelker, 1996). A written instruction and advice sheet is helpful.

It is essential to check that the patient can get out of a chair, in and out of bed and up and down stairs unaided before discharge. Difficulties may be resolved by teaching helpful strategies, such as not choosing too low an armchair, and getting out of it once an hour.

Zeiderman et al. (1990) found that the increased cardiorespiratory effort and reduced muscular efficiency associated with low-intensity exercise could limit mobilization after surgery and contribute to a greater feeling of fatigue. A balance has to be developed between excessive rest, which will increase catabolism, and gently increasing exercise, which can, over time, enhance energy levels.

The patient should be encouraged to do a little more each day to promote the return of strength, suppleness and stamina. This could be by walking increasing distances daily or climbing more stairs, depending on home circumstances. Improvements in stamina (endurance fitness) are best achieved by, for example, walking a little harder and faster each time. The goal is to sustain 20–30 minutes of moderate-to-brisk exercise five times a week. It may take up to 3 months to achieve this level – more if the patient was sedentary pre-operatively. Swimming and cycling are particularly encouraged. Jogging, squash and aerobics tend to be recommended only beyond 3 months post-surgery.

Older patients, men and women alike, may benefit from an exercise prescription to arrest bone reduction from osteoporosis. Goodman (1985) offers a programme to build up reserve bone mass.

It is important to incorporate additional activity into the daily routine, initially as a conscious decision. Taking the stairs instead of the lift, getting off the bus one stop early and cycling to work are a few examples. The reward will be that exercise will become an almost automatic habit, not needing the tremendous motivation of exercise that is performed exclusively to feel more fit. If positive, precise and focused advice is received and acted upon, the goal of recovery of pre-operative fitness may not only be achieved more quickly, but even exceeded (Wilson-Barnett and Fordham, 1982).

Follow-up

The patient may see the surgical team at an outpatient appointment to monitor progress, or follow-up may be with the GP. It must be clear to the patient which system will be used. Some units have a letter for the patient to deliver to her GP; others send one on later. The support of a clinical nurse specialist, such as a stomatherapist, may continue after leaving hospital. The patient needs to have a telephone number to ring if she is worried or needs further information.

Food and fluids

The pre-operative work of enhancing the patient's knowledge of a balanced diet can be reinforced. The convalescent phase can lay down good eating habits; the 'tilted plate' formula (see p. 10) is likely to be easy to apply. Over and above this, there are the increased metabolic requirements of surgery, fasting and healing. The importance of enough protein and vitamin C can hardly be overstated.

Infection, surgical stress and trauma increase the activity of the sympathetic nervous system, which increases the secretion of catabolic hormones such as cortisol, glucagon and the catecholamines adrenaline and noradrenaline, while inhibiting anabolic hormones such as insulin and testosterone. This chain of events leads to loss of body nitrogen, indicative of a net loss of protein. The breakdown of muscle throughout the body is enhanced (Adam and Oswald, 1984). The patient needs to be reminded to drink about 1.5–2.0 L of fluid (excluding alcohol) daily to replenish body water levels. A useful rule is to drink enough to keep the urine 'pale and plentiful'.

Hobbies

For some, the recovery period can be enjoyably productive, with time to pursue a hobby. Others may take up a new one, such as learning a new language. If used positively, a sense of achievement can be a real boost to the morale at a time when it is much needed. It also provides a distraction from feeling unwell and worrying about every ache and pain. The tendency to vegetate is to be discouraged, except in the very short term.

Housework

The convalescent phase may present the patient with an opportunity to rethink how the housework is organized, as she will initially be unable to do much unaided. Those tasks involving stretching and bending, such as bed-making and cleaning the bath, will need to be avoided for up to 3 months, as will using a vacuum cleaner and carrying a full load of wet washing or shopping. Other problem areas are those involving standing for long periods, such as preparing vegetables, washing-up and ironing. If help is not available in the first 2 weeks after discharge, the patient might be better off staying with someone else or doing the absolute minimum, sitting down as much as possible.

Probable progress through convalescence

Convalescence after surgery is characterized by a period of fatigue, the duration of which is unrelated to the seriousness of the operation. For example, one-third of those who had had abdominal surgery felt tired throughout the first post-operative month, while the rest returned to pre-operative fitness in 3–4 weeks (Zeiderman et al. 1990). It is therefore reasonable for the patient to feel tired when she leaves hospital and for a while thereafter.

The expectations of the patient and her family may not match, so it can be helpful to brief both. Expected landmarks and changes can be noted in writing, so that progress and complications can be distinguished.

Rest and sleep

The patient may initially feel like taking after-noon naps when she gets home; these will help to restore her probable sleep deficit (Closs, 1988). Sleep shifts the balance in favour of anabolism: deep sleep is the normal stimulus for the release of growth hormone, which increases protein syn-thesis and releases free fatty acids to provide energy, thereby saving amino acids for anabolism (Adam and Oswald, 1984).

Sexuality

The classical advice in this area is non-existent or, rarely, 'take it easy'. The advice really needed is when usual sexual activity can be safely resumed (Vaughan and Taylor, 1988). In some ways, the patient is the best judge of this, as she must be feeling better to feel like resuming it. Some units suggest that the time she restarts work is reasonable.

Some recommendations can prevent unneces-sary discomfort. If the patient has had abdominal or pelvic surgery, she will be more comfortable on top of her partner or in a side-lying position. This can be an opportunity to change some stale or unsatisfactory habits by giving her a licence to ask for what she wants.

The male patient may encounter a short-term loss of libido after surgery as a reflection of the trauma. He needs reassurance that this is tem-porary and that recovery will mirror his general physical improvement. When he feels like resum-ing his sex-life, the suggestion will be 'carefully', as he will have residual aches from the area of surgery. After an inguinal hernia repair, for ex-ample, he has to allow the area to heal and gain strength, so very vigorous activity may be ruled

out for as long as 6 weeks to 3 months. Following pelvic or abdominal surgery, it is recommended that he adopt an on-top or side-lying position to avoid pain. Some operations cause impotence or retrograde ejaculation; some drugs also cause impotence. The team needs to be honest with the patient about this from the start. Resumption of contraception, especially the oral contraceptive pill, needs discussion.

Specific recommendations or prohibitions

There are likely to be some very precise 'dos and don'ts' for many operations (*see* the specialist chapters in Part Two). As part of their convales-cence, patients may arrange a holiday, but the health hazards of air travel are not always appre-ciated by the lay public or even health profession-als. It is necessary to ensure that flying is not contraindicated by the patient's condition. Low-ered atmospheric pressure and hypoxia during the flight can cause problems such as gangrene in a plastered limb. If the patient is already anaemic from surgery, the hypoxia could trigger serious problems. Other effects may be caused by gases expanding; for example, the expansion of a pocket of gas in the small intestine may lead to discomfort, nausea, vomiting, severe pain or even fainting (a vasovagal syncope): 'In theory, the expansion would be sufficient to rupture a dis-eased part of the intestine, in particular in the presence of colitis, septic or duodenal ulcers and recent abdominal surgery' (Kahn, 1990). Long-haul flights increase the risk of deep vein throm-bosis, even in healthy passengers.

Support system

A sense of supportive camaraderie (Wilson-Barnett and Fordham, 1982) among the occupants of the ward may be greatly missed by the patient when she goes home. Part of planning for dis-charge will be to mobilize her support system in terms of family, friends and neighbours in real-istic anticipation of the amount of help needed. The support can then be reasonably 'shared out' without the patient feeling a burden to any particular individual. It is necessary to involve the key member of the patient's family in generating a realistic plan for discharge, as the expectations are then more likely to match.

Patient comments

'My husband thought that I would come home and go straight to bed for a week. He was surprised that I could move around much better than he expected.'

'My girlfriend was great! She bullied me into doing the right exercises for my knee, and wouldn't let me walk badly. I hated it at the time, but I'm so grateful now, as I'm sure it kept me going.'

Weightlifting

Classical advice to the post-operative patient is 'do not lift any heavy weights' but what constitutes a heavy weight may not be clearly specified. After abdominal or pelvic surgery, the initial amount should not exceed 1 kg (2.2 lb) – the equivalent of a full kettle of water. The advice here is to take the water to the kettle cupful by cupful, as the walking will be better for the patient. Static or isometric exercises such as lifting heavy weights induce increases in blood pressure and intra-abdominal pressure. Infected wounds and those subjected to the high pressure stress of coughing are more likely to burst (Wilson-Barnett and Fordham, 1982). If serious weightlifting is a part of the patient's life this will have been elicited at interview and the safest progression discussed with the patient, for example not resuming weightlifting for 6 weeks after an uncomplicated appendicectomy, and slowly building up from very light weights.

Work

Time to return to work is a reasonable indicator of recovery from surgery; it depends upon the physical nature of the job. Those with sedentary jobs or flexible work activities can probably return to work by 6 weeks after, for example, an

inguinal hernia repair. If there are no 'light duties', the patient may have to stay off for longer. (*See* the specialist chapters in Part Two for some indication of convalescent times.)

Wound care

With the increasing trend towards early discharge and day case surgery, the patient needs to be well-informed about the progress of wound healing, and many will go home with sutures or clips still in place. An appointment must be made to have these removed at a time dictated by the likely rate of healing, as assessed pre- and post-operatively. Suture removal may take place on the ward, in the OPD, at the local health centre or at home. It can be a useful chance for the patient to raise any queries she may have and for the health-care professional to check progress.

The patient's concerns are likely to include the wound's appearance, odd sensations, pain and soreness, whether it is healing as it should and the hardness of the scar (Vaughan and Taylor, 1988).

The appearance of the wound will vary as healing progresses. It will look red (densely black in black skins) and swollen when the patient first sees it. The healing process takes up to 2 years, gradually rendering the scar flat and silvery white (or black).

Sensations are related to the fact that the sensory nerves are cut at operation. Some areas will be numb, others exquisitely sensitive. The patient will be reluctant to touch the scar, and it will feel alien to her.

Pain and soreness are related to the bruising sustained at operation, the oedema of the inflammatory process and the stitches.

The feeling of hardness in the scar due to replacement by fibrous tissue can be disconcerting.

Wounds may itch, which is part of the normal process. It is better to slap the wound than scratch it.

The patient can help the normal process of healing and simultaneously incorporate the new scar into her body image in a positive way. Unlike normal skin, fibrous tissue has no sebaceous glands to moisturize the surface. For the same reason, no hairs grow on the scar itself. From 24 hours after the sutures or clips are removed, the patient should lightly moisturize the scar after bathing or showering with any lotion that she regularly uses elsewhere. A few weeks later, when she is ready, she can use a thicker cream and more firmly massage the scar and surrounding tissues to prevent adhesions and encourage a smoother, flatter, more comfortable scar. This is especially important if the scar is over bone. The procedure should be carried out daily for 3–9 months after surgery, depending on the results. Having to touch the scar is helpful to adaptation. Thereafter, the occasional use of moisturizing lotion will keep the scar comfortable, but it will always be drier and more sensitive than the surrounding healthy skin. For at least the first year following surgery, sunblock must be used if the scar is exposed to sunlight. Healing is the process of laying down and remodelling the collagen in the scar; sunlight destroys the collagen structure of the skin.

Overgrowth of the scar occasionally occurs, leading to a raised, broad, red (or black), itchy scar – a keloid – particularly seen in those with black skins. This manifests itself after some months as a widening, spreading scar, when the healing process appears to be on schedule. The regions most at risk are the chest and shoulders. The problem is referred to a plastic surgeon. Seek help if:

- the pain in the wound markedly increases;
- the amount of redness and/or swelling increases;
- there is any unexpected discharge from the wound.

'Do not be afraid to ask for advice, however small your worry may seem. A few words can often save a lot of anxiety' (Vaughan and Taylor, 1988).

Summary

1 The patient is anxious.

2 An operation and anaesthetic carry risks.

3 The aims of care are to find out as much as possible about patients, identify their risks and reduce those risks to a minimum.

4 Accurate information must be constantly conveyed to the team and the patient.

5 The period of hospitalization can offer health promotion opportunities.

6 Planning for discharge begins on admission.

7 A calm, well-informed and well-prepared patient will be at a lower risk of complications.

8 The patient is monitored most closely during anaesthesia, less so during recovery, and so on, down or up a sliding scale, according to her progress.

9 The aim of post-operative care is to maximize the patient's progress towards independence.

CASE HISTORY

Mrs Stagg, aged 73, is being admitted for elective surgery on a large swelling on her upper arm: she lives alone very competently but is anxious at the prospect of the anaesthetic, and the implications of the operation. The last time she was in hospital was 20 years ago.

What strategies would you employ to reduce Mrs Stagg's anxiety and keep her safe?

Review Questions

1 What are vital signs observations and how do they differ from neurovascular observations?

2 Identify the risk factors that may delay wound healing.

3 Explain the difference between acute retention of urine and acute renal failure.

4 How would you assess a patient's comprehension while you are explaining an investigation to her?

5 Why and where are skin clips used instead of stitches?

6 What is secondary haemorrhage?

7 List three things you could do to keep your patient orientated.

8 Why does long-distance flying increase the risk of deep vein thrombosis?

9 How would you detect shock or haemorrhage?

ACKNOWLEDGEMENTS

Many thanks to many, many students nurses, including Sue Sills and Natalie Rutherford, and colleagues such as Anne Armstrong, Lesley Chislett, Penny Joyce, Deirdre Keeble and Jan Soley who all reviewed and criticized successive drafts, offering useful comments and suggestions that were much appreciated.

References

Adam, K. and Oswald, I. 1984 Sleep helps healing. *British Medical Journal* **289**, 1400–1.

Aggleton, P. and Chalmers, H. 1986 *Nursing models and the nursing process.* Basingstoke: Macmillan.

Alderson, P. 1995 Consent to surgery: the role of the nurse. *Nursing Standard* 9(35), 38–40.

Allan, D. 1988 Making sense of infusion pumps. *Nursing Times* 84(35), 46–7.

Bass, C. and Kerwin, R. 1989 Rediscovering monoamine oxidase inhibitors. *British Medical Journal* **298**, 345–6.

Behi, R. 1986 Look after yourself. *Nursing Times* Sept 10, 35–7.

Bibby, B.A., Collins, B.J. and Aycliffe, C.A. 1986 A mathematised model for assessing the risk of postoperative wound infection. *Journal of Hospital Infection* **1**, 31–9.

Bond, D. and Barton, K. 1994 Patient assessment before surgery. *Nursing Standard* 8(28), 23–8.

Bone, M.E., Wilkinson, D.J., Young, J.R., McNeil, J. and Charlton, S. 1990 Forum: Ginger root – a new antiemetic. The effect of ginger root on postoperative nausea and vomiting after major gynaecological surgery. *Anaesthesia* **45**, 669–71.

Boore, J. 1978 *Information – a prescription for recovery.* London: RCN.

Booth, J.A. (ed.) 1983 *Handbook of investigations.* London: Harper & Row.

Brennan, S.S., Foster, M.E. and Leaper, D.J. 1984 Adverse effects of antiseptics on the healing process. *Journal of Hospital Infection* 5(suppl. A), 122.

Buchanan, M. 1995 Enabling patients to make informed decisions. *Nursing Times* 91(18), 27–9.

Bysshe, J.E. 1988 The effect of giving information to patients before surgery. *Nursing* 3(30), 36–9.

Campling, E.A., Devlin, H.B., Hoile, R.W. and Lunn, J.N. 1992 *The report of the National Confidential Enquiry into Peri-Operative Deaths.* London: NCEPOD.

Caprini, J.A., Scurr, J.H. and Hasty, J.H. 1988 Role of compression modalities in a prophylactic program for deep vein thrombosis. *Seminars in Thrombosis and Hemostasis* **14** (suppl.), 77–87.

Carter, M. 1989 Effects of anaesthesia on mental performance in the elderly patient. *Nursing Times* (Occasional Paper) 85(4), 40–2.

Channer, K. 1985 Stand up and take your medicine. *Nursing Times* 81(28), 41–2.

Chapman, A. 1996 A study of preoperative fasting. *Nursing Standard* 10(18), 33–6.

Clark, C.R. & Gregor, F.M. 1988 Developing a sensation information message for femoral arteriography. *Journal of Advanced Nursing* 13, 237–44.

Classen, D.C., Evans, R.S., Pestotnik, S.L. *et al.* 1992 The timing of prophylactic administration of antibiotics and the risk of surgical-wound infection. *New England Journal of Medicine* 326(5), 281–6.

Closs, J. 1988 Patients' sleep–wake rhythms in hospital. Parts 1 and 2. *Nursing Times* 84(1), 48–50; 84(2), 54–5.

Coe, A.J. and Laurent, S. 1989 Rediscovering monoamine oxidase inhibitors. *British Medical Journal* 298, 671.

Creagh, T. 1988 Nasogastric warnings. *Nursing Times* 84(7), 46–7.

Cruse, P.J.E. and Foord, R. 1980 The epidemiology of wound infection – a ten year study of 62,939 wounds. *Archives of Surgical Clinics of North America* 60(1), 27–40.

Cushieri, A. 1994 *Minimal access surgery.* Report from a working group chaired by Professor Alfred Cushieri. Edinburgh: HMSO.

Dossey, B. 1991 Awakening the inner healer. *American Journal of Nursing* 91(8), 30–2.

Evans, A. (1991) Sensible stockings. *Nursing Times* 87(51), 40–1.

Firth, F. 1991 Pain after day surgery. *Nursing Times* 87(40), 72–6.

Gaffney, L. and Jones, M. 1988 Knotted tubes. *Nursing Times* 84(7), 48.

Glide, S. 1992 Cleaning choices. *Nursing Times* 88(19), 74–8.

Goodman, C.E. 1985 Nutrition and exercise regime that reverses bone loss. *Geriatric Medicine* 15(11), 14–20.

Gould, D. 1994 Understanding the nature of bacteria. *Nursing Standard* 8(28), 29–31.

Greenland, S. 1995 A review of the uses of epidural analgesia. *Nursing Standard* 9(32), 32–5.

Griffiths, C., Whyman, M., Bassey, E., Hopkinson, B. and Makin, G. 1989 Delayed recovery of grip strength predicts postoperative morbidity following major vascular surgery. *British Journal of Surgery* 76, 704–5.

Haines, N. and Viellion, G. 1990 A successful combination: preadmission testing and preoperative education. *Orthopaedic Nursing* 9(2), 53–7.

Hall, J.C., Tarala, R.A., Tapper, J. and Hall, J.L. 1996 Prevention of respiratory complications after abdominal surgery: a randomised clinical trial. *British Medical Journal* 312, 148–53.

Hayward, J. 1975 *Information – A prescription against pain.* London: RCN.

Hecker, J. 1988 Improved technique in IV therapy. *Nursing Times* 84(34), 28–33.

Hind, M. 1994 An investigation into factors that affect oesophageal temperature during abdominal surgery. *Journal of Advanced Nursing* 19, 457–64.

Holden, U. 1995 Dementia in acute units: confusion. *Nursing Standard* 9(17), 37–9.

Holmboe, J. and Williams, I. 1990 Conscious and unconscious awareness during anaesthesis – how deep is the patient's sleep? *Tidsskr-Nor-Laegeforen* 110(27), 3506–8.

Holmes, S. 1985 Drug–nutrient interactions. *Nursing Mirror* 160(12), 43–4.

Holmes, S. 1986 Nutritional needs of medical patients. *Nursing Times* 82(17), 34–6.

Kahn, F.S. 1990 *The curse of Icarus: the health factor in air travel.* London: Routledge.

Kurz, A., Sessler, D.I and Lenhardt, R. 1996 Perioperative normothermia to reduce the incidence of surgical-wound infection and shorten hospitalisation. *New England Journal of Medicine* 334(19), 1211–14.

Lamb, J. 1995 Peripheral IV therapy. *Nursing Standard* 9(30), 32–5

Landford, R. 1996 The hole truth. *Nursing Times* 92(40), 46–7.

Law Commission 1991 *Mentally incapacitated adults and decision making: an overview.* Law Commission Consultation Paper No. 119. London: HMSO.

Lennard-Jones, J.E 1992 *A positive approach to nutritional treatment.* London: Kings Fund.

Lloyd, S. 1989 Better blocking agents? *Nursing Standard* 16(3), 31–2.

Long, B.C. and Phipps, W.J. 1985 *Essentials of medical-surgical nursing: a nursing process approach.* St Louis: CV Mosby.

McCaffery, M. 1983 *Nursing the patient in pain.* London: Harper & Row.

McGarvey, H. 1990 Making sense of endotracheal intubation. *Nursing Times* 86(42), 35–7.

Markanday, L. & Platzer, H. 1994 Brief encounters. *Nursing Times* 90(7), 38–42.

Martin, D. 1996 Pre-operative visits to reduce

patient anxiety: a study. *Nursing Standard* **10**(23), 33–8.

Mason, P. 1992 Starving amidst plenty. *Nursing Times* **88**(7), 21.

Milne, C. 1988 Anaesthetics. *Nursing Standard* **2**(28), 22–3.

Mirakhur, R.K. 1991 Preanaesthetic medication: a survey of current usage. *Journal of the Royal Society of Medicine* **84**, 481–3.

Moody, M. 1992 Looking for non-adherence. *Nursing Times* **88** (19), 65

Morison, M.J. 1992 *Colour guide to nursing management of wounds.* London: Wolfe. Cited in RCN Nursing Update: Wound care – a problem solving approach. *Nursing Standard* **8** (19), 7.

Moynihan, P. 1994 Special nutritional needs of surgical patients. *Nursing Times* **90**(51), 40–1.

Nightingale, K. 1989 Making sense of wound drainage. *Nursing Times* **85** (27), 40–2.

Nursing Times 1992 Nurses have much to contribute to audits into peri-operative deaths in that they could shed further light on how and why patients die after an operation. *Nursing Times* **88**(18), 3, (comment, editorial).

Phair, L. 1996 Dementia: professional issues, professional development. *Nursing Times*, **92**(26), 9–12.

Pinfold, C. 1991 Patient consent. *Senior Nurse* **11**(5), 25–7.

Robson, R. 1994 Refusing treatment. *Nursing Standard* **8**(29), 23.

Rowbotham, D. 1995 Recognising risk factors. *Nursing Times* **91**(28), 44–6.

Scanlon, F., Dunne, J. and Toyne, K. 1994 No more cause for neglect: introducing a nutritional assessment plan. *Professional Nurse* **9**(6), 382–5.

Scurr, J.H., Coleridge-Smith, P.D. and Hasty, J.P. 1988 Deep venous thrombosis: a continuing problem. *British Medical Journal* **297**, 28.

Seropian, B. and Reynolds, B.M. 1971 Wound infections after pre-operative depilatory versus razor preparation. *American Journal of Surgery* **121**, 251–4.

Sessler, D. 1988 Quoted in: Why such a lotta shakin' going on? *New Scientist* **117**(1602), 44.

Shanks, J. 1992 Where have all the clients gone? *Nursing Times* **88**(18), 34–5.

Spencer, K.E. & Bale, S. 1990 A logical approach: management of surgical wounds. *Professional Nurse* **5**(6), 303–8.

Stotts, N.A. 1992 Nutritional factors associated with wound healing in the elderly: the role of specific nutrients in the healing process. *Diabetes Spectrum* **5**(6), 354–5.

Strathern, D. 1996 Epidural analgesia: educating patients and nurses. *Nursing Standard* **10**(25), 33–6.

Strong, C. 1979 Informed consent: theory and policy. *Journal of Medical Ethics* **5**, 196–9.

Thomas, E.A. 1987 Pre-operative fasting – a question of routine? *Nursing Times* **83** (49), 46–7.

Thomas, N. 1995 Patient-controlled analgesia. *Nursing Standard* **9**(35), 31–5.

Tudor, R. and Gupta, R. 1992 Healing physiology. *Nursing Times* **88**(19), 70–4.

Vaughan, B. and Taylor, K. 1988 Discharge procedures: homeward bound. *Nursing Times* **84**(15), 28–33.

Voelker, R. 1996 DVT collision course. *Journal of the American Medical Association* **275**(12), 901.

Warwick, P. 1992 Making sense of the principles of patient controlled analgesia. *Nursing Times* **88**(41), 38–40.

Wicker, C.P. 1990 A reassuring presence. *Nursing Times* **86**(29), 59–61.

Williams, A., Hind, M. and Sweeney, B. 1994 The incidence of postoperative nausea & vomiting in patients exposed to positive intraoperative suggestions. *Anaesthesia* **49**(4), 340–2.

Wilson-Barnett, J. and Fordham, M. 1982 *Recovery from illness.* Developments in Nursing research, Vol. 1. Chichester: John Wiley & Sons

Wood, B.M. 1987a *Anaesthetics for O.D.A.'s and theatre nurses.* West Bromwich: Sandwell District General Hospital.

Wood, B.M. 1987b *Pharmacology for the O.D.A.* West Bromwich: Sandwell District General Hospital.

Zeiderman, M.R., Welchew, E.A. & Clark, R.G. 1990 Changes in cardiorespiratory and muscle function associated with the development of postoperative fatigue. *British Journal of Surgery* **77**(5), 576–80.

Further reading

Booth, B. and Kumar, A. 1989 Surgery for elderly patients; a new speciality? *Nursing Times* **85**(29), 26–30.

Cornock, M. 1996 Making sense of central venous pressure. *Nursing Times* **92**(40), 3–39.

Cradock, S. 1989 Surgery in patients with diabetes. *Surgical Nurse* **2**(4), 22–4.

Currie, L.E.S. and Simpson, P.J. 1989 *Understanding anaesthesia*. London: Heineman.

Drain, C. and Shipley Christoph, S. 1987 *The recovery room*. New York: WB Saunders.

Droogan, J. and Dickson, R. 1996 Pre-operative patient instruction: is it effective? *Nursing Standard* **10**(35), 32–3.

Evans, C. and Richardson, P.H. 1988 Improved recovery and reduced postoperative stay after therapeutic suggestions during general anaesthesia. *Lancet* **ii**, 491–2.

Fawcett-Henesy, A. 1995 All right on the day? Viewpoint: Healthy debate. *Nursing Standard* **9**(43), 52.

Hamilton-Smith, S. 1972 *Nil by mouth*? London: RCN.

Holmes, S. 1986 Nutritional needs of surgical patients. *Nursing Times* **82**(19), 30–2.

Jordan, S. 1992 Drugs for severe pain. *Nursing Times* **88**(2), 24–7.

Lamb, J. 1993 Peripheral IV therapy. *Nursing Standard* **7**(36), 31–5.

Moran, S. and Kent, G. 1995 Quality indicators for patient information in short-stay units. *Nursing Times* **91**(4), 37–40.

Phillips, K. 1996 Issues of quality in minimal access surgery. *Nursing Standard* **11**(3), 52–3.

Rigge, M. 1995 All right on the day? Viewpoint: Healthy debate. *Nursing Standard* **9**(43), 52.

Taylor, S. and Goodinson-McLaren, S. 1992 *Nutritional support: the team approach*. London: Wolfe.

Tortora, G.T. and Anagnostakos, N.P. 1984 *Principles of anatomy and physiology*. London: Harper & Row.

Wicker, P. 1994 Local anaesthesia in the operating theatre. *Nursing Times* 90, 46, 34–35.

PART TWO

Surgery and the elderly patient

2

Vivienne Mathews

Introduction

The population of elderly people in the UK, especially those classified as the 'very elderly' (over the age of 75 years) is anticipated to expand into the 21st century (Central Statistical Office, 1993). The period of old age may now even extend to over 100 years of age.

This wide age range clearly includes people who are chronologically old but biologically healthy, the chronically sick and those who have become frail through advancing chronological years. The changes of ageing affect everyone who lives long enough, altering the function of many organs and resulting in characteristic changes in body composition and metabolism. Thus, in any one elderly person, the co-existence of age-related physiological changes, chronic disease processes, the use of medication and social and environmental factors, such as bereavement and isolation, can influence health status (National Dairy Council, 1992). There are often precarious social circumstances exacerbating the ageing process, so that elderly people are more susceptible to acute illness than any other group of the population (Brocklehurst and Allen, 1987).

The object of surgery for an elderly person is not always to save life; it may be to improve quality of life by pain relief, to increase mobility or to enable an elderly person to enjoy a greater degree of independence.

Incidence of surgery in the elderly

Fifty per cent of all those over the age of 60 require surgery before they die (Jackson, 1988), and 40% of all elderly people admitted to acute care hospitals will require surgery before they are discharged (Miller, 1981).

As emergency operations carry added risks, even for younger, fitter patients, it follows that elderly people are at a particular disadvantage. The older the patient, the more likely it is that surgical admission will be on an emergency, rather than an elective, basis (Seymour, 1986), this rising sharply with age. Age by itself should not preclude surgery: an elderly patient has as much right to the latest surgical and anaesthetic techniques as does the younger patient.

The decision to operate on an elderly patient is affected by four major considerations:

1 *Pathological factors.* Not only the surgical disease, but also any coincidental illness complicating either surgery or recovery should be considered.

2 *Physiological decline.* The impaired homeostasis that tends to accompany ageing may reduce the ability to cope with the additional stresses of surgery and anaesthesia.

3 *Social factors.* For example, the current attitude towards surgery in the elderly is that it should be reserved for the person who is 'healthy', described as being 'reasonably active, over 65 years of age and without symptoms of cardio-pulmonary disease' (Crawford, 1985). This perspective may have a marked influence on the number and type of patients referred for surgery.

4 *Length of hospitalization.* 'Although the mean average stay in hospital for all surgical patients is 7.2 days, patients between 65 and 74 years of age increased their period of hospitalization to an average of 11 days, whilst patients over the age of 85 years stayed in hospital an average of 19 days' (Carter, 1989). Social and economic factors may contribute to an extended stay in hospital for some elderly patients, but it has been well recorded that recovery after surgery is markedly delayed in the elderly.

Decline in elective admissions in old age

Elective surgery admissions reach a peak between the ages of 30 and 65 years and then decline rapidly in older age groups. Why should this be?

First, it can be claimed that some elderly people may have been denied elective surgery, for example by long waiting lists. Second, elderly people may not bring a condition to the GP's attention because of embarrassment or a false belief that they are 'too old' for surgery. Third, it is possible that an elderly person may not recognize the significance of symptoms until late in the disease process. In the past, surgery may not have been recommended for elderly people because of the anticipated risk of complications. Recent studies show that delay, or reluctance to perform elective surgery, may lead to increasingly frequent emergency procedures, which places the elderly person at much greater risk (Dean, 1987).

Improved surgical procedures, knowledgeable pre-and post-operative care given to elderly people and a greater percentage of elderly patients undergoing surgery have resulted in a change in attitudes towards surgery and the elderly person, although there continues to be a risk of complications associated with anaesthesia. The elderly both tolerate and respond well to surgical intervention, but speed is an essential factor, as the longer the elderly patient remains in hospital, the more difficult will be discharge at the original level of independence (Devas, 1977).

Pre-operative nursing assessment

The value of making a full, detailed and careful nursing assessment is nowhere more important than when assessing an elderly patient. Nursing care of an elderly person is no different from that of any other surgical patient, except that it may need more information, more concentration and the highest possible calibre of nursing input.

If realistic planning for rehabilitation to former health levels is to be achieved, a comprehensive physical examination, health history and mental state check, including pre-operative mobility and activity levels, the degree of social interaction, the significant relationships of the patient and the depth of family support, is essential. Identification of the key family member through whom information can be channelled is important. Elderly people may resent questioning, especially of a personal nature, so tact and privacy are vital. Some elderly people view admission to hospital as the first step towards being institutionalized, so are afraid to answer questions relating to their ability to cope with activities of daily living, their finances or their support system. Elderly people have been identified as being capable of self-deception and will often present a 'rose-tinted' account of their social resources and activities.

Areas requiring education should be outlined during initial planning, so that cohesion and continuity of care can be established throughout hospitalization. Sensory impairment should be assessed; economic resources and home environment should be discussed, as should the availability of community resources to provide support after discharge. Prosthetic aids, their care and usage, should be recognized.

Stress, such as recent bereavement or financial distress and lack of family support, should be noted.

Carrick (1982) has emphasized that questioning the patient about previous illnesses, such as angina, myocardial infarction, asthma, diabetes and transient ischaemic attacks (TIAs), is of great importance, as pre-operative evaluation is a team effort requiring special skills in order to differentiate between normal changes of ageing and pathology.

Figure 2.1 lists a number of pre-operative baseline observations that can be used for post-operative comparisons.

Information-giving should be considered to be a two-way process – from nurse to patient and patient to nurse. It is important that elderly people know exactly what is happening to them. It has been well documented that exchange of information prior to surgery has a clear link with the degree of recovery and the extent of co-operation to be expected in elderly patients (Bysshe, 1988). Give as much information as the patient can cope with and, whenever possible, involve him in any decision-making about his care. Deafness, anxiety, fear or pain may prevent or limit an elderly person's response to questions asked or advice given, and confusion may compound this. The elderly person will be more responsive if treatment is known, expectations fulfilled and outcomes explained.

- Blood pressure
- Pulse
- Temperature
- Weight
- Respiratory rate
- Urine analysis
- Medication regimens
- Dietary considerations
- Mobility level
- Elimination patterns
- Skin colour and condition

Figure 2.1 Preoperative base line observations that could be used for post-operative comparisons

Other types of assessment

Drug history

A drug history and assessment on admission is essential. Over-the-counter drugs are frequently taken by elderly people but may not be regarded as medication as they have not been prescribed by the doctor. Elderly people may not be able to remember, or pronounce correctly, the names of the drugs they are taking, or state when they last took them. If possible, ascertain, from family, friends or neighbours what prescription or non-prescription drugs the patient has been taking. Sedatives, hypnotics, tranquillizers and alcohol may cause confusion and disorientation.

Respiratory assessment

Respiratory complications are the most common cause of death in elderly patients during the post-operative period (Jackson, 1988). Nursing assessment of respiratory state includes the ability to speak in sentences without difficulty or, if mobile, walk a reasonable distance without becoming dyspnoeic.

The effect of muscle relaxants, antidepressants (e.g. amitriptyline and imipramine) and anaesthesia given per-operatively further reduces the already reduced oxygenation of elderly tissues. Elderly patients will benefit from pre-operative physiotherapy, encouraged and maintained by nursing staff. Deep breathing exercises and correct positioning should be taught to minimize pain and aid breathing. Assurances of adequate pain relief should be given at all times.

Fluid and electrolyte assessment

Fluid and electrolyte status tends to be unbalanced in the elderly. Because of changes in skin elasticity and turgor, much drier mucous membranes and a diminished sense of thirst, the degree of hydration is often difficult to determine in elderly people. A major factor in detecting under hydration and poor renal function is urinary output, which may be pale and plentiful but, conversely, may be concentrated, a darker colour and of scant amount.

Input and output recording, especially in an emergency situation, should begin as soon as the patient is admitted to hospital and be accurately continued throughout the pre- and post-operative periods.

Integumentary assessment

Alterations in skin colour, condition and turgor may give the first indication of pre-operative complications, including adverse reactions to drugs. A baseline assessment of skin colour, the presence of bruises and ulcers, peripheral vascular circulation condition and oedema should be completed. The maintenance of skin integrity and of the patient's own degree of hygiene during hospitalization is of supreme importance.

The cost of treating pressure sores is escalating, figures being given in the region of £1–1.5 million per health authority and rising at an estimated rate of 13% per annum (Waterlow, 1991). A pressure sore risk calculator, such as the Waterlow or Norton Score, should be a vital part of pre-operative assessment. Deterioration of existing pressure sores can be judged by the use of pressure sore calculators. Although risk assessment calculators cannot replace good nursing observations and care, it is recognized that they provide valuable help during assessment.

STUDENT ACTIVITY

Find the assessment tool used in your unit to assess the risk of pressure sores. Look up another and compare the two. Which is more suitable for use with elderly patients and why?

Nutritional assessment

It has been reliably reported that the elderly are generally deficient in protein, vitamins A, C, D and E, thiamine, folic acid and iron (Palmer, 1990).

Five days is considered to be the maximum that an elderly patient should remain without nutritional support following surgery (Holmes, 1986). Surgery causes severe stress upon nutritional reserves, so good nutrition is required to promote healing, maintain organ function, reduce post-operative morbidity and improve immunocompetence. Unfortunately, many operative regimens require the patient to be starved for investigations and to be nil by mouth pre- and immediately post-operatively and the patient also may not be capable of eating a full and well-balanced diet for several more days post-operatively, amounting to much more than the recommended 5 days. It has been estimated that elderly patients in hospital need an average of 2000–2500 calories per day, 3500 calories post-operatively and even more in cases of sepsis or burns.

Any recent weight loss of 2.5 kg or more may be indicative of poor nutritional status in an elderly person. Lack of plasma proteins, proteins and vitamins will delay wound healing and may increase the risk of infection (Sullivan, 1990).

An oral examination may reveal the presence of mouth ulcers, gingivitis, stomatitis, advanced caries and ill-fitting dentures, which may be the cause of poor food and fluid intake. A detailed dietary history should be taken, so that likes and dislikes can be catered for promoting the best possible nutritional state before surgery.

Prior to admission, a period of nausea, vomiting and diarrhoea or blood loss will have adverse effects on the elderly patient's nutritional state. Diagnostic procedures, particularly those involving colonic clearance, may further compound this. Parenteral fluids given pre-operatively may not meet the nutritional needs of the body, as there are very few nutrients in a litre of intravenous fluid.

It should be possible to anticipate problems that may arise from such long-standing, chronic disorders as anaemia, obesity and diabetes, and to make nutritional adjustments to supply the increased levels of proteins and vitamins needed for recuperation.

The nutritional nurse specialist, now seen in many hospitals, will in co-operation with the dietitian, advise and co-ordinate the management of elderly patients who may require specific additional nutritional support.

Pre-operative care

Psychological factors

Elderly patients who are highly motivated to be independent and have positive expectations of their surgical outcomes will be able to cope successfully with the stress of surgery. They may have a significantly lower rate of post-operative complications and disability than those who feel they have no function left in life, perceive their illness as a punishment for past transgressions and have high levels of pre-operative anxiety. Elderly patients who have some degree of mental impairment and those who are admitted from an institutional setting may represent a high risk.

Plans for family members and friends to be with the patient pre-operatively, the sensitive use of touch and an awareness of the elderly patient's cognitive impairments in the area of communication (Fig. 2.2) may well be effective in decreasing anxiety and reducing stress levels for elderly patients.

Where possible, establish patterns of eating and sleeping, and encourage elderly patients to use their own personal possessions. An admission several days prior to elective surgery should

- Intellectual loss
- Short-term memory loss
- Confusion
- Dementia
- Impaired
  - Concentration
  - Comprehension
- Mood swings
- Learning difficulties
- Disorientation

Figure 2.2 Cognitive impairments to communication

be aimed for to acclimatize the patient to ward routines and altered meal and bedtimes.

There has, in the past, been less than efficient pre-operative communication between ward staff and theatre teams, leading to a lack of vital nursing information about the elderly patient, for example on a back problem resulting from osteomalacia, unrelated to the present surgical incident but exacerbated by poor positioning during surgery.

All patients, whatever their age, will benefit from pre- and post-operative counselling, with its attendant opportunity to ask questions and express fears relating to anaesthesia or the likelihood of post-operative pain and its relief.

As well as the usual theatre checklist, establishing the time of premedication, position of dental crowns and absence of jewellery, make-up and prostheses, the visiting theatre nurse may make use of a pre-operative assessment sheet. This information-collecting tool will help to identify difficulties and concerns, allow amendment of planned care and establish individual needs so that both patient and nurse benefit from a mutual exchange of information.

Consent

When medical staff are obtaining an elderly patient's consent for surgery, the nurse should be aware of the family and patient's need for information, not only about the level of risk, but also about the level of comfort and quality of life that

can be expected post-surgery. The decision to carry out surgery can be a difficult one for elderly patients and their families.

Drugs

Pre-operative drug levels may impose an unpredictable risk in elderly patients. High levels of unbound drugs in the elderly person's systems are caused by a combination of factors:

- a decreased rate of excretion;
- decreased plasma binding of drugs;
- changes in drug metabolism owing to liver atrophy;
- decreased body fluid level and lean body mass;
- a decreased number of tissue receptors;

all of which may prolong and potentiate the effects of drugs.

STUDENT ACTIVITY

Identify a drug commonly taken by elderly patients and list all its known side-effects and interactions.

Increased sensitivity to drugs may also occur in the brain as a result of neurofibrillary tangles. Patients who are taking digitalis may develop digoxin toxicity because of the changes in electrolyte balance that usually accompany surgery. The signs and symptoms of digoxin toxicity in the elderly may include:

- nausea and loss of appetite (early symptoms);
- a pulse rate below 60 beats per minute;
- headache and drowsiness;
- coupled beats, owing to ventricular extrasystols following normal beats;
- vomiting, due to stimulation of the vomiting centre in the medulla by digitalis;

- rarely, visual disturbances, for example hazy or blurred vision, difficulty in red–green colour perception and difficulty in reading.

It is important to consider all drugs that must be continued during the pre-operative period, especially those drugs taken for diabetes, cardiac conditions and rheumatoid arthritis, as well as some forms of diuretic therapy.

Medication such as morphine, scopolamine and barbiturates given in their usual doses may cause confusion and disorientation in the elderly patient.

Emotional support

Pre-operative emotional support is extremely important for all patients about to undergo surgery; for the elderly, it is vital. A hospital may be seen as a frightening, anxiety-provoking place from which one might not emerge unscathed, where confusion and loneliness contrast with the hustle and bustle of a home environment. The perceived hostile environment may begin to appear less impersonal if nurses take the time to furnish care and reassurance.

Premedication

Premedication is usually given 1.0–1.5 hours pre-operatively. Every elderly patient should, by this time, have been assessed for weight, general health and age, which may indicate that a reduction in drug dosage is required. All patients must be assessed according to their condition, so the frail elderly may have their drug dosage reduced to half the normal adult dose.

Channer (1985) claimed that it is doubly important for elderly patients to be given oral premedication with a drink. He felt that a 60 ml bolus of water given with a tablet, even if the elderly patient were being starved for surgery, was desirable and without harmful effects, as the stomach produces approximately 125 ml/hour of gastric juice regardless of the amount of fluid drunk. This simple measure, Channer stated, would prevent delayed oesophageal transit of tablets, in which the tablet may possibly 'get stuck' just above the oesophageal sphincter and the drug remain unabsorbed. The smaller the amount of fluid taken with the tablet, the smaller the wave of peristalsis produced to propel the tablet onwards.

Intra-operative considerations

According to Mason (1976) and Sikes and Detmer (1979), the safest surgery is 'that which is elective, short, away from the diaphragm, requires a minimum of post operative sedation, has little accompanying pain and allows for early ambulation', but this sort of surgery rarely takes place in the elderly person. Surgery of longer than 2.5 hours is not tolerated well by the elderly patient.

Anaesthetic

The effects of anaesthesia on the elderly surgical patient have been poorly researched, but, as with other drugs, both increased and delayed responses should be expected. Many elderly patients express fears about the effects of anaesthesia centering on going to sleep and possibly never waking up, or on the fear of paralysis following spinal anaesthesia.

An important effect of anaesthesia in the elderly is a sudden dose-dependent fall in blood pressure, which may be correlated to increased mortality in the elderly. This sudden drop is to be avoided because of the danger of deep vein and other thrombosis, as well as a reduced amount of oxygen that will be transported to the vital organs.

Because of decreased cardiac output, lower circulating plasma volume and decreased peripheral resistance with decreased vasomotor tone, the elderly are specifically prone to:

- hypotension;
- hypothermia;
- cerebral oedema;
- hypoxaemia;

after an anaesthetic (Miller, 1981). Some anaesthetic agents cause severe problems in the elderly person; for example, methoxyflurane has been implicated in renal failure. Unfavourable anaesthetic drugs interact with other medication; for example, tricyclic antidepressants interact with halothane and can cause serious cardiac arrythmias (Miller, 1981).

Positioning

Post-operative joint pain unrelated to the site of operation may result from poor positioning of arthritic joints and limbs during surgery. The lithotomy position, for example, will be extremely uncomfortable for patients with an arthritic lumbosacral spine and hip joints. Tissue necrosis may be greatly increased owing to the loss of subcutaneous fat, poor peripheral circulation, prolonged periods of immobility and trauma to the extremities. Operating room nurses have a duty to check that the elderly patient's limbs are in relaxed alignment to the body and that the appropriate amount of padding and air cushions is used. Last, the patient's operation notes should detail the

exact time that the patient has remained in one position, which may help to reduce the incidence of pressure sores following surgery (Mason, 1976).

Temperature

The temperature in operating theatres is generally between 36°F and 38°F which can place elderly people at risk of hypothermia. Hypothermia has been seen as a major intra-operative concern for elderly patients and may have several causes, for example medication, spinal and general anaesthesia, low room temperature and/or cold intravenous fluids. These low temperatures cause shivering, which increases the body's oxygen demand by as much as 300–500%. This leads to increased cardiac output and ventilation, which may cause tissue ischaemia in the heart and brain. The lower the body temperature, the more the delay in the return of reflexes and arousal. Elderly patients have a lowered ability to combat hypothermia, so it will take longer for their body temperature to return to normal. Harmful cooling can be prevented by: first, warming intravenous fluids before use; second, using anti-hypothermia (space) blankets; third, placing a heating pad under the patient; and, fourth, warming any exposed limbs.

Post-operative care

Infection

It has been said that the longer the patient is in hospital prior to surgery, the higher the probable rate of infection, because of exposure to various bacteria present in the ward environment (Farrell, 1990). Elderly patients, because of decreased effectiveness in the immune system, poor metabolic function and other factors (Fig 2.3), are highly prone to infection. Urinary tract infections are twice as common in the elderly as

in the middle-aged adult, in direct proportion to the incidence of catheterization (Jackson, 1988).

Because of age-related changes in the body's temperature control system, the elderly person's temperature may not increase in the presence of infection, and only excessive restlessness and/or confusion may indicate a possible infection. Aseptic technique must be used for all dressing changes and invasive procedures. Avoid placing a pre-operative patient in the same room as one with an infection.

- Decreased resistance to infection
- Poor nutritional state
- Lowered immune response
- Presence of residual urine
- Poor peripheral circulation
- Fragile skin
- Increased likelihood of allergic response to tape and dressings

Figure 2.3 Increased risk of infection in the elderly patient

Pain

'pain is whatever the experiencing person says it is, existing whenever the person says it does.' (McCaffery, 1979)

Most elderly patients are remarkably stoic in the amount of pain that they experience without complaint, but they should not be expected to tolerate pain for longer than younger people. Undue complaints of pain from an elderly patient should be investigated immediately, as they are often an indication of complications arising from surgery.

Pain relief from analgesics is important as there is a narrow margin between adequate pain control and the start of complications such as confusion, loss of balance, hypotension and incontinence. Analgesic doses should consist of the lowest possible dose compatible with effective pain control over a 24 hour period and with an acceptable level of side-effects. It should be adequate enough to control incisional pain and allow deep breathing and coughing exercises. Non-verbal expressions of pain may be the best indicator of the effectiveness of analgesia.

STUDENT ACTIVITY

Identify an analgesic drug commonly used after surgery and identify its known side-effects and interactions. What is the standard adult dose and the dose for the elderly patient?

Complementary pain relief therapies, such as relaxation techniques, aromatherapy, imagery, reflexology, hypnotism and massage, have now become acceptable.

Respiratory complications

During the critical immediate post-operative period, the elderly patient should be observed continuously. The risk of regurgitation and aspiration is increased because of decreased airway reflex activity and the increased incidence of hiatus hernia in the elderly.

Early mobilization, with its attendant deep breathing, will help to increase lung capacity and may assist in the prevention of deep vein thrombosis, but it may prove too difficult if the patient or family is apprehensive of falls or believes that bedrest is synonymous with healing. It is vital that the importance of early ambulation is stressed.

Pulmonary complications may be prevented by coughing and deep breathing exercises. Because of the high risk of infection in elderly patients, inhalation equipment must be kept meticulously clean and free from residual moisture.

Cardiovascular complications

Monitoring an elderly person's cardiac function, blood pressure, fluid levels and chest sounds is critical post-operatively. Because there is an increased risk of atherosclerosis, the presence of other cardiovascular pathology, such as injury to veins following lengthy surgery, the use of venous catheters, inflammatory reactions and immobility, means that elderly patients are at risk of venous thrombosis, with its concomitant risk of pulmonary embolism. Once again, the most favoured post-operative preventive action is that of early ambulation. Other measures include active and passive exercises of the extremities, anti-embolic stockings (put on before the patient puts a leg out of bed) and elevation of the foot of the bed.

Incontinence

Incontinence has been considered to be a major post-operative complication for many elderly patients. The problems of frequent bedpan use may be exacerbated by:

- inappropriate placing of the nurse call bell;
- onerous procedure when using a bedpan;
- inability to find the toilet;
- insufficient nursing staff;
- inability to move quickly enough;
- the use of sedation;
- restrictions on the patient's mobility.

The psychological overtones of incontinence may cause depression and lead a family to decide that they cannot cope with the elderly patient's return home.

Pre-operative assessments of elimination patterns may enable appropriate bladder and bowel training programmes to be initiated. Most elderly patients regain control of their bladder within a short time of their operation, but it has been noted that one-third of elderly surgical patients remain incontinent for longer. The most appropriate way to restore bladder and sphincter control is to encourage mobility and walking to the toilet as soon as possible.

STUDENT ACTIVITY

Outline a planned programme of teaching pelvic floor exercises to post-operative surgical patients. How would you modify your programme to take account of advanced age?

Confusion

The incidence of post-operative confusion is higher in elderly people than any other age group (Holden, 1995). Contributing factors include:

- drugs;
- hypothermia;
- anaesthesia;
- decreased cerebral perfusion;
- pain;
- stress and anxiety;
- infection;
- a full bladder;
- an unfamiliar environment.

It has also been found that loss of personal space can cause elderly people to withdraw or exhibit other confusional characteristics. If patients can own their 'locus of control', they become reorientated to time, place and person more readily than if they feel they have no control over their identity. Elderly patients may shout, become unco-operative and generally behave in an antisocial way if they feel disorientated, lack sleep, are in pain or feel alone in strange surroundings. The nurse may often, with the use of touch and a calm manner, reassure an elderly person, and regular visiting by patients' relatives can help to decrease confusion and prevent depression.

Hearing aids, dentures, hair pieces and other prostheses should be worn as soon as possible after surgery in order to preserve self-respect and dignity.

Information-giving has an important role in keeping patients in touch with reality. Although many elderly patients will not ask direct questions, they should nevertheless be kept informed of their treatment and progress. It is important to keep explanations short because of short-term memory loss and to repeat information as often as necessary to reduce anxiety. Relatives may also need information to make realistic plans for the future. Early mobility, preventing demineralization of bone, circulatory complications and skin breakdown, will also provide a sense of progress, control and increased self-esteem.

Day surgery

It has been stated by Markanday and Platzer (1994) that day surgery is an economical, efficient and effective use of surgical resources. It reduces waiting list times and last minute cancellations, and allows those who prefer aftercare to be given at home to choose this.

Because of the increasing complexity of day surgery and the increase in number to a suggested target of 346 cases per bed per year (Audit Commission, 1990), it has become increasingly obvious that not all people requiring treatment are suitable candidates for it. Many hospital trusts have policies discriminating against elderly people. A 'suitable candidate' has been described as one who is under 65 years of age and generally fit, has a responsible adult to collect and care for them for at least 2 days after surgery, has access to a telephone and is ideally living within 1 hour's drive of the hospital. Setting an upper age limit of 65 years of age fails to take into account the fact that good health is compatible with normal ageing (Squires, 1988). Everyone should be given the chance of day surgery, especially as day care surgery of the elderly patient has been proved to be successful by Lieber et al. (1990), who states that it was routinely safe and feasible if appropriate precautions were undertaken and common sense used. It can be argued that iatrogenic complications associated with the hospitalization of many elderly people may make day surgery safer than a stay in hospital (Gillick et al. 1982).

Following its success in America, day care cataract surgery was introduced in the UK in the 1970s as the risks of eye surgery in the elderly proved to be low and could be performed on all but the most debilitated of patients (Traynor and Ingram, 1991).

The few hours required in hospital for the operation and the consequent minimal disruption to the patient's way of life will help to maintain independence, reduce disturbances of routine and lessens anxiety for both patient and relatives.

It is undeniable that a number of diseases causing disability become more common with advancing age (Shaw, 1984). Perhaps the most significant problem of ageing is that of diminished functional independence, so good home support is essential. The type of accommodation, level of carer support and amount of understanding to enable compliance with treatment need to be very carefully considered when planning ambulatory surgery. It is of the utmost importance to plan correctly right from the start.

Conclusions

Adverse reactions to surgery are rarely due to age alone, but elderly patients have fewer reserves than younger patients in coping with the multiple stresses associated with surgery. The reality of the loss of independence and control, the fear of pain, the loss of a spouse and/or friends, and the additional fear of possible admission to a long-term care facility, bring extra stresses that may not be necessarily present in a younger patient.

Porter (1991) sees pre- and post-operative visiting by theatre staff as an important part of holistic individualized care for an elderly surgical patient. Explanations from theatre staff can reduce anxiety and provide reassurance, in turn leading to a reduction in pain and facilitating an uneventful recovery.

Some elderly patients die. Most, however, because of the nurse's scrupulous attention to detail, enlightened knowledge and specialist skills, will recover and be discharged into their own environment, but, as the demography of the population continues to change, the number of very elderly patients undergoing surgery will continue to rise.

By developing an increasingly large body of knowledge about the elderly surgical patient and the nursing care needed, elderly patients can expect surgery not only to prolong life, but also to give meaning, comfort and dignity to their remaining years.

Summary

1 There are four major factors to be considered when contemplating surgery for an elderly person: pathological factors, physiological decline, social factors and intended length of hospital stay.

2 Pre-operative nursing assessments, with information-giving on both sides, is nowhere more important than for the elderly surgical patient.

3 Assessments of drug history, respiratory function, skin condition, nutritional status and electrolyte and fluid balance are of vital importance for an elderly person undergoing surgery, in order to anticipate problems that may arise from longstanding pathological conditions.

4 Specific pre-operative care should focus on positive issues to enhance independence, give informed consent, continue drug regimens, contribute emotional support and administer correct amounts of premedication.

5 Intra-operative factors, such as correct positioning, adequate temperature control and knowledge of the effects of anaesthesia, can greatly reduce the risks of surgery for elderly people.

6 Infection, pain, respiratory and cardiovascular complications, the danger of incontinence and confusion are potential post-operative complications that are added hazards for the elderly surgical patient.

7 For elderly people, day surgery decreases the risk of infection, holds minimal disruption and will enhance independence by lessening anxiety for patients and their relatives.

CASE HISTORY

Mrs Lee lives alone in sheltered accommodation. She is 85 years old and is being admitted for planned surgery to her knee. She takes drugs for hypertension and arthritis, and enjoys a glass of sherry before meals. Using your favoured nursing model, make a checklist of the areas that will be included in her pre-operative assessment, giving a reason for each.

Review Questions

1 How can the risk of pressure sores be calculated in the elderly surgical patient? Why is this relevant?

2 What is the absolute maximum number of days that an elderly patient can be left without nutritional support post-operatively?

3 How many kilocalories are there in a litre of 5% dextrose?

4 Why are there likely to be high levels of unbound drugs in the elderly person's body systems, and what are the implications of this?

5 What measures can you take to calm and reassure an elderly patient during a stay in hospital?

References

Audit commission 1990 *A short cut to better services: day surgery in England and Wales*. The Audit Commission for Local Authorities and the NHS in England and Wales. London: HMSO.

Brocklehurst, J.C. and Allen, S.C. 1987 *Geriatric medicine for students* 3rd edn. Edinburgh: Churchill Livingstone.

Bysshe, J.E. 1988 The effect of giving information to patients before surgery. *Nursing* 3(30), 36–9.

Carrick, L. 1982 The older adult and drug therapy, consideration for the older surgical patient. Part 2 *Geriatric Nursing* 3(1), 43–7.

Carter, M. 1989 Effects of anaesthesia on mental performance in the elderly. *Nursing Times* (Occasional Paper) 85(1), 40–2.

Central Statistical Office 1993 *Social trends 23*. London: HMSO.

Channer, K. 1985 Stand up and take your medicine. Progress of a tablet through the oesophagus. *Nursing Times* 81(28), 41–2.

Crawford, F.J. 1985 Ambulatory surgery: the elderly patient. *AORN Journal* 41(2), 356–9.

Dean, A.F. 1987 The ageing surgical patient: historical overview, implications and nursing care in the ambulatory setting. *Perioperative Nursing Quarterly* 3(1), 1–7.

Devas, M (ed.) 1977 *Geriatric orthopaedics*. London: Academic Press.

Farrell, J. 1990 *Nursing care of the older person*. Philadelphia: JB Lippincott.

Gillick, M.R., Serrell, N.A., Gillick, L.S. 1982 Adverse consequences of hospitalisation in the elderly. *Social Science and Medicine* 16(10), 1033–8.

Holden, U. 1995 Dementia in acute units: confusion. *Nursing Standard*, 9(17), 37–9.

Holmes, S. 1986 Nutritional needs of the surgical patient. *Nursing Times* 82(19), 30–2.

Jackson, M.F. 1988 High risk surgical patients. *Journal of Gerontological Nursing* 14(1), 40–2.

Lieber, C.P., Seiniqe, U.L. and Sataloff, D.M. 1990 Choosing the site of surgery, an overview of ambulatory surgery in geriatric patients. *Clinical Geriatric Medicine* 6(3), 493–7.

McCaffery, M. 1979 Nursing management of the patient with pain, 2nd ed. Philadelphia: JB Lippioncott.

Markanday, L., Platzer, H. 1994 Brief encounters. *Nursing Times* 90(7), 38–42

Mason, J.H. 1976 The care of the geriatric patient in general surgery. In: Steinburg, F.U. (ed.), 5th ed. Missouri: CV Mosby.

Miller, R.D. (ed.) 1981 Anaesthesia for the elderly. In: *Anaesthesia*, Vol. 2. New York: Churchill Livingstone.

National Dairy Council 1992 Nutrition and elderly people. Factfile No. 9 London: NDC.

Porter, L. 1991 Theatre nursing: patient visiting – an essential role. *Nursing Standard* 6(2), 54–5.

Seymour, D.G. 1986 *Medical assessment of the elderly surgical patient*. London: Croom Helm.

Shaw, M.W. 1984 *The challenge of ageing*. Melbourne: Churchill Livingstone.

Sikes, E.D. Jr and Detmer, D.E. 1979 Ageing and surgical risk in older citizens of Wisconsin. *Wisconsin Medical Journal* 78(7), 27–30.

Squires, A.J. 1988 *Rehabilitation of the older patient*. London: Croom Helm.

Sullivan, D.H. 1990 Impact of nutrition status on morbidity and mortality in a select population of geriatric rehabilitation patients. *American Journal of Clinical Nutrition* 51(5), 749–58.

Traynor, M. and Ingram, R. 1991 Visionary work: Day care cataract surgery. *Nursing the Elderly* 3(5), 28–30.

Waterlow, J. 1991 A policy that protects: the Waterlow pressure sore prevention/treatment policy. *Professional Nurse* 6(5), 258, 260, 262.

Further reading

Irvine, R.E. and Strouthide, T.M. 1977 *Medical care in geriatric orthopaedics*. London: Academic Press.

Palmer, M.A. 1990 Care of the older surgical patient. In: Eliopoulous, C. (ed.), *Caring for the elderly in diverse care settings*. Philadephia: JB Lippincott.

Salmond, S.W. 1982 Recognising protein caloric malnutrition. *Critical Care Update* 9(1–5), 5–8.

3 Neurosurgical nursing principles

Anne Murray

Introduction

As investigative, diagnostic and neurosurgical procedures develop, so does the field of neurosurgical nursing. Although many patients requiring neurosurgical intervention are cared for in specialist units, few nurses will go through their training or professional careers without encountering patients with problems resulting from disease of or trauma to the nervous system.

This chapter cannot possibly cover the complexities of the nervous system and the wide range of patients' problems, surgical procedures or nursing care. Its purpose, therefore, is to give the reader an insight into caring for the patient undergoing neurosurgical procedures.

Surgical approaches to the brain and spinal cord are many and varied, so only the most common are discussed here. Recent advances have reduced the need for open surgical techniques such as those employed in treating cerebral aneurysms. An effort has thus been made to select areas of care and treatment that will give the reader an understanding of some of the key issues.

The nervous system (along with the endocrine system) controls and integrates the functions of the body. As a highly efficient communications network, it is the body's most rapid means of maintaining homeostasis. The gross structures involved are the brain, spinal cord and cranial and peripheral nerves.

Nerve cells (neurones) consist of a cell body and myelinated or non-myelinated fibres (axons and dendrites), which can be divided into three main groups: sensory, association and motor. Broadly speaking, sensory information is relayed along afferent pathways to the central nervous system (CNS) (the brain and spinal cord), where it is processed. Motor information is relayed along efferent pathways away from the CNS to stimulate muscle and/or glandular tissue (Tortora and Anagnostakos, 1990).

Lesions that interfere with the functioning of the nervous system, such as abnormalities of the cerebral blood vessels, benign or malignant tumours of the meningeal or glial (support) cells or lesions that disrupt the flow of cerebrospinal fluid (CSF), often arise from tissues other than nervous tissue.

Lesions within the nervous system can affect an individual's ability to function mentally and/or physically and, if not dealt with promptly, can have devastating consequences. Displacement or distension of nervous tissue or ischaemia owing to interruption of the blood supply may initially produce problems specific to that particular part of the brain or spinal cord, for example pain and sensory disturbance in relation to the distribution of a peripheral nerve pathway in the case of a spinal lesion, or loss of the ability to move one side of the body (hemiplegia) with a cerebral lesion. However, because the skull and spinal vertebrae are rigid structures, the brain or spinal cord becomes compressed as the lesion grows and/or the area around it becomes oedematous, and the effects of local lesions extend much further. For example, a lesion within the spinal column may eventually result in paralysis with loss of bladder and bowel control. If the lesion is within the cranium, the intracranial pressure (ICP) may begin to rise, and eventually the whole brain becomes compressed (Jennett and Galbraith, 1994).

Raised intracranial pressure

It is extremely important for the nurse to be able to recognize the most common signs and symptoms of raised ICP as they indicate a series of events that threaten a patient's life, although the list below is by no means definitive:

- early morning headache;
- vomiting occurring with the headache;
- deterioration in the level of consciousness;
- alteration in pupil size and reaction to light;
- a slowed pulse;
- an increase in systolic blood pressure;
- changes in the rate, depth or rhythm of respiration;
- abnormal posturing of the limbs;
- hemiplegia/hemiparesis.

The rate and the order in which these findings occur vary from patient to patient, depending upon the position of the offending lesion and its rate of growth (Allan, 1988; Jennett and Galbraith, 1994). For example, a haematoma developing within the cranium may cause rapid deterioration, the patient becoming unconscious within hours or even minutes. In contrast, a patient may have an equally large tumour but be conscious, if a little confused and complaining of headache. This difference arises because the brain tissues have had time to compensate for the added mass, which is not possible when the lesion develops rapidly.

Neurological observations

In order to monitor the neurological status of patients, an internationally accepted, objective set of criteria – the Glasgow Coma Scale (GCS) (Teasdale, 1975) – has been established. The observation chart that subsequently developed has been adapted for use by both doctors and nurses in a variety of settings (Fig. 3.1)

Not all charts have the same format, but the principles remain the same, the observations being broken down into four sections:

- conscious level;
- pupil reactions;
- vital signs;
- limb movements.

Conscious level

Changes in level of consciousness are the earliest and most sensitive indicator of a change in neurological status, (Hickey, 1992; Jacobs, 1995).

Conscious level is assessed using the 'coma scale', divided into three sections:

- eye opening;
- best verbal response;
- best motor response.

EYE OPENING

Eye opening is closely linked to being awake and alert (Frawley, 1990), but, although eye opening is a normal response to sound stimulation, it does not necessarily imply awareness.

		Score
Spontaneously	The patient opens his eyes without any prompting from the nurse	4
To speech	The patient opens his eyes when addressed by the nurse	3

To pain	The patient opens his eyes when a peripheral painful stimulus is applied (*see* p. 000)	2
None	No response	1

Eye opening:

- If there is any trauma or swelling around the patient's eyes, this response is not assessed and is simply recorded as 'C' for closed

- Use a peripheral painful stimulus as a central stimulus may cause the patient to grimace and therefore close his eyes

- The patient may have a hearing impairment

- If the patient's eyes are open, observe whether they focus on you and follow your movements

Patient comment

'It was so confusing, I could hear people talking around me but couldn't seem to make contact with them.'

BEST VERBAL RESPONSE

This section assesses the patient's ability to make sense of sensory information and respond appropriately.

		Score
Orientated	The patient knows his name, where he is and the month. It is not reasonable to expect the exact date as anyone can forget this (Teasdale, 1975)	5

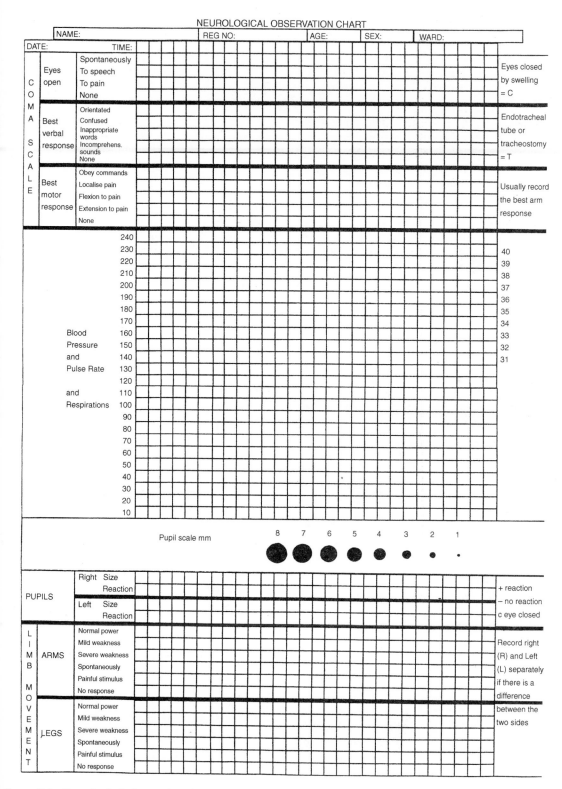

Figure 3.1 Neurological observation chart

Confused	The patient gets one or more of the above wrong and, while able to converse, is not replying correctly	4
Inappropriate words	The patient replies with obscenities or using only one or two words; he does not converse or answer the question	3
Incomprehensible sounds	Words cannot be identified; the patient usually merely grunts or moans in response to a painful stimulus	2
None	No response	1

		Score
Obeys commands	The patient will perform simple voluntary movements on request, for example lift an arm or move the fingers	5
Localize to pain	The patient moves a hand towards the source of the central painful stimulus	4
Flexion to pain	The patient's elbow bends and the patient's hand pulls away from the source of the painful stimuli	3
Extension to pain	The patient's elbow extends, often accompanied by flexion of the wrist	2
None	No response	1

Best verbal response:

- The patient may have a hearing impairment

- The patient may not understand English

- The patient may have an endotracheal or tracheostomy tube in situ, recorded as 'T'

- The patient may have a speech problem inhibiting the ability to give a correct response

Patient comment

'It got very irritating being asked the same questions every half an hour throughout the night, when all I wanted to do was sleep'.

Best motor response:

- The response is always assessed using the arms, as spinal reflexes in the legs can mislead

- If there is a difference in response from the right and left arm, the best response is always recorded

- The patient is never asked to squeeze the assessor's hands, as the simple action of placing a hand in the patient's may elicit a reflex grip

- If the patient is unable to move his limbs, for example when trauma to the spinal cord is also present, record the best response that could be reasonably expected from the patient, such as opening and closing the eyes.

BEST MOTOR RESPONSE

This is generally considered to be the most sensitive parameter. To obey commands, the patient must be able to make sense of the instructions given.

Coma score

In some neurosurgical and A&E departments, patients are given a coma score. Each response within the scale is given a number (*see* above). At the end of the assessment, the response numbers are totalled. The score ranges from 3 = no responses, to 14 (in some areas 15) = fully awake and orientated (Jennett and Galbraith, 1994; Jacobs, 1995).

Painful stimuli:

- A painful stimulus is used only when other stimuli have failed to elicit a response

- The usual methods of administering painful stimuli are by applying pressure to the:

  - nail bed, using the smooth edge of a pen. This is known as a peripheral painful stimulus
  - supraorbital ridge (inner aspect of the eyebrows) using the thumb, or pinching the trapezius (shoulder) muscle. These are known as central painful stimuli

- The patient is localizing to painful stimuli when he attempts to remove the source of the stimulus. Central painful stimuli are usually employed for this purpose. The patient should move his hand(s) at least as far as either the shoulder or chin

- Painful stimuli are only applied once during a set of observations, at which point eye opening, verbal and motor responses are observed for

- Damaged nail beds and injured limbs must not be used

Pupil reactions

As a result of a generalized rise in ICP or direct pressure caused by a lesion in the region of the oculomotor nerve, abnormalities may be observed in the patient's pupils. The two most important questions are:

- Are the pupils equal?
- Are they both reacting to light?

The nurse first looks at both eyes simultaneously to assess whether or not the pupils are equal in size; the number corresponding to the pupil size is then charted. Then, using a bright pen torch with a narrow beam of light, the nurse brings the light in from the temple, thus avoiding shining the light in both eyes at the same time, and notes the reaction of each pupil to light. Pupil constriction is recorded as a positive (+) reaction. Lack of constriction is recorded as a negative (−) reaction.

STUDENT ACTIVITY

In a dim light, stand close to a mirror. Using a pen torch, move the beam in from the temporal side and note the pupil reaction. Try the opposite side. Do the two pupils react equally to light?

Pupil reactions:

- Unequal pupils may indicate a neurological emergency and should always be reported immediately

- If the patient is particularly sensitive to light (photophobic) it may be decided, after discussion with other members of the team, that it is kinder to omit this test

- If there is any eye trauma or orbital swelling, a 'C' for closed is recorded

- Occasionally, particularly in individuals with brown eyes, it is difficult to be sure whether a pupil is reacting to light. If in doubt, get someone more experienced to check your observation

Patient comment

'Strangely, the photophobia was made worse by contrasting colours rather than bright lights.' (Vaughan, 1995)

Vital signs

When assessing a patient's neurological status, vital signs observations are important additions. Any changes outside normal limits may be significant.

Vital signs:

Temperature

- Temperature is recorded in the axilla, never orally, as patients with neurological problems may have seizures, altered consciousness or reduced facial muscle tone

- An increase in body temperature will result in an increase in cellular metabolic requirements, thus decreasing the amount of oxygen available to the brain. A rise in ICP may also occur. Thus every effort must be made to keep the temperature within normal limits

Pulse and blood pressure

- A slowing pulse, a widening of the pulse pressure (the gap between diastolic and systolic blood pressures) and a general increase in blood pressure may indicate a raised ICP. In the case of raised ICP, these are generally late changes, and the patient's conscious level will already have deteriorated. (Remember, if the patient's blood pressure or pulse is slightly raised, the patient may be in pain or have a full bladder)

Respiration

- Changes in the rate, depth or rhythm of respiration may indicate a rise in ICP and/or problems associated with gas exchange in the lungs, for example an obstructed airway

Limb movements

The nurse is primarily observing for a difference between the left and right sides of the body in the power or reaction of the limbs. Normal power or mild or severe weakness is usually detected following a verbal request, for example asking the patient to raise his legs against either gravity or a little counterpressure.

Spastic flexion or extension may be observed without any stimulation or in response to peripheral painful stimuli.

Neurological observations – general points

- Neurological assessment forms only part of the overall nursing assessment

- All the observations are important

- These observations should not be the sole source of information about the patient: the nurse's general powers of observation are also important. During her observations, she may note, for example, the patient's skin colour, any abnormal movements or subtle changes in the patient's breathing

- Continuity is important. On each shift, one nurse should be responsible for the patient's observations and handover given on a one-to-one basis

- Accuracy is vital. If in doubt, ask a more senior colleague to check your observations

- Always ask, 'Why am I carrying out these observations?'

Pre-operative care

In many instances, patients are admitted to neurosurgical wards as emergencies, often necessitating rapid assessment and investigation immediately prior to surgery. However, if the patient's status allows, he is admitted several days before to surgery to allow detailed assessment by appropriate members of the multidisciplinary team, more time to orientate the patient, answer his questions, give explanations and allay fears, and more time to involve patients and their relatives in decision-making.

The prospect of neurosurgery is frightening, and all efforts must be made to establish relationships based on empathy and trust.

Neurological examination

The doctor will perform a general examination of the body systems. Of particular importance is the neurological examination, involving assessment of the level of consciousness as well as a detailed examination of:

- mental state, with reference to the patient's behaviour, mood, degree of orientation, memory and intellectual abilities;
- speech, in terms of the patient's ability to understand what is said and express himself. Problems such as dysphasia and dysarthria may be identified at this stage;
- cranial nerve functions, assessing the patient's vision, ocular movements, pupil reactions, facial reflexes, sense of taste, gag and swallowing reflexes, hearing, balance and other relevant motor and sensory functions;
- motor system – movements in relation to power, posture, co-ordination and spinal reflexes;
- sensory system – the patient is assessed for signs of paraesthesia and/or abnormalities in relation to touch, pain, temperature, pressure, vibration and joint position (proprioception).

STUDENT ACTIVITY

Look up and write down the cranial nerves and their functions. Make a phrase of their initial letters to help you remember them.

This examination often enables the doctor to identify the approximate locality of the causative lesion and make a diagnosis. Obviously, in order to perform such an examination, the patient's co-operation is required. If he is unconscious, the doctor may be able to test only the patient's reflexes.

Investigations

These will be determined by the surgeon to confirm diagnosis and/or provide guidance during surgery. Commonly performed investigative procedures include (Verran and Aisbitt, 1988; Quigley *et al.*, 1989):

- *Plain skull/spinal X-rays* – to identify fractures, other bony abnormalities or areas of calcification. The findings may help in localizing and identifying the nature of the lesion. For example, certain tumours calcify.

- *Lumbar puncture* – contraindicated if raised ICP is suspected and may be impossible if there is spinal deformity. However, in a neurosurgical setting, it is performed to, for example, establish a diagnosis of subarachnoid haemorrhage or meningitis.

- *Computerized axial tomography (CAT scan)* – to locate and identify space-occupying lesions. The CAT scan produces pictures that demonstrate differences in the density of tissues. The less the density of the tissue, for example CSF, the darker it appears on the picture. The greater the density, the whiter the area appears. Tumours often appear very much whiter than the greyish areas of brain tissue around them.

- *Magnetic resonance imaging (MRI)* – the uses being very similar to these of the CAT scan; however, it produces very detailed, clear pictures of the nervous system and is noninvasive. It is used when other investigations have failed to produce the degree of detail required or when other methods are contraindicated because of their invasive nature.

- *Electroencephalography* – records the electrical activity of the brain. In a surgical setting, it may be performed again to assist in the localization and diagnosis of specific lesions. It is of particular importance when the presenting problem is largely one of epileptic seizures.

- *Angiography:* – is an invasive procedure performed under local or general anaesthetic, usually to establish the location of an aneurysm or the nature of an arteriovenous malformation. Radio-opaque dye is injected directly or indirectly into the cerebral circulation and X-rays taken, giving clear pictures of the arterial blood vessels.

- *Myelography and radiculography* – in order to establish the existence of a space-occupying lesion, a contrast medium is introduced via lumbar puncture into the subarachnoid space, and X-rays are taken. These give a clear outline of the spinal cord (myelography) and nerve roots (radiculography).

Patient comment

'The investigations were far more frightening than the prospect of the surgery.'

The patient

What the patient is able to do while awaiting surgery will depend upon the degree and type of neurological problem and any restrictions imposed as a result of investigations. Patients are generally encouraged to do whatever they can within the confines of the admission, unaided or with assistance. When appropriate, the rehabilitation process, which may involve the planning and implementation of physiotherapy, occupational and speech therapy programmes, is commenced.

Nursing care will be determined by individual needs. The patient may be unconscious and require considerable care, or may be relatively independent, requiring very little nursing intervention.

Patients and their relatives must be given time to express their anxieties, kept informed and provided with explanations.

As an essential part of the medical and nursing assessment, neurological observations are commenced. The regularity with which these are performed will depend upon the patient's neurological status and its expected rate of change.

Preparation for theatre

The operation is explained to the patient by the surgeon, and consent obtained, although surgery may proceed without it in life-threatening situations in which it cannot be gained. When a patient's cognitive function is impaired, consent is obtained from the relatives. Patients in a neurological setting are often extremely anxious and/or have neurological problems affecting their ability to understand or remember what is said. It is, therefore, advisable for a nurse to be present when doctors give explanations so that she may reinforce these, answer any subsequent questions (Craddock, 1989) and explain what can be expected post-operatively.

The anaesthetist will visit the patient to confirm fitness for a general anaesthetic (certain neurological procedures may be performed under local anaesthetic), and, whenever possible, the recovery nurse will also visit.

In an emergency situation, the anaesthetist will need to know when the patient last ate or drank; otherwise, the patient is nil by mouth for approximately 4–6 hours pre-operatively. Premedication or night sedation may not be prescribed to patients undergoing cranial surgery as both may interfere with the patient's level of consciousness.

Drugs that may be prescribed pre- and post-operatively include:

- a mild hypnotic – for an anxious patient as night sedation;
- cortico steroids – dexamethasone, to reduce oedema and/or inflammation; hydrocortisone,

prophylactically to patients undergoing surgery on or near the pituitary gland;

- anticonvulsants – either prophylactically or as continual therapy;
- antibiotics – prophylactically;
- an osmotic diuretic – for example mannitol to reduce ICP.

Physical preparation is as for any other surgical procedure. Those undergoing cranial surgery should have special attention paid to their hair, which should be washed with an antiseptic shampoo. It is unusual nowadays for a full-head shave to be performed unless the patient requests one. Usually, only a small area around the operation site is removed, this being done in the anaesthetic room after the patient has been anaesthetized (James, 1990).

Peri-operative care

During anaesthesia, controlled ventilation is maintained. Measures may be taken by the anaesthetist to reduce intracranial or arterial pressure at the surgeon's request, and hypothermia may be induced. A nasal endotracheal tube will be used if it is felt that elective artificial ventilation will be required after surgery.

Burr hole

This is for tissue biopsy, removal of haematoma or insertion of a ventriculo-atrial or peritoneal shunt. The patient is usually positioned in the lateral or three-quarter prone position.

- A small incision is made in the scalp, exposing the skull.
- A hole approximately 1 cm in diameter is made in the bone.
- The outer covering of tbe brain (dura mater) is then opened.
- A small quantity of tissue is removed for biopsy (Fig. 3.2), or the haematoma is aspirated or the shunt inserted.
- The dura is then sealed and the skin sutured.

Supratentorial exploration (craniotomy)

Craniotomy is performed in order to approach lesions within the anterior and middle fossa of the cranium, in the region of the cerebral hemi-

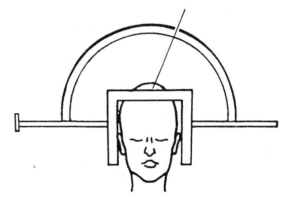

Figure 3.2 A metal stereotactic frame may be used to ensure accurate placement of a brain cannula. Specific reference points are determined by computer using, for example, CAT scan (adapted from Arbour, 1993)

spheres. The patient is usually positioned on the operating table in the lateral or three-quarter prone position.

- An incision, usually semicircular, is made in the scalp in order to preserve the blood supply and within the hairline, for cosmetic reasons.
- The scalp is gently elevated from the skull by dissection.
- A series of burr holes is made in the skull.
- The bone is cut between the burr holes and a fairly circular piece of bone removed or turned back (Fig. 3.3).
- The dura mater is opened and the offending abnormality dealt with.
- The dura mater is then closed, the bone placed back in position and the scalp sutured.

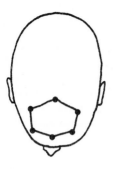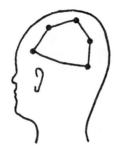

Figure 3.3 Examples of craniotomy sites

- A drainage tube may be inserted under the scalp to prevent a subcutaneous haematoma.

Posterior fossa exploration (craniectomy)

Craniectomy is usually performed to approach lesions within the posterior fossa involving the cerebellar hemispheres or brain stem (Fig. 3.4). The patient may be operated on prone or in a sitting position. If the sitting position is used, in order to maintain venous pressure and prevent air embolism, a pneumatic counterpressure device, 'G' suit or anti-embolic stockings are used (Atkinson, 1992).

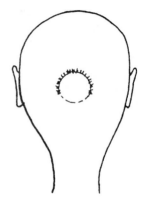

Figure 3.4 Example of a craniectomy site

- A suboccipital midline or lateral vertical incision is made in the scalp.
- A hole is made in the skull, which is then enlarged to provide access.
- The dura mater is opened.
- The offending abnormality is dealt with, and then the dura, muscle and skin are resutured.
- A drain may be inserted under the scalp to prevent haematoma formation.

A bony defect will be left, but this is not a concern as the strong muscles of the neck afford sufficient support and protection.

Post-operative care

Following surgery, the patient may be cared for in the neurosurgical ITU or recovery ward for approximately 24 hours. The prepared bed should be placed in an easily observable position near to post-operative and emergency care equipment, set up and ready for use, including:

- suction equipment;
- oxygen equipment;
- resuscitation equipment with emergency drugs;
- an artificial ventilator;
- specialized monitoring equipment as required;
- observation equipment and charts;
- the care plan.

The approximate times spent in theatre are:

- burr hole: 1 hour;
- supratentorial exploration: 2–3 hours;
- posterior fossa exploration: 2–4 hours.

The patient is transferred to the recovery area, accompanied by the anaesthetist, who will relay any special instructions to the recovery nurse. The patient is usually nursed in a semiprone position. The head of the bed may be raised 30°, helping to reduce ICP by aiding venous return.

If surgery was performed with the patient sitting, he will be nursed in this position post-operatively. The head and neck should be well supported by pillows.

During certain procedures, a ventricular catheter may have been inserted in order to allow post-operative drainage of CSF. The catheter is connected externally to a reservoir attached to the head of the bed, level with the patient's head. If the ICP rises, CSF will be pushed out into the system, thus reducing the pressure.

An intravenous infusion will be in progress to prevent dehydration, replace blood loss (although heavy loss is rare) and/or administer intravenous medication. This will continue as prescribed until the patient is taking adequate oral fluids.

Immediate accurate assessment of the patient's neurological status is essential. Therefore, anaesthetic techniques allow for this, and patients recover from the effects of the anaesthetic very quickly. Neurological observations are initially made every 15 minutes, the subsequent frequency depending on the patient's condition and progress.

If hypothermia was induced intra-operatively, measures may be needed to raise the patient's temperature if it is below 36°C.

The nurse must also observe for seizures. The risk of epilepsy, although minimal, is a complication in itself or may indicate, for example, a developing haematoma. The seizures may be major convulsions or simply twitching of one side of the mouth. Anticonvulsant therapy will be prescribed, and a patient with suspected haematoma may be returned to theatre for re-exploration.

An osmotic diuretic may have been administered during the operative period, resulting in a temporary increase in urinary output, necessitating the passage of a urinary catheter. This may still be in situ and can be removed as soon as the patient is able to use a bottle or bedpan.

Diabetes insipidus (high urinary output with a low specific gravity) can occur following intracranial surgery, particularly on or around the pituitary gland and hypothalamus. Fluid replacement is essential, and treatment with an antidiuretic agent may be necessary.

The wound site should be observed for any sign of swelling or leakage of blood or CSF. The wound drainage tube should be observed for patency and the volume drained recorded. Minimal amounts of blood loss will be expected. The surgeon should be asked how much she would consider acceptable, and any excess is reported. The drain is usually removed 24–48 hours post-operatively. If a CSF leak is observed (clear fluid demonstrating a positive glucose reaction when tested with a glucose test stick), the doctor should be informed; she may prescribe prophylactic antibiotics or re-explore the wound site in order to resuture the tissues.

Bruising and/or oedema around the eyes can occur following supratentorial exploration. The patient and relatives should be warned pre-operatively and reassured that it will settle down; it can be eased with eye toilet and cool compresses.

STUDENT ACTIVITY

Try putting witch hazel into the fridge and using it for cool compresses for oedematous eyes.

Patient comment

'Those cool compresses felt so good and helped my headache too.'

If it is suspected or known that the patient's ICP is above normal limits, nurses and physiotherapists need to co-ordinate their efforts. Suctioning, chest physiotherapy or even simply turning the patient may cause a further increase in pressure. Therefore, these activities need to be planned and implemented in such a way as to cause the patient the least amount of disturbance (Lee, 1989; Rising, 1994).

The surgeon may decide to place the patient on artificial ventilation post-operatively. This allows the doctor to sedate the patient without risk to respiratory function, if she suspects a high risk of seizures or wishes to, for example, hyperventilate the patient. Controlled hyperventilation may be used to reduce ICP (Jennett and Galbraith, 1994).

The patient may complain of headache or pain from the wound site. If appropriate, a pain assessment tool should be used and action taken accordingly. The analgesic of choice is usually one that will have minimal effect on the patient's level of consciousness or vital signs, for example codeine phosphate, 30–60 mg 4–6 hourly. Simple actions such as a cool flannel on the forehead or turning off bright lights may also help.

Patient comment

'If only the nurses had turned the light off over the bed. It was so irritating.'

Specific post-operative considerations

Following posterior fossa exploration, the patient is kept nil by mouth until the swallowing reflexes have been tested as pressure affecting the glosso-pharyngeal, vagus and hypoglossal nerves may interfere with swallowing. The gag reflex is usually tested by the doctor using a tongue depressor. When touched, the soft palate should move upwards, and touching the pharyngeal wall should cause contraction. The reflex is tested on both sides. An absent or diminished reflex will determine the type of fluids and diet the patient is able to take orally; nasogastric feeding may be needed (DiIorio and Price, 1990).

Patient comment

'It was so frightening not being able to swallow and I would have loved a cup of tea.'

Facial paralysis, a rare and often transient complication following surgery at or near to the facial nerve, may cause difficulties for the patient when speaking, eating and drinking. The main problem is initially one of communication. The nurse should allow the patient time to form words, keep his mouth moist and clear of excessive secretions and, if difficulties arise, use aids such as a word board. The expertise of the speech therapist is essential in the management of speech and swallowing problems.

Patient comment

'It was just so frustrating not being able to make myself understood and the nurses always seemed in such a hurry.'

Rehabilitation

Rehabilitation following cranial surgery is highly individual. Problems faced by patients can be complex and varied, and patients' responses to the same problem differ. However, uneventful recoveries are common and general principles can be applied:

- As soon as the patient feels able, he may eat and drink, except when a diminished swallowing reflex is suspected.

- Most neurosurgical units encourage a modified form of open visiting, so patients may have visitors once they have recovered from the anaesthetic and circumstances allow.

- Mobilization will commence as soon as possible. For example, if not contraindicated, the patient may be encouraged to sit up in bed the first post-operative day, and sit out of bed in a chair and walk short distances the second day.

- It takes approximately 48 hours for a full and comprehensive analysis to be made on tissue taken for biopsy. Results are therefore usually available on approximately the second post-operative day.

- Sutures used in supratentorial exploration are removed post-operatively on the fourth or fifth day, and for posterior fossa explorations between 7 and 10 days post-operation.

- Steroid therapy may dictate that the sutures remain in situ for 1 or 2 days longer, as healing may be inhibited.

- Wigs can usually be arranged; however, many patients, once their dressings have been removed, prefer to wear headscarves or hats. Hair will grow back more quickly if the head is left uncovered for at least part of the day.

Patient comment

'The main problem is with the scar and the short cropped hair. People look at you as if you are about to do something crazy.'

- Patients who experienced post-operative seizures may be prescribed prophylactic anticonvulsant therapy for up to a year. The patient or appropriate relatives and/or friends will be educated in the management of seizures and medication, and advised on legal regulations for driving. At present, individuals are required to be seizure-free, when awake, for 2 years. Specific lifestyle adjustments may be needed (Readman, 1990).

If a full recovery is made, patients are discharged between 1 and 3 weeks after surgery. If full recovery does not occur, for example the pre-operative deficits remain or there are post-operative problems, the skills of the multidisciplinary team in supporting both patient and relatives may be required for many months or years, or there may be referral to specialist rehabilitation units. The goals are to assist the patient to reach her maximum potential, adapt to limitations and attain the greatest possible degree of independence.

STUDENT ACTIVITY

What are the first aid principles for an epileptic fit? What should you avoid doing?

Spinal surgery

The spinal cord is protected by the bony vertebral column. Any changes in its structure may compress the spinal nerve roots and, in some instances, the spinal cord (Fig. 3.5). Degenerative changes involving the intervertebral discs of the lumbar spine are common. Cord compression may also be caused by a space-occupying lesion such as a tumour or haematoma.

Spinal cord compression may result in problems related to the loss of motor, sensory and autonomic function below the level of the lesion. In nerve root compression, motor and sensory function may be affected, but severe pain along the related nerve pathway is usually the most prominent feature (Jennett and Galbraith, 1994).

Common causes of change to the vertebral column

- Cervical spondylosis;
- Disc prolapse;
- Rheumatoid arthritis;
- Fractures;
- Congenital abnormalities;
- Tumours.

Spinal surgery may be performed as an elective or an emergency procedure. It is usually indicated if the patient is experiencing continued pain or is developing a neurological deficit such a limb weakness. It is considered an emergency if there is disturbance of bowel and bladder control or rapid neurological change.

The most commonly performed procedures within a neurosurgical setting are lumbar laminectomy and anterior cervical spinal fusion (Atkinson, 1992).

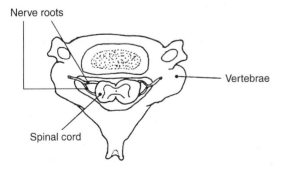

Figure 3.5 Spinal cord, peripheral nerve roots and vertebrae

Pre-operative considerations

Preparation of patients in a neurosurgical setting is very similar to that outlined in Chapter 12. Individualized assessments occur and investigations, including X-ray, lumbar puncture, CAT scan, myelography and radiculography, are carried out. The aims of surgery are to relieve symptoms and prevent deterioration; it is important to note that spinal surgery does not always cure and a patient may still have his presenting deficits.

Patients are taught deep breathing exercises, which are particularly important prior to surgery on the cervical and thoracic spine as pain may inhibit the patient's breathing post-operatively. When a cervical spinal fusion is to be performed, patients are also instructed on the range of neck movement allowed post-operatively; movement is restricted in order to allow the bone graft to fuse. Patients undergoing surgery on the thoracic and lumbar spine are taught techniques for turning in bed and getting in and out of bed appropriately, which are designed to ensure normal spinal alignment.

The most common causes of spinal problems tend to be chronic conditions so patients frequently present with not only physical signs, but also psychological and social problems. Their concerns focus on such issues as job security, finance, role changes and relationships; these should be addressed when assessing needs and planning care. The prospect of spinal surgery, whether for a prolapsed intervertebral disc or a spinal tumour, will provoke some degree of anxiety. Time must be taken to listen to patients' concerns and convey information.

In some instances, patients have already tried other treatments, such as bedrest, traction or osteopathy, and surgery is viewed as a final option. Post-operative pain is often worse, as a result of localized swelling.

Intra-operative period

The most commonly performed procedures carry no special considerations concerning anaesthetic protocol. Positioning on the operating table varies according to the surgeon's preference and the position of the lesion within as well as along the length of the vertebral column, i.e. cervical, thoracic or lumbar region.

The time spent in theatre will again depend on the type of lesion. The removal of a prolapsed intervertebral disc or a straightforward cervical fusion may take only about 1.5 hours, but exploration and removal of a spinal tumour may take between 4 and 6 hours.

Recovery and rehabilitation

SPECIFIC CONSIDERATIONS

Post-operative patients are normally nursed in a supine position for approximately 2 hours, to minimize any strain on the wound site and keep the spine in alignment. When allowed to turn, a patient may be reluctant to move from side to side owing to pain or fear of damaging the spine. Reassurance and pain management are needed.

Following lumbar surgery, patients remain flat in bed for 24–48 hours and are normally allowed to stand with supervision, on the second or third post-operative day. Sitting is not usually allowed until the sutures have been removed, although this differs from unit to unit. Mobilization will not begin until any wound drains have been removed.

Following cervical surgery, patients are usually allowed to sit up on the first post-operative day, after a neck X-ray confirming that the operative site is stable. The patient should be instructed not to use his arms to pull himself up in bed, as this will place considerable strain on the wound. A soft foam collar, to restrict neck movement, is normally worn until the first out patient appointment, when its continued need will be assessed.

Again, following cervical surgery, the patient's breathing must be closely monitored, as the phrenic nerve, responsible for controlling the diaphragm, may be affected by localized swelling, leading to hyperventilation. There is also the potential risk of a haematoma, which may result in pressure on the airway. Equipment should be readily available to remove either clips or sutures. The obese patient may have difficulty with inspiration as the ability of the diaphragm to descend on inspiration can be inhibited in the supine position. The head of the bed may be raised to ease pressure on the diaphragm, but the neck must remain well supported and aligned. The patient must also be pain-free and encouraged regularly to take deep breaths.

Neurological assessment is important and should include assessment of motor (power and muscle tone) and sensory function. It should be compared with the pre-operative assessment and any changes immediately reported to the appropriate senior nurse and/or doctor.

Retention of urine or incontinence should also be reported. Elimination may be a problem if use of a bedpan is impossible or contraindicated. Sitting on the commode is usually permitted.

Eating and drinking when lying flat are generally a problem; after the first 24 hours bedrest, patients who have had lumber spinal surgery usually find it easier to stand for meals.

Pain may initially be worse post-operatively owing to localized swelling. Patients should be reminded that this does not mean that the operation has been a failure. The additional problem of muscle spasm following surgery on the lumbar spine is often relieved when the patient is instructed to flex his hips and knees. Pain should be assessed using an appropriate tool, prescribed analgesia administered and its effectiveness monitored. Patient-controlled analgesia (PCA) has become increasingly popular. The patient will be asked pre-operatively if he would prefer this method, and if so, will then be instructed in its use. If a spinal fusion has been performed and a bone graft used, the patient may suffer the added problem of pain from the donor site. Pain is a good indicator of degree of mobility; if pain occurs during mobilization, the patient should be encouraged to rest.

If the patient has sensory loss (paraesthesia), the involved skin areas should be checked for signs of inflammation; special care should be taken when handling and positioning the patient.

The principles of wound care are as for any wound, but particular attention should be paid to signs of CSF leakage. If it occurs, the wound may need resuturing and antibiotics may be prescribed prophylactically to prevent meningitis.

Suture removal will depend on the status of the individual patient and the site and type of surgery. It ranges from 7 to 14 days post-operatively.

Prior to discharge, patients are advised not to drive for a minimum of 6 weeks and are instructed in lifting and handling techniques. Return to work will depend largely on the surgery performed, individual progress and the type of work.

Conclusions

Nursing patients undergoing neurosurgical intervention demands highly developed observational skills, the ability to work closely with other disciplines, the patience necessary to help individuals, for example, learn to speak again, and, in contrast, the ability to act swiftly and decisively when faced with critical changes in a patient's neurological status. It is an exciting and rewarding specialty.

Summary

1 Raised ICP is life-threatening but may have a fast or slow onset, depending on its cause.

2 Neurological observations concentrate on level of consciousness, pupil reactions, vital signs and limb movements. They may need to be repeated frequently to assess patient progress.

3 Where possible, rehabilitation is commenced while investigations and preparation for surgery are taking place. The hair must be washed prior to cranial surgery.

4 Common cranial operations are used to illustrate the principles of care, including controlled ventilation during surgery.

5 Post-operative care can identify areas of particular concern, such as observing for seizures.

6 Rehabilitation continues in the post-operative phase, with early mobilization usually encouraged. The team may include the physiotherapist and speech therapist.

7 The patient undergoing spinal surgery will be taught techniques for turning and getting in and out of bed in order to secure normal spinal alignment.

8 Immediately post-operatively, the pain may be worse as a result of swelling and muscle spasm. The patient must be prepared for this before spinal surgery.

CASE HISTORY

Mr Swanstone, aged 45, has undergone planned cranial surgery. What trend in his neurological observations would indicate that he might have a haematoma?

Review Questions

1 List the signs and symptoms of raised ICP. Why is this dangerous?

2 What is included in a set of neurological observations?

3 What is the difference between vital signs observations and neurological observations?

4 Explain the Glasgow Coma Scale to a junior student.

5 What is the reaction of CSF on a glucose test strip?

6 Look up the formation and circulation of CSF.

7 Look up the pathways of the optic and oculo motor nerves and try to explain why the pupil reaction shows what is happening within the skull.

ACKNOWLEDGEMENTS

With thanks to Thomas Aird, Lecturer at South Bank University, London.

References

Allan, D. (ed.) 1988 *Nursing and the neurosciences.* London: Churchill Livingstone.

Arbour, R.B. 1993 Stereotactic localization and resection of intracranial tumors. *Journal of Neuroscience Nursing* **25**(1), 14–21.

Atkinson, L. 1992 *Operating room technique,* 7th edn. London: Berry & Kohn's.

Craddock, E. 1989 Psychological care before brain surgery. *Nursing* **3**(46), 17–19.

DiIorio, C. and Price, M. 1990 Swallowing: an assessment guide. *American Journal of Nursing* **90**(7), 38–43.

Frawley, P. 1990 Neurological observations. *Nursing Times* **86**(35), 29–34.

Hickey, J.V. 1992 *The clinical practice of neurological and neurosurgical nursing.* Philadelphia: JB Lippicott.

Jacobs, B.B. 1995 Emergent neurologic events. *Critical Care Nursing Clinics of North America* **7**(3), 427–44.

James, A. 1990 Why perpetuate the shaving ritual? *Nursing Times* **86**(41), 37–8.

Jennett, B. and Galbraith, S. 1994 *An introduction to neurosurgery,* 5th edn. London: Heinemann.

Lee, S. 1989 Intracranial pressure changes during positioning of patients with severe head injury. *Heart and Lung* **18**(4), 411–14.

Quigley, J., Marshall, C., Reaveley, C., Page, P. and Kenny, J. 1989 Neurological investigations. *Nursing* **3**(46), 17–19.

Readman, S. 1990 The challenge of epilepsy. Part 2: Patient education. *Practice Nurse* **3**(4), 219–22.

Rising, C.J. 1994 The relationship of selected nursing activities to ICP. *Journal of Neuroscience Nursing* **25**(5), 302–9.

Teasdale, G. 1975 Acute impairment of brain function Part 2: Observation record chart. *Nursing Times* **71**, 972–3.

Tortora, G. and Anagnostakos, N.P. 1990 *Principles of anatomy and physiology.* London: Harper & Row.

Vaughan, R. 1995 High anxiety. *Nursing Times* **91**(12), 54–5.

Verran, B.A. and Aisbitt, P.E. 1988 *Neurological and neurosurgical nursing.* London: Edward Arnold.

4 Ophthalmic surgery

Penelope Simpson

Introduction

Admission to hospital for an eye operation, even as a day case, is likely to cause considerable anxiety. The eye is delicate and sensitive, and there is the fear of pain and discomfort, if not blindness. As many ophthalmic patients are elderly, it is worth noting that ophthalmic surgery and nursing care have progressed dramatically in recent years. Patients can be reassured that their experience will probably be far better than they anticipate. Many will be home the same day or within a few days.

The ophthalmic nurse must possess gentleness and manual dexterity to reduce fear of the eye being touched. She must also have a thoughtful approach to the person with a visual handicap. The subtle use of touch, introducing herself each time she approaches and indicating when she is leaving, will enhance the patient's dignity. The nurse should approach the patient from the side with the better vision, if this can be determined. Describing the layout of the ward or unit while showing the patient around can aid orientation. Describing the contents of a plate of food, using the 'clockface' technique, can be useful, as may a plate guard. Shouting must be avoided; the person who is visually handicapped is not necessarily deaf as well.

Patient education, which aims for a better-informed client, is very important in the nursing care of ophthalmic surgery patients. It is anticipated that some teaching will take place in the OPD or pre-surgical assessment clinic, reinforcement and follow-up occurring on the ward. It is worth establishing the patient's beliefs and knowledge in order to know how best to present new information and in what quantity.

Examination and treatment can be hindered by the fact that many people dislike having their eyes touched; some may feel faint, or actually faint, during some procedures. Thus thoughtful positioning of the patient on the chair or couch will prevent harm.

Pre-admission clinics are now widely established, ensuring that the patient is suitable and well prepared for the proposed surgery. Macleod (1994) discusses the value of this service for patients undergoing corneal grafting, for example in terms of their feeling that their questions were adequately answered.

The surgical eye department will most frequently deal with:

- cataract extraction;
- correction of squint;
- repair of retinal detachment;
- surgery for glaucoma;
- corneal grafting;
- trauma;
- enucleation (removal of the eye).

Anatomy

Figure 4.1 and the following description of the anatomy of the eye may enable the patient to understand her condition. A model may be useful.

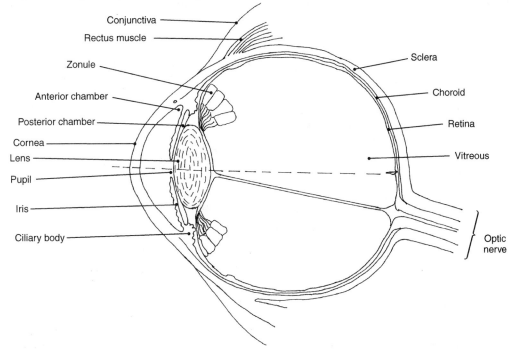

Figure 4.1 Section through the eye

Each eyeball lies in a bony socket (orbit) in the front of the skull, mostly surrounded by a bed of fat. The eyeball is almost round in shape and has three coats. The outermost is the tough sclera, which is the 'white' of the eye; the middle choroid layer has many blood vessels and contains pigment; and the inner surface is the retina, onto which light rays fall. The muscles that move the eye are attached to the outside of the sclera, a little way back from the edge of the cornea.

The clear 'window' at the front of the eye is the cornea, through which can be seen the coloured portion of the eye, the iris in the centre of which is the hole known as the pupil. Behind the pupil lies the lens, which helps to focus light rays. The area between the cornea and the iris is the anterior chamber; between the iris and the lens is the posterior chamber, both of these are filled with fluid called aqueous humour. Jelly-like vitreous humour fills the rest of the space. The conjunctiva, a thin layer of tissue, lines the upper and lower eyelids and covers the sclera up to the edge of the cornea.

Stollery (1987) contains a more detailed anatomy and physiology of the various structures.

Issues common to all eye operations

Admission and assessment

The patient is usually admitted less than 24 hours before surgery unless there is a medical condition needing monitoring pre-anaesthesia. Eighty per cent of ophthalmic surgery is performed under local anaesthetic and as day case work. A pre-admission clinic system may be in operation.

It is important that the time before operation is used to orientate the visually impaired person to her new surroundings and the people caring for her. Patient co-operation during and after surgery is of paramount importance, so hearing aids need to be retained, and the patient's ability and willingness to instill eye drops for several weeks will be assured. The nursing staff will teach the patient the necessary technique.

This teaching is best started pre-operatively as most inpatient stays are very short, with limited time to learn much that is new post-operatively.

It is useful for the patient to bring something to while away the time waiting for surgery and distract the mind.

Patient comment

'Waiting for my operation was a nasty combination of boredom and anxiety. I couldn't concentrate on much.'

Talking books can be helpful, and hobbies are beneficial if they do not require much equipment.

Mobility must be encouraged until just before the operation. It is useful to wash the hair shortly before surgery, as this may later be restricted.

The visual acuity of the patient will be recorded as part of the overall patient assessment, which will generate a focused nursing care plan for the duration of the patient's stay and give pointers to the support and education she will need on returning home.

Pre-operative preparation

Some eye operations are performed under local anaesthesia. The choice of general or local anaesthetic is made in the light of the patient's general condition.

All patients need sensory as well as process information to tell them what they are likely to feel and hear during the induction and per- and post-operatively. This can reduce fear and anxiety and increase co-operation (Dobson, 1991). Hearing aids should be left in place. They are only removed for general anaesthesia during which they are stored in dry, labelled pots to protect them from damage by fluids and then reinserted immediately post-operatively to facilitate communication (Dobson, 1991).

In addition to the pre-operative care for the type of surgery and anaesthetic (as outlined in Part One), there are likely to be topical prepara-

Instillation of own eye drops

1 Wash the hands thoroughly

2 Check the bottle for correct drug, eye, timing, expiry date and dose

3 Shake the bottle

4 Remove the lid

5 Invert the bottle

6 Use the ipsilateral hand (the same side as the eye to be treated) to hold the bottle, part of hand resting on forehead, if necessary to steady it

7 Use the contralateral (other) hand to hold a paper tissue, if necessary resting part of the hand against the upper jaw for steadying

8 Tilt the head back

9 Open the eye wide

10 Look up

11 Do not blink

12 Use the finger or thumb of the contralateral hand to ease the lower eyelid down very gently

13 Let the drop fall into the centre of the lower conjuctival sac (**never** onto the cornea)

14 Do not allow the dropper to come into contact with anything at all as this will contaminate the dropper and eyedrops

15 Replace the lid

16 Allow at least 5 minutes before instilling any other drop to the same eye. (One drop is usually 50 µl and will overload the average conjunctival sac, which has a capacity of 25 µl).

17 Use paper tissue to dab gently any overflow

18 Record that the drop has been given.

tions, depending on local policy, which may include:

- taking conjuctival swabs for culture and sensitivity;
- trimming the eyelashes for intra-ocular surgery;
- instilling prophylactic antibiotic drops (e.g. chloramphenicol) in such regimens as four times daily for 1–2 days;
- lacrimal (tear duct) syringing;

- marking which eye is to be operated on. This procedure varies from unit to unit.

Details of these procedures may be found in Stollery (1987) and your unit's nursing procedure book. Wells (1993) points out that many units are phasing out swab-taking, trimming lashes and the routine use of antibiotic drops, reserving them for clearly defined circumstances.

The patient, when mentally and physically prepared for the operation, will usually be prescribed a systemic premedication, given orally or by injection. In addition to this, ophthalmic premedication may be given, for example:

- Chloramphenicol drops intensively, every 15 minutes in the 2 hours immediately prior to surgery.

- Mydriatic (pupil-dilating) drops intensely, immediately before cataract extraction or retinal detachment surgery, for example, every 15 minutes for 1–2 hours pre-operatively.

- Local anaesthetic drops for the patient having an operation under local anaesthesia, for example cocaine hydrochloride or amethocaine hydrochloride, given every 5–15 minutes for up to an hour before surgery, as prescribed. The anaesthetized eye needs to be covered with a cartella shield for safety. Wicker (1994) outlines the side-effects of local anaesthetic drugs.

The patient undergoing local anaesthesia will have an intravenous cannula for safe access and may possibly be given an intravenous sedative and amnesiac such as diazepam. The surgeon will then inject local anaesthetic into the skin below the lower lid and at the side of the face (facial block) to numb the eye.

Once the patient is placed supine on the table, her head must, for ease of access and minimum movement, be correctly positioned on a horseshoe sandbag, Ruben's pillow, or head ring for a child.

Peri-operative care

For the patient undergoing local anaesthesia, it is important for a nurse to sit and hold her hand throughout for emotional and physical support (Wicker, 1994). This also allows the nurse to monitor the patient's condition by:

- taking her pulse;
- noting the colour of her fingernails;
- observing chest movements.

The nurse will agree with the patient that she will squeeze her hand when she wishes to speak, as the head invariably moves during speech. The tightness with which the patient holds the nurse's hand will indicate the degree of pain, discomfort or tension being suffered by the patient, her face being hidden by the theatre drapes. Per-operatively, the patient may experience disorientation or claustrophobia as she will not only have her face covered by a sterile towel, but may also have the unaffected eye taped shut. This will make head movement more likely during the operation. Oxygen and air are usually administered via a facemask.

Post-operative care

Patients having local anaesthesia can usually get up immediately after surgery; some units even have 'walk-in, walk-out' theatres.

Once back in the ward, the patient who has had a general anaesthetic will usually spend the rest of the day quietly in bed, resting and sleeping. She may be placed lying on her side with the operated eye uppermost, reducing trauma to the eye and relieving the pressure applied to the body's dorsal regions in theatre. Prescribed medication will be available for pain and nausea, and the eye should not be touched. It is frequently covered by an eyepad and/or cartella shield, which must be left undisturbed.

If the patient is sufficiently recovered, she can start drinking and then eating approximately an hour after her return.

During the first 24 hours post-operatively, the patient may have visitors and will be encouraged to mobilize in readiness for going home unless this is contraindicated by the particular surgery.

The operated eye will be examined, after explanation and consent, using a good pen-torch or slit lamp. The patient sits facing the lamp, resting her chin on a little shelf opposite the examining nurse or doctor. The eye is usually checked systematically from outside to the inside:

- The *pad* (if worn) is inspected for blood and discharge.
- The *eyelids* will be checked for swelling, discolouration, discharge, crusting and entropion (an eyelid turned in owing to, for example, poor padding technique or age-related laxity of the lid muscles, allowing the lashes to rub against the globe of the eye).
- The *conjunctiva* will be checked for injection (redness), subconjunctival haemorrhage (bright red), oedema, an intact suture line and iris prolapse.
- The *cornea* will be checked for clarity and abrasions.
- The *anterior chamber* will be assessed for depth: it should be deep but needs to be compared with the other eye. Also check for hyphaema (blood in the anterior chamber), hypopyon (pus in the anterior chamber) and an implanted lens (following implant surgery).
- The *iris* may be checked for peripheral iridectomy/iridotomy (a small hole/incision at the outer edge of the iris to promote the flow of fluid between the anterior and posterior chambers; this is rarely performed) and iridodonesis after cataract surgery (the iris, now unsupported by the lens, shimmers and wobbles).
- The *pupil* will be assessed for shape (a peaked pupil may indicate an iris prolapse), size (it may be dilated with mydriatics, or constricted – miosed – with miotics), reaction (none if mydriatics or miotics are being used) and colour (it should be black, but the red reflex may be noted).

Following examination of the eye, it is gently bathed with sterile normal saline, according to local policy. The eye is usually first cleansed closed, using each eye swab (non-linting) once only, and working from the inner to the outer margin of the eye. The patient is asked to look up, her lower lid is everted and the lower margin is cleansed with a fresh swab, working from nasal to temporal. As many swabs as are required to clear crusting and discharge are used. The upper lid margin is then attended to by asking the patient to look down as the nurse gently elevates the lid away from the globe and swabs in the usual direction. This should be repeated if necessary. Stubborn discharge loosens if a damp swab is placed over the eye for a few minutes. The frequency of eye bathing, anything from once to four times a day, depends on local policy. Drops will be given after eye bathing.

Eye drops will be prescribed for instillation several times a day. As with any other drug, there will be variations in local policy and procedure. The basic principles are:

1 Identify the patient, explain the procedure and gain her consent.
2 Cross-check the drops and the eye to be treated against the prescription sheet.
3 Ask the patient to look upwards.
4 Evert her lower lid.
5 Put one drop into the centre of the lower fornix (conjunctival sac).
6 Ask the patient to close the eye gently without squeezing.
7 Wipe away any excess.
8 Sign for the drug.

Only one drug at a time will be instilled. The prescribed regimens are likely to include:

- antibiotic drops, ranging from hourly or 2 hourly to four times a day;
- steroid drops;
- mydriatic drops;
- eye ointment, which may be applied at night.

The principles, for use of the latter are the same as for the instillation of drops, except that point 5 will be: squeeze 6.4 mm ($\frac{1}{4}$") of ointment along the lower fornix, from the nose outwards.

Eye protection may be needed. This will consist of a cartella shield, worn at night for up to 2 weeks to prevent accidental trauma. If necessary, the patient may have to wear a 'drip pad' of gauze taped to the cheek to absorb tears. When no other eye protection is being worn, dark glasses are advised for patients with dilated pupils to prevent photophobia.

Mobilization is encouraged, aiming at growing independence to perform activities of daily living either unaided or to the pre-operative level. The patient is taught not to bend down below the level of the waist. The actual length of her stay is related to the type of surgery performed and the abilities of the patient and her family to perform the necessary follow-up care.

Advice and education

The main areas of advice with particular reference to the treated eye concern:

- the instillation of eyedrops;
- cleaning the eye;
- eye protection activities;
- medical follow-up;
- convalescence.

EYEDROPS

The patient will need to be reasonably proficient at eyedrop instillation by the time she goes home. Explaining the actions of and reasons for the drugs is time well spent in terms of gaining co-operation. It is worth teaching another member of the immediate household at the same time in case there are problems. A large-print written summary of instillation times or, if vision is severely impaired, audiotapes help to increase compliance. Consider using an autodropper device.

CLEANING THE EYE

The affected eye may be sticky in the mornings and need cleaning, using cool, boiled water and damped cotton wool or gauze. Dry cotton wool should never be used near the eye, for example to remove make-up, as loose fibres can enter it. This may also be written down as a reminder for the patient.

EYE PROTECTION

For the first 2 weeks after surgery, the patient has to behave in a way that protects her eye from trauma and anything likely to raise intra-ocular pressure. She is reminded not to bend down below waist level, lift anything heavy, get constipated, smoke or do anything that makes her cough or sneeze violently, or travel on jerky, unpredictable forms of transport. She will also need to have her hair washed backwards over a basin. Patients should check about resuming sexual activity since there is the risk of increasing intra-ocular pressure and/or damaging the eye (Kelly, 1994).

Avoiding such activities will protect against haemorrhage or iris prolapse and increase the likelihood of success. If there are any unexpected events or problems, the patient needs the ward's telephone number in order to obtain advice from the nursing staff. An A&E department attendance might also be needed. The specific advice sheet for the particular operation should list what to expect and what to report.

MEDICAL FOLLOW-UP

An outpatient appointment is usually made for approximately 2 weeks from the date of discharge. The patient is not allowed to drive until reviewed by the outpatient consultant. At this appointment, the eyedrop regimen may be changed or discontinued.

CONVALESCENCE

Convalescence will be relatively short, as this is not classified as major surgery in terms of its physiological impact. For most patients, even the aged, a couple of weeks of a quieter than normal life, with a little extra support, may be sufficient. The psychological boost of the prospect of improved sight means that these patients, on the whole, 'bounce back' from surgery very well.

Driving

To be able to resume driving the patient must be able to

- read to a level of 6/9 on the Snellen chart

If they have only one functioning eye, they may be allowed to drive if:

- the insurance company is aware, and
- they have a period of adaptation

The ophthalmologist may not be happy with the above criteria, or may feel that the vision in the operated eye will change as healing occurs, affecting the patient's visual judgement. In such circumstances, permission to resume driving will not be given.

Squint correction

A squint (strabismus) is caused by malfunction of the eye muscles, each eye having six. This results in deviation of one or both eyes in an inward, outward, upward or downward direction. Corrective surgery involves an operation, lasting 30–45 minutes, on one or more muscles to straighten the affected eye.

Pre-operative care

The squint will have been assessed on more than one occasion by an orthoptist in the OPD prior to admission. Consultations demand patient concentration for several minutes while eye position and movement are measured. The tests may be performed again on the day before and the day after surgery. For a detailed description of these tests, see Stollery (1987). The post-operative test may be uncomfortable, but the other sensations and requirements will be familiar to the patient.

The patient may require careful explanation of why the 'good' eye needs an operation and needs to be prepared for at least a week's convalescence.

Post-operative care and discharge advice

The eye is not usually padded post-operatively and is likely to look very red (conjunctival injection and subconjunctival haemorrhage). Antibiotic and steroid drops are prescribed.

The pain and nausea associated with this surgery need to be treated with regular medication.

Children are advised not to go back to school for 2 weeks. Orthoptists will advise on whether close work or television is permissible. Swimming must be avoided for 1 month.

Some adult patients have adjustable sutures that are repositioned the day after surgery. The patient may feel nauseated during this until the sutures are finally tied.

Eye redness is likely to persist for about a fortnight, settling down as healing progresses.

Liaison with the orthoptic department is necessary to determine whether non-surgical treatments such as glasses or occlusion need to be continued and to make a follow-up appointment.

Complications

These include:

- stitch abscess, which will cause the patient to experience much-increased pain in the affected region;
- the muscle slipping away from its new position because the sutures have broken; the patient may complain of severe double vision or more pain;
- failure of the operation to produce binocular single vision when this is the aim;
- poor cosmetic result;
- overcorrection of the squint.

The patient should be given a telephone number in case she is worried or needs advice.

Retinal detachment

The retina consists of several layers; the separation of these layers is termed 'retinal detachment'. The patient may complain of:

- flashes of light caused by the separating layers stimulating the rods and cones that convey visual information to the optic nerve;
- 'floaters', caused by small haemorrhages, usually from the retinal vessels;
- 'cobwebs' or 'curtains', which are loss of vision (field loss) in the area affected by the separation.

There are no outward signs of the condition, so diagnosis largely depends on a patient's symptoms or incidental discovery by an optician or doctor.

Pre-operative care

Bedrest is usual initially to prevent further detachment. It may be necessary to wait until any haemorrhage inside the eye has ceased and cleared for adequate examination. In this case, the patient can sit up with her back, head and shoulders supported by pillows. Care must be taken to minimize possible complications of bedrest by ensuring regular changes of position, adequate nutrition and hydration, and deep breathing and leg exercises. This needs to be carefully explained to the patient and reinforced. The patient is likely to be frightened by the thought of losing her sight, yet feel perfectly well in herself and be irked by the restrictions.

Prescribed mydriatic drops are instilled into both eyes. Indirect ophthalmoscopic examination of the affected eye will be performed by the medical staff and an accurate diagram drawn of the retina, showing holes, tears, attached and detached areas and the presence of subretinal fluid to aid the surgeon. The unaffected eye will be checked for any problems, which can be dealt with at the same time.

It may be necessary in exceptional circumstances to have both eyes padded to rest the eye and prevent movement 'stirring up' the bleeding. This may be difficult to tolerate so any way in which the nurse can increase the patient's understanding will help her to cope better. This state is likely to be tedious, so the patient needs distraction with a radio, talking books or personal stereo. Conversation and visitors will be welcomed. Pads are removed for eating, drinking and visits to the toilet. If there is no haemorrhage, surgery can be performed earlier.

Dependent positioning or 'posturing' will be prescribed by the medical staff if warranted by the nature of the detachment. The rationale is to position the patient so that the detachment lies dependently against its underlying layer, encouraging the subretinal fluid to reabsorb and re-attachment to occur. The eye will be regularly inspected to determine progress, which involves the lids being handled. Some patients find this, and the bright lights from the examination equipment, unpleasant. Examination is performed with the patient lying on a couch or bed. The mydriatic drops dilate the pupil to facilitate retinal examination but cause further blurring of vision. If this is not explained, it may generate further anxiety.

Types of surgery

For all types, except vitrectomy, the eye is not opened. The approach is from the outside, over the sclera.

Cryotherapy, laser or photocoagulation

Intense local cold or heat is used to seal tears and holes by setting up a local inflammatory reaction, preventing fluid seeping between the retinal layers.

Plombage or scleral buckling

In this procedure, a silastic sponge or plomb (a small rectangle of inert material) is stitched onto the sclera, causing an indentation over the site of the hole and bringing the separated layers of the retina together.

Encirclement

A silicone strap is positioned around the outside of the eyeball, underneath the extra-ocular muscles. This enables greater indentation to take

place and is performed where there is a large area of detachment or multiple holes.

Drainage

Drainage of subretinal fluid must be carried out as part of each procedure outlined above to allow the separated layers to realign.

Vitrectomy

Vitrectomy is the removal of the vitreous in cases in which vitreous traction has caused the detachment. The underlying detachment is then operated on, using one of the above methods. Air can be used to replace the vitreous, but it is absorbed within 24–36 hours. A slower absorption rate is achieved by mixing air with an inert gas (such as sulphahexafluoride: SF6). Silicone oil can also be used to replace the vitreous, but it can cause cataract formation and glaucoma. The 'bubble' caused by the replacement substance is used to assist re-attachment of the retina.

The combination of surgical interventions used is likely to result in a treatment duration of 1–2 hours, so a general anaesthetic is most often employed.

Post-operative care

The patient will be positioned in order to ensure drainage of the subretinal fluid.

The eyelids and conjunctiva are usually swollen after surgery because of the amount of handling and movement of the eye.

The cornea must be checked for clarity. Cloudiness may indicate ischaemia of the anterior segment of the eye, caused by the encirclement band being too tight.

The pupil will remain dilated.

Drops will be instilled:

- an antibiotic, e.g. neomycin;
- a mydriatic, e.g. atropine or cyclopentolate;
- a steroid, e.g. betamethasone.

The patient may need to be nursed in a dependent position following surgery, especially after vitrectomy. This is important because the injected gas or air bubble must be uppermost to put pressure onto the detached area of retina. This 'posturing' may need to be continued for several days. The majority of the patient's time will be spent in the required position, with short breaks for drinks, meals and toiletting.

Ocular pain is a feature of retinal detachment surgery for most patients. A prescribed analgesic will need to be given regularly.

Complications

- Subretinal fluid continuing to collect between the retinal layers must be removed to:
  - prevent further detachment;
  - aid re-attachment.

- An encirclement strap that is too tight will result in ischaemia of the anterior segment of the eye, shown by a cloudy cornea and increased pain. It will need urgent loosening or replacement.

- The plomb or encircling band may become infected, requiring its removal.

- The plomb may become loose and work its

way to the surface, extruding under the conjunctiva.

Progress

Visual improvement takes place slowly, depending upon the severity of the detachment and how effective the repair has been. Ninety per cent of detachments need only one operation to achieve reasonably good vision. Only 6% of the remaining 10% will benefit visually from further surgery (Stollery, 1987).

Discharge advice

As the patient is likely to have been subjected to a lengthy general anaesthetic, and still has a degree of visual impairment, she must not drive until she has formally been passed as fit to do so. She should not drive for a minimum of 2 weeks following surgery.

The patient will feel tired and must rest when she first returns home, indulging in only light physical activity. She must not fly if SF6 gas has been inserted, until the gas disappears, usually at about 2 weeks post-surgery.

Cataract extraction

A cataract is a lens opacity that prevents light rays reaching the retina and thus limits the patient's ability to see. It tends to be progressive, but many people cope with the painless blurring of their vision, reduced ability to focus and perceive colour, and increased glare from lights for years before requiring removal of the lens because of virtual blindness. A cataract is said to be immature when only part of the lens is opaque. When all of the lens is opacified, and possibly swollen, it is termed 'mature'.

The types of cataract are congenital (e.g. owing to rubella), familial, senile, traumatic, toxic (e.g. owing to radiation), secondary to existing eye disease or associated with systemic disease such

as diabetes. Smoking, too much alcohol, poor nutrition, myopia, steroid use (Kelly, 1994) and exposure to ultraviolet light are also risk factors.

The timing of cataract removal depends upon the patient's lifestyle and the degree of incapacity caused. Old age is no bar to removal, as surgery can enhance the person's independence and quality of life (Mangione et al. 1994).

Pre-operative care

The operation may be performed under local or general anaesthetic, as an inpatient or as a day case. Crick (1991) describes the last in useful detail. The patient undergoing local anaesthesia needs to be able to lie flat and still for 30 minutes, so anyone with confusion or tremor is unsuitable (Ralph *et al.*, 1995).

The pupil of the affected eye is dilated before surgery, which lasts from $\frac{1}{2}$ to 1 hour. Removal of the cataract is usually followed by implantation of a plastic lens. This is calculated by the medical staff or biometrist and discussed with the patient beforehand.

Types of operation

The method of extraction depends on the age of the patient and whether an intra-ocular lens is to be implanted. The incision will be either limbal, under a conjunctival flap or via a peripheral corneal approach.

Needling or lens aspiration

This is performed on patients under the age of 15 years. The soft cortex (coat) and nucleus (centre) of the lens are irrigated out through an incision in the anterior lens capsule, leaving the posterior capsule behind.

Lensectomy

'Lensectomy' also known as phacofragmentation, involves removing the whole lens, including the capsule, using a special irrigation/cutting/aspiration probe. This appears to have a lower complication rate than needling and is also used for young eyes.

Intracapsular lens extraction

This procedure involves removal of the entire lens plus its capsule. Once the eye is opened, the enzyme chymotrypsin is introduced into the eye to dissolve the zonular fibres. The lens, once free of attachments, can be removed by cryoprobe (intense cold) or forceps. An anterior chamber intra-ocular lens is usually implanted, or a contact lens or glasses will be needed. This is still the favoured operation in developing countries.

Extracapsular lens extraction

The anterior lens capsule, cortex and nucleus are removed, leaving the posterior lens capsule in place to support the anterior face of the vitreous humour. A posterior chamber intra-ocular lens is usually implanted. This sits in the posterior capsule and has hairlike plastic loops that tuck into the muscle ring at the root of the iris to keep it in place. This operation has largely superseded intracapsular extraction in developed countries.

Phacoemulsification

In phacoemulsification, ultrasonic vibration is used to break up mature lens fibres. The liquid lens matter is then sucked out in an action similar to that of a vacuum cleaner. This means a smaller scleral or corneal incision, generally no sutures and therefore less post-surgical astigmatism. It may be particularly suitable for patients undergoing anticoagulant therapy, as this does not need to be interrupted (Kammann *et al.*, 1994). This technique lends itself to day case surgery under local anaesthetic (Fischel and Lipton, 1996).

Post-operative care and discharge advice

If a lens has been implanted, its position needs to be checked:

- An anterior chamber intra-ocular lens will be seen in place in the anterior chamber.
- A posterior chamber intra-ocular lens can be seen reflected through the pupil, which may or may not be dilated.
- An iris clip lens (the least commonly used type) can be noticed by its reflection through the pupil, which must not be dilated or the lens will dislocate. The pupil may be miosed.
- With no intra-ocular lens, or an anterior chamber lens, the pupil may be dilated to rest the eye post-operatively.

Patients with implant lenses are referred to as pseudo-aphakic. They do not have their own lens, but they do have a pseudo or artificial lens.

Antibiotic and steroid drops will be instilled regularly as prescribed, usually four times a day. This will continue at home. Some ophthalmic departments have specialist nursing staff to examine patients at home (Sanders *et al.*, 1994).

Many patients note a dramatic improvement in their sight at the first eye dressing, 24 hours post-operatively. As the cataract may have imparted a brownish or yellowish cast to their vision, the blue end of the spectrum is particularly appreciated. This is most noticeable in those who have received implants.

Patient comment

An artist patient with bilateral cataracts complained after the first extraction that the surgeon was depriving her of her ability to see 'true' colours, perceiving the implant as having a blue tint.

Pre-existing mascular degeneration may preclude a good visual result. This can be bitterly disappointing to the patient with high expectations of the surgery, so good pre-operative preparation is needed (J. Sheppard, personal communication, 1996).

Restrictions on activities apply for only 2 weeks, although heavy lifting and return to work must be avoided for 6 weeks.

Patients who have an implant may still require spectacles for reading. These are prescribed 6 weeks post-operatively. Temporary aphakic glasses will be given to the patient if no intraocular lens has been implanted. They do not help if the patient is very short sighted or has unilateral aphakia with reasonable eyesight in her other eye. Getting used to these aphakic glasses will take some time, and she will need encouragement to persist.

Those without implants may notice distorted vision, such as doorways looking 'coffin-shaped'. The improvement in vision is slower and less dramatic following correction of the aphakia with permanent spectacles or a contact lens, which will be prescribed about 6 weeks after surgery. Until the contact lens is fitted, the patient with only one cataract removed will complain of double vision, and the aphakic eye may have to be occluded.

Complications

Wound breakdown may be caused by faulty technique or trauma, such as rubbing the eye, and may be associated with iris prolapse. The patient will need to return to theatre for wound repair under local anaesthetic. The earlier this can be performed the better as, in a very recent prolapse, the iris can literally be pushed back into position. Over 12 hours, the prolapsed iris becomes necrotic and has to be excised, leaving the patient with a very broad, almost funnel-shaped pupil. The use of a Cartella shield at night for 2 weeks may reduce the risk of such a prolapse.

After all cataract surgery except intracapsular extraction, the remaining posterior lens capsule often scleroses, causing visual impairment. This is treated on an outpatient basis by capsulotomy, a small incision in the capsule usually made by YAG laser, enabling light rays to pass through.

Intracapsular lens extraction may carry an increased risk of retinal detachment compared with extracapsular extraction.

Anterior chamber introcular lens implantation may be associated with corneal pathology. The lens may touch the inner surface of the cornea, rubbing off cells, which will not be replaced. The implant then has to be removed.

Chronic low-grade endophthalmitis may also require explantation of the intra-ocular lens (Busin *et al.*, 1994). The appropriate antibiotics are administered intravenously, subconjunctivally or even into the vitreous if they are not toxic to the retina (Perry and Tullo, 1995). Steroids may also be given.

Hypopyon and acute endophthalmitis may increase the possibility of losing the eye. The patient is admitted, and intravenous antibiotics are used in conjunction with intensive topical treatment, involving half-hourly eye drops both day and night. If this proves ineffective, the eye may have to be eviscerated.

Glaucoma

Glaucoma is a rise in intra-ocular pressure, which is determined by the balance between the rate of production and the rate of drainage of aqueous fluid within the eye. The two main types of glaucoma are:

1 acute/closed angle/congestive glaucoma;
2 chronic/open angle/simple glaucoma.

Acute glaucoma occurs in patients with shallow anterior chambers, which have narrow angles. Owing to various causes (*see* Stollery, 1987, for details), the angle becomes blocked so that the aqueous cannot drain away, and, as aqueous production continues, pressure builds up within the eye. This causes congestion of the structures surrounding the anterior and posterior chambers.

Chronic glaucoma has an insidious start and is slowly progressive. It affects 2% of the population at the age of 40, rising to 70% over the age of 75. People with close relatives with glaucoma, diabetics and Afro-Caribbeans are more likely to develop it. It may not be noticed by the patient until she has a marked degree of tunnel vision.

Both types of glaucoma lead to loss of visual acuity. The optic nerve is the first structure to be affected by the raised intra-ocular pressure, causing the nerve fibres to atrophy and producing loss of vision in the affected area.

STUDENT ACTIVITY

Read up, in an anatomy and physiology textbook, the formation and circulation of aqueous humour.

The patient with acute glaucoma will probably need surgery following an acute attack, characterized by:

- severe headache and pain in the affected eye;
- nausea and vomiting;
- abdominal pain and generally feeling unwell;
- a red, swollen eye with a hazy cornea, and a 'muddy', swollen iris;
- a pupil that may be fixed, dilated and oval in shape;
- a shallow anterior chamber;

- raised intra-ocular pressure;
- rapidly reduced visual acuity, with haloes seen around lights.

The immediate care needed is admission to hospital for reduction of pressure, relief of symptoms and, later, preparation for operation. The patient will be feeling very unwell and fearing for her sight, so she will require constant explanation of what is being done and why.

- She needs to be horizontal, in a quiet, dark place, with a cold compress on her forehead and access to a vomit bowl and call bell.

- Intravenous acetazolamide will be given as prescribed to reduce the production of aqueous humour.

- Pilocarpine drops will be instilled intensively to constrict the pupil and draw the bunched iris away from the drainage angle. The other eye will probably also be prescribed miotic drops to prevent an acute attack.

- If pain and nausea continue despite treatment, analgesic and anti-emetic therapy will be commenced.

- If the pressure does not reduce, more energetic treatment such as mannitol, an intravenous diuretic, may be administered.

- Acetazolamide will be prescribed to continue orally four times a day.

Once the intra-ocular pressure has returned to normal, the patient will need laser treatment or surgery to improve drainage of the eye.

Pre- and per-operative care

PERIPHERAL IRIDECTOMY

This will be performed (often under local anaesthetic) on the affected eye. The pupil must be constricted as part of the preparation. The operation creates an artificial opening in the iris, allow ing an increased amount of aqueous to flow into the anterior chamber. This causes the iris to fall backwards away from the drainage angle, thus relieving the obstruction.

As acute glaucoma is a bilateral condition, the other eye needs a prophylactic iridectomy, usually carried out a few days later.

Peripheral iridotomy, performed by means of a laser, uses the same principle as iridectomy. Local anaesthetic and miotic drops are part of the preparation. The patient may be sent home with instructions after this procedure.

Post-operative care

At the first dressing, the peripheral iridectomy will be noticed; an iridotomy will not be visible to the naked eye. The anterior chamber will remain shallow, but the cornea should be clear and bright.

Mydriatic, antibiotic and steroid drops will be prescribed for initial instillation four times daily. It is important to check that the mydriatic drops are instilled only into the operated eye as in the unoperated eye, they could provoke an acute attack of glaucoma.

The patient can probably go home 1–3 days after her last eye operation, depending on her overall condition and home circumstances.

Discharge advice

If intra-ocular pressure is still raised, the patient will be prescribed acetazolamide orally four times a day. She must be warned of the side-effects of tingling in the extremities, nausea, loss of appetite and fatigue. Potassium chloride is usually prescribed to counteract these unwanted effects.

Drops that the patient needs to learn how and when to administer may include:

- timolol maleate to reduce the production of aqueous fluid. This must be given strictly 12-hourly; after several weeks' use the outflow of aqueous is increased;
- mydriatic, antibiotic and/or steroid, which will continue until an OPD follow up appointment, when they may be reviewed or stopped.

Complications

Those failing to respond to treatment will experience recurring acute attacks, which may lead to other complications:

- cataract formation;
- the root of the iris adhering to the posterior surface of the cornea, obliterating the drainage angle;
- visual field loss occurring increasingly with each attack;
- a blind, painful eye as the end result of failed treatment. Enucleation (removal) or injections of alcohol to eliminate the pain may be needed. The eye can become smaller and atrophy, and the degenerating cornea ulcerate and perforate.

The cause of chronic simple glaucoma is thought to be an initial degeneration of the trabecular meshwork and the canal of Schlemm, which normally drain the aqueous fluid away. The intra-ocular pressure rises, causing a typical loss of vision in at first the nasal peripheral field. It causes loss of night vision and then progressive loss of the remaining peripheral field if the patient is not treated or if treatment is unsuccessful, often resulting in marked tunnel vision. Those with relatives with glaucoma need an ophthalmic check-up every 3–5 years. Once detected, medical treatment will be given to preserve what sight is left. Oral drugs and eye drops are given to reduce the production of aqueous humour and increase its drainage. Beta-blocking drops can be useful as long as side-effects (such as breathlessness) are not too severe. Cannabis is said to have an effect but is not yet legal in the UK (Curtis, 1995).

If medical treatment cannot control the pressure and further visual loss occurs, surgery is planned. Glaucoma surgery is also performed when patients demonstrate difficulty in complying with treatment, for example if it is hard to find the time at work to instill drops.

TRABECULECTOMY

Trabeculectomy is usually performed under a general anaesthetic. A scleral flap is made, and a strip of trabecular meshwork removed from below this flap, which is then sutured back into place. It heals incompletely, forming a fistula through which the aqueous can drain. Lying under the conjunctiva, the bulge over the scleral flap is known as a 'bleb'.

Post-operative care

Patient comment

'The stitch under my eyelid felt like a brick in my eye.'

At the first eye dressing, the bleb will be noticed under the conjunctiva. The anterior chamber should be shallow. Eyedrops will be antibiotic, steroid and mydriatic.

Complications

A flat anterior chamber is due to too much aqueous draining via the bleb. The doctor is informed and may request that a firm eyepad and bandage be applied to seal the bleb. In some instances, a sponge of mitomycin or an injection of fluorouracil is used to prevent fibrosis of the bleb.

Hyphaema is common in the early post-operative period owing to the sudden alteration in intra-ocular pressure.

Discharge advice

The most important aspect to stress is the careful instillation of the correct drops to the correct eye, as the operated eye may be receiving a mydriatic

and the other eye a miotic as treatment for chronic glaucoma.

TRABECULOPLASTY

Lasers are used, so the patient can be treated as an outpatient under local anaesthesia. The laser beam bombards the trabecular meshwork, and the resultant scarring opens up the meshwork to improve aqueous drainage.

Peri-operative care

The patient's consent and co-operation are gained, and local anaesthetic drops instilled. The patient must look at one spot for what will feel like a long time while experiencing repeated flashes of very bright light.

Post-operative care

The patient is made comfortable at rest, and the intra-ocular pressure is checked 2 hours after the procedure. If it is raised, acetazolamide will be prescribed for immediate intravenous administration, and oral treatment will follow four times a day for 2 days.

Discharge advice

This is as for trabeculetomy. Restrictions apply for only the first 2 weeks.

Complications

These are as for acute glaucoma.

Corneal grafting

Corneal opacity prevents light rays entering the eye, rendering the patient virtually blind. It can arise as a result of trauma or chronic infection or irritation, and may be associated with less than meticulous contact lens care. Corneal disease may cause thinning and threat of perforation, so a patch is needed to strengthen the eye.

The problem is treated by removing a disc of opaque cornea and replacing it with one the same size from a donated cornea, stitched into place.

Corneal transplant surgery involves the use of donated tissue and can be regarded as a semi-urgent procedure. Where eye banks are set up, it is possible to some extent to plan surgery, and patients can be given a potential admission date (Macleod, 1994). Corneal tissue taken after death into culture medium can be stored at body temperature and remains suitable for grafting for up to 1 month (Frith et al., 1994).

Pre-operative care

All graft material is tissue-typed and the donor tested for HIV. Some of the preparation can be achieved on an outpatient basis while the patient is on the waiting list for a 'match', of which she will be informed by telephone. If donor material storage facilities are not available, the problems inherent in emergency surgery arise. The patient also needs to be informed, preferably in writing, about the follow-up appointments and eyedrops necessary for many months after surgery (Perry and Tullo, 1995).

The patient is usually admitted the day before surgery, and general anaesthesia is preferred because the operation lasts about 1.5 hours.

The relatively large wound area involved in a penetrating graft requires a longer healing time, so the patient may need to stay in hospital for up to 7 days, being well briefed about what to expect during that time.

Types of operation

Corneal grafts may be full thickness (penetrating) or, more rarely, lamellar (partial thickness) keratoplasty.

Post-operative care

The patient will be on bedrest for the first 24 hours post-operatively to allow recovery from the anaesthetic and to prevent pressure on the corneal wound. She will need to be reminded not to lean over the side of the bed or to touch or rub the eye dressing (Perry and Tullo, 1995). The operated eye will probably be sore for some days until corneal epithelium has grown over the stitches.

The first dressing will be performed the day after surgery, observing particularly for:

- loose sutures;
- leaking wound;
- a shallow or flat anterior chamber;
- hazy donor tissue;

any of which must be reported to medical staff at this stage or at subsequent dressings (Perry and Tullo, 1995).

Some form of visual assessment, even if it is only hand movements, will be made on the first post-operative day.

Until epithelialization has taken place, the eye will probably be covered with an eyepad or shield. By 48 hours post-surgery, a shield only will be worn at night to protect the eye.

It is normal for vision to be blurred during healing and while eyedrops are being instilled. The patient should be assisted with hygiene and gentle mobilization in the early stages of healing and reminded not to touch the eye if it waters. A clean tissue should be used to wipe the cheek rather than the eye.

The patient and carer need to be taught before discharge how to instill drops. If this is not possible, the district nurse may need to supervise or perform both drop instillation and eye hygiene. The regimen will usually include a combination of antibiotic, anti-inflammatory and mydriatic drops.

Discharge advice

The patient will go home about 3–4 days after surgery. Early follow-up at weekly to fortnightly intervals is essential because of the risk of graft rejection. If the patient suffers from unusual pain, increasing ocular discomfort, red eye, sensitivity to light, watering or decreased vision, she must seek medical attention urgently. The risk of rejection is highest in the early months but continues at a low level for years. These patients take steroid drops long term, or indefinitely if rejection has already occurred.

The sutures will remain in place for approximately 6 months, depending on how healing progresses. Vision will be assessed at a later date, when the condition has settled. The patient may

Rejection

Corneal graft rejection (Frith *et al.*, 1994) may cause:

- aching pain;
- photophobia;
- reduced vision.

be impatient while waiting, imagining that the graft has been a failure.

The patient must avoid rubbing or wiping the eye, heavy lifting and driving. The surgeon will advise on resumption of driving (not for at least 2 weeks) and return to school, college or work (usually at about 6 weeks). Hobbies and sports need to be discussed. Weightlifting or contact sports should be avoided as they lead to raised intraocular pressure, thus increasing the strain on the sutures. Constipation must for the same reason be avoided.

The patient will be followed up regularly for 12–18 months to assess the progress of the graft accurately. Investigations and tests will be performed on each visit.

Complications

Graft rejection or graft failure may occur. The signs of rejection are explained at each appointment. Should problems arise, patients are advised to telephone their ward or attend an ophthalmic A&E department.

Trauma

Many eye injuries can be caused by using high-speed tools or chemical substances without adequate eye protection, by direct contact with a squash or golf ball, which fits neatly into an eye socket, or by a boxing glove creating damaging pressure changes. In serious physical trauma to the eye, the iris may be ruptured, the lens dislocated and the retina bruised or torn, and there may be intra-ocular haemorrhage or traumatic glaucoma.

The patient should take things easy for about 2 weeks but may need from 6 weeks to 3 months for full recovery.

An apparently trivial injury to the eye can cause more serious trouble years later, so the patient should be followed up.

Enucleation

This is removal of an eye that is blind, painful, damaged or posing a threat to the patient's life, health or sight in the other eye.

One reason is retinoblastoma, a malignant tumour of the retina affecting young children, mostly in the first 3 years of life. It is usually diagnosed when large enough to cause a white pupil (Perry and Tullo, 1995).

Another cause is sympathetic ophthalmitis – inflammation of one eye secondary to disease or injury of the other, usually occurring more than 2 weeks after injury. For this reason, severely damaged eyes with no hope of useful vision should be removed within 10–12 days of injury (Perry and Tullo, 1995).

Pre-operative care

The patient will need psychological support to cope with the anticipated drastic change in her body image, perhaps being distressed and depressed about the change in her appearance

(Perry and Tullo, 1995). She will need to grieve and express her anger, and may wish to talk to a person who has already experienced this operation. Failing that, a tape-recording of what to expect could be borrowed.

Patient comment

'It feels so very final.'

It can be helpful for the ocular prosthetist to visit to offer practical support, discussion of fears and information on how soon the artificial eye can be fitted. The cosmetic results are likely to be fairly pleasing, but patients may expect to have gaping holes where their eyes have been (Beed, 1991).

The patient may be frightened of the wrong eye being removed. Constant reassurance, coupled with careful checking, is needed, and the affected side must be clearly marked with indelible pen by the surgeon. At all stages, the information in the notes is cross-checked with the patient and the skin marking.

Type of operation

A general anaesthetic is needed as the extraocular muscles and optic nerve are cut. In some cases, a plastic implant, which restores some volume to the orbit, is stitched to the muscles within the orbit, and conjunctiva is sutured over it. The coral-derived hydroxyapatite sphere is a popular, integrated orbital implant, designed to provide improved motility of the ocular prosthesis. Without an implant, the conjunctiva is stitched together and forms a smooth pink healthy pouch or socket resembling the inside of the mouth (Frith et al., 1994).

Post-operative care

The patient will return from theatre with an eyepad and possibly a bandage over the affected eye. She will be nursed on the affected side to maximize pressure on the dressing. The eye will look like a black eye immediately post-operatively, the wound not being obvious.

The pad and socket will be observed for haemorrhage or discharge every half hour during the first 4–6 post-operative hours and at each dressing. Observed clots must not be dislodged, in case of further bleeding. Excess or fresh bleeding or discharge is reported to medical staff. The original dressing is not removed, but extra firm padding and bandaging is applied over the top.

As there is a potential risk of infection in the socket:

- Aseptic technique is used.
- Sterile saline is used to bathe the socket.
- Antibiotic drops/ointment may be prescribed.
- The patient is educated to avoid touching or rubbing her lids, particularly with dirty hands or tissues (Perry and Tullo, 1995).
- The patient is taught to wash her hands prior to dealing with the affected socket.

Steroid drops are usually prescribed for their anti-inflammatory properties.

Patients will wear dark glasses for psychological comfort. Safety glasses may be recommended particularly to people under 21 years old, to protect the remaining eye once home (Drack et al., 1994).

The first prothesis or shell is fitted 2–3 days post-operatively, once any swelling around the socket has settled. The moulded shell, rather like a large, thick, hard contact lens, is placed behind the lids to help maintain normal contour (Frith et al., 1994). This initial fitting is often carried out by the ophthalmic nurse (Perry and Tullo, 1995). The patient will be taught how to insert, remove and clean the shell before she is allowed home and must be as competent as possible as shell-care must be performed daily to avoid infection. Further community or hospital staff support may be needed before the patient becomes proficient.

The patient will be discharged home as soon as possible following enucleation to enable her to resume her life with minimal disruption. Continuing psychological support will be needed to cope with the changed body image and altered vision. A young child may be more adaptable than an adult, who may need advice concerning employment if the loss of an eye affects her work. Driving should be avoided, as after any operation, and vision should be checked with respect to safety before driving is resumed. It will take a while to adjust to unilateral vision, although this is, of itself, no bar to driving.

Discharge advice

The parents of a child or the partner of an adult (as well as the patient herself if she is capable) will be taught how to care for the socket and to insert and remove the prothesis with confidence unsupervised before she goes home.

To insert the shell or prosthesis:

- The patient must have her head well supported and be lying flat or sitting up.
- Hands should be freshly washed before cleaning the socket and shell with saline.
- The patient looks upwards.
- The upper lid is lifted and the shell gently pushed up into the socket.
- The lower lid should blink into position over the lower edge of the shell.
- Check for comfort and wash the hands.

To remove the shell or prosthesis (Perry and Tullo, 1995):

- An extractor is used.
- The tip of the extractor is touched onto the shell.
- The lower lid is pushed down with the extractor until it is underneath the edge of the shell, the handle being brought down until it is nearly flat against the cheek.
- The patient looks upwards and then downwards; the shell should come out normally.

Written instructions should be provided, in large print if necessary. The ward telephone number should also be included. Swimming is not advised for a few weeks, and patients may prefer not to return to work until they have been fitted with an artificial eye, at approximately 6 weeks; the time of return will depend on the patient's acceptance of her changed body image.

At about 4 weeks post-operatively, follow-up appointments with the ocular prosthetist will be made for fitting an artificial eye, once the patient and/or her carers are confident with the shell and there is no discomfort or infection. The artificial eye is similar to the glass shell, made of hard plastic, with iris detail hand-painted onto it to match the other eye (Frith *et al.*, 1994). One naval patient had a series of artificial eyes made with progressive degrees of bloodshot effect to match his 'good' eye on a heavy evening out. The final eye had a Union Jack painted where the iris usually was.

The patient who has received a natural coral implant, which allows blood vessels to grow through it, will have the artificial eye secured at about 6 weeks following surgery by a pin drilled into the coral. This gives a good cosmetic effect and a more permanent feeling of a secure prosthesis.

Complications

Infection or discomfort of the socket may occur if it is not kept sufficiently clean. The patient may be encouraged to regard the prosthesis rather like dentures, a removing and cleaning them at the same time. If a well-fitting artificial eye is achieved, and the patient's other eye is healthy, no ophthalmic follow-up is required (Frith *et al.*, 1994).

Retinoblastoma may be bilateral, so close monitoring of the other eye will be arranged. Other children in the family will have to be screened, and genetic counselling will be necessary. The local address of self-help groups and clubs can be obtained from the unit (Perry and Tullo, 1995).

The coral-derived implant may be associated with:

- conjunctival thinning, which is managed by observation and prosthesis adjustment;
- conjunctival erosion, treated by combinations of scleral patch graft, conjunctival flap and prosthesis adjustment;
- orbital infection, which will respond to intravenous antibiotics (Shields *et al.*, 1994).

Summary

1 The eye is delicate and patients fear blindness, so a gentle, informative approach is essential.

2 The shortness of the patient's stay means that patient teaching, supported by large-print or taped material, is part of all nursing care.

3 Patient co-operation is vital, particularly during local anaesthesia, so psychological, ophthalmic and systemic assessment and preparation must take place.

4 Post-operatively, anything that 'makes the eyes bulge', i.e. raises intra-ocular pressure, must be avoided.

5 Patients must not drive after eye surgery until given formal clearance.

CASE HISTORY

Mrs Lorenz, aged 82, has bilateral cataracts and lives with her daughter. She is admitted as a day case for her first cataract extraction. What advice, support and teaching will she and her daughter need before she may safely be discharged home?

Review Questions

1 How would you recognize a detached retina?

2 Why should patients be discouraged from carrying heavy weights post-operatively?

3 Why is only one eyedrop instilled at a time?

4 What are the signs of rejection of a corneal graft?

5 Why are eyedrops placed in the centre of the conjunctival sac, and why can the patient taste the drops?

ACKNOWLEDGEMENTS

With many thanks to Joy Sheppard for rigorous and untiring advice, and Barbara Marjoram for reviews.

References

Beed, P. Losing her eyes. *Nursing Times* **87**(47), 26–8

Busin M. Meller, D., Cusumano, A and Spitznas, M. 1994 [Chronic low grade endophthalmitis. A growing indication for explantation of intraocular lens.] *Ophthalmoge* **91**(4), 473–8.

Crick, E. 1991 Day case cataract surgery – the patient's choice. *British Journal of Theatre Nursing* **1**(Jul), 10–12.

Curtis, N. 1995: ACTing for change. *Nursing Standard* **9**(37), 18–20.

Dobson, F. 1991 Perioperative care of the visually impaired. *British Journal of Theatre Nursing* **1**(4), 8–9.

Drack, A., Kutsche, P.J., Stair, S and Scott W.E. 1994 Compliance with safety glasses wear in monocular children. *Journal of Ophthalmic Nursing and Technology* **13**(2), 77–82.

Fischel, J.D and Lipton, J.R. 1996 Cataract surgery and recent advances: a review. *Nursing Standard* **10**(41), 39–43.

Frith, P., Gray, R., MacLennan, S and Ambler, P. 1994. *The eye in clinical practice.* Oxford: Blackwell Scientific.

Kammann, J., Dornbach G., Linares, I. and Schuttrumpf, R. 1994 [Lens implantation in patients treated with anticoagulants.] *Ophthalmologe* **91**(4), 486–9.

Kelly, J. 1994 Nursing intervention in the treatment of cataracts. *British Journal of Nursing* **3**(12), 602–6.

Macleod, J. 1994 Pre-admission clinics for corneal graft patients. *Nursing Times* **90**(26), 35–6.

Mangione C.M., Phillips, R.S., Lawrence, M.G., Seddon, J.M., Orav, E.J. and Goldman, L. 1994 Improved visual function and attenuation of declines in health-related quality of life after cataract extraction. *Archives of Ophthalmology* **112**(11), 1419–25.

Perry, J.P. and Tullo, A.B. 1995 *Care of the ophthalmic patient: a guide for nurses and health professionals,* 2nd edn. London: Chapman & Hall.

Ralph, J., Otero, C. and Hammond, B. 1995 Operation cataract. *Nursing Standard* **9**(34), 18–20.

Sanders, R., Bennett, N. and Docherty, P. 1994 Evaluating home visits in cataract day surgery. *Nursing Times* **90**(1), 11.

Shields, C.L., Shields, J.A., De Potter, P. and Singh, A.D. 1994 Problems with the hydroxyapatite orbital implant: experience with 250 consecutive cases. *British Journal of Ophthalmology* **78**(9), 702–6.

Stollery, R. 1987 *Ophthalmic nursing.* Oxford: Blackwell Scientific.

Wells, H. 1993 Pre-operative ophthalmic procedures: ritualistic or necessary? *British Journal of Nursing* **2**(15), 755–62.

Wicker, P. 1994 Local anaesthesia in the operating theatre. *Nursing Times* **90**(46), 34–5.

Further reading

Phillips, C. 1991 An eye-opening experience. *British Journal of Theatre Nursing* **1**(Jul), 14–15.

Ear, nose and throat nursing

5

Barbara Richards, Helen Fawcett-Adamson and
Marva D.F. Brown

Introduction

Otorhinolaryngology is the study of the ear and its function in hearing and balance, including conditions that affect the nose and sinuses, the throat and speech; it also encompasses head and neck surgery. Most of the work is elective, although there are a number of emergency situations, including acute airway obstruction, sudden total deafness, epistaxis and peritonsillar abscess (quinsy).

Surgery ranges from minor procedures such as insertion of a small tube (grommet) into the tympanic membrane to treat deafness, to major ear operations and head and neck surgery. Some major surgery can be disfiguring.

For this reason, nurses working within this specialty need to adopt a positive yet sensitive approach to the care of patients and their families.

The hearing-impaired patient

Difficulty with hearing and communication can cause confusion and embarrassment. When talking to a hearing impaired person, it is essential to speak clearly and slowly without shouting, which can cause discomfort, particularly if a hearing aid is worn. Many people with hearing loss are helped by a hearing aid and sometimes lip reading. Severe congenital deafness may be managed by sign language and mouthing words. Some severely deaf people have a speech impairment as they have never heard speech. It may be necessary to write information down for a patient with acquired severe deafness, if understanding cannot be achieved in any other way.

Environmental aids, such as flashing lights connected to the telephone or door-bell, can be provided in the home. There are telephones specifically adapted for use by persons with a hearing aid. The telephone system Minicom can be used by the severely and totally deaf.

People living on their own may benefit from having a 'hearing dog for the deaf'. These have proved to be great companions and invaluable in emergencies, such as fires, when they have been known to lead their owners out safely.

STUDENT ACTIVITY

Do your usual grocery shop using heavy duty earplugs.

Hearing aids

Every hearing aid consists of a microphone that picks up sound, an amplifier to increase the sound and an earphone to deliver this to the ear through a mould fitting the contours of the patient's ear. Most hearing aids are worn behind the ear, although more sophisticated ones are now available which fit the ear canal itself.

Some elderly people with hearing impairment and limited manual dexterity gain more benefit from a body-worn aid that clips onto a lapel or can be placed in a pocket or around the neck. Malfunction of hearing aids often results from impaction of ear wax in the ear mould or from batteries needing to be changed. Elderly patients with both poor sight and poor manual dexterity may require assistance in rectifying these problems. Technical advances mean that the more sophisticated types of hearing aid (bone-anchored hearing aids implanted over the mastoid area during surgery) are now available.

Communal areas, such as lounges, outpatient waiting areas and wards, which are shared by both the hearing and the hearing impaired, should have a loop system allowing the volume on radios and televisions to be turned down.

Moving texts – lighted signs giving continuous information that can be quickly updated – can be very helpful.

Patients with hearing aids should be encouraged to use them. Poor mould fittings and faulty connections should be dealt with promptly. Inability to hear can lead to feelings of isolation, vulnerability and loneliness, particularly in an unfamiliar environment.

Sleep–wake disorders

The study and treatment of obstructive sleep apnoea has become an extension of the specialty of ENT.

The patient often snores, is restless while sleeping, has poor memory and concentration, and shows irritability and personality changes that can lead to relationship problems. Employment often suffers, sometimes resulting in job loss. Drivers may fall asleep at the wheel, with serious implications.

These patients should be seen, studied and treated by a dedicated team of specialists. The patient's partner should be present at the consultation. Investigation is in designated sleep laboratories fitted with infra-red video equipment to record full polysomnography. Patients should be followed up with a multidisciplinary consultation in which future management and planned treatment are discussed and agreed.

- Sleep apnoea is cessation of airflow
- Some patients' blood oxygen level falls below 80%
- The condition can be life-threatening
- CPAP can be employed as short-or long-term medical treatment

Treatment includes:

- continuous positive airway pressure (CPAP)
- sleep nasendoscopy study;
- uvulopalatopharyngoplasty (UVPP);
- tracheostomy.

CPAP

The CPAP machine supplies positive airway pressure via the nose and is used at night to maintain the opening in the upper airway.

SLEEP NASENDOSCOPY

The patient is admitted as a day case and studied under sedation. During sleep, the airway is visualized using the rhinopharyngolaryngoscope. The doctor is then able to pinpoint the exact site of obstruction (Camillieri *et al.*, 1995).

UVPP

This is the surgical removal of extra tissue in the soft palate, the lateral pharynx being trimmed and tightened. If appropriate, it can be performed by laser surgery, which is a less painful procedure (Whinney *et al.*, 1995) but sometimes leaves patients feeling as though 'they have tissue paper in the throat because it is so dry'.

Day surgery

The past 15 years have seen a surge of new techniques and anaesthesia, with better tolerance and fewer side-effects, resulting in an increase of the range of operations suitable for day case surgery. In ENT, the laser has revolutionized the surgeon's work. However, not all patients are suitable for day surgery and not all types of surgery are appropriate, so definitive criteria are usually drawn up (Morallee and Murray, 1995).

- Following general anaesthetic or sedation, driving or operating machinery must be avoided for 48 hours
- Patients need good post-operative instructions, and the GP must be aware that the procedure has taken place
- The GP must take responsibility for aftercare, and the community health-care team should provide back-up if necessary
- Travelling time (from hospital to home) is a major consideration

Endoscopy

Endoscopy allows direct examination of the pharynx, larynx, trachea and oesophagus. In many specialist centres, it is now possible to examine the sinuses endoscopically.

Advanced technology has produced a rigid fibrescope (Hopkins' rods) that uses light fibres to give a clear view of the antrum and sinuses following local application of an anaesthetic spray. The flexible fibreoptic endoscope permits examination of the pharynx, larynx and trachea via the nasal passageway, with good patient compliance, in an outpatient setting (Spraggs and Harries, 1995). This has greatly reduced the number of inpatient procedures.

Direct laryngoscopy – passage of the laryngoscope over the epiglottis to examine the larynx – is the most common of such procedures.

Bronchoscopy involves passing the bronchoscope through the vocal cords, into the trachea and then into each main bronchus.

Oesophagoscopy permits visualization of the oesophagus and sometimes the upper part of the stomach.

Pre-operative care

Patients requiring endoscopic procedures may be admitted to hospital on the day of operation or the previous day and are fasted for 6 hours beforehand.

The procedure

The endoscope is introduced into the oral cavity and guided down to the area to be examined; a small tissue sample may then be obtained using biopsy forceps.

Post-operative care

Patients sometimes experience throat discomfort caused by passage of the endoscope. Mild analgesics, such as soluble paracetamol, can be administered as prescribed. Caution is necessary if local anaesthetic has been used as this can impair the gag reflex and result in aspiration of fluids taken too soon. Blood pressure, temperature and pulse should be recorded for the first few hours after endoscopy. Any complaints of pain or temperature elevation should be reported to the doctor immediately, since one complication of this procedure is a tear in the tissue of the neck.

Patients can normally eat and drink as soon as they feel able, although the surgeon sometimes prohibits this until the next day. In such cases, intravenous fluids provide hydration.

Voice rest is sometimes advocated for 24–48 hours after direct laryngoscopy.

Discharge advice

Patients normally go home on the day of the operation or the following day, and an outpatient appointment is required 1 or 2 weeks later. Histology will be available by this time, and a decision can be taken on any further treatment required.

Normal work can usually be resumed immediately, although the surgeon may advise against this until after the outpatient appointment.

Lasers

The use of lasers is a well-established technique becoming increasingly common in the ENT department. Laser stands for Light Amplification by Stimulated Emission of Radiation. A beam the thickness of a human hair delivers a controlled high-precision cutting action of great intensity, which creates a bloodless field. This is vital when working in confined spaces such as the larynx. As

a result of this advance, patients with recurrent papillomata of the larynx now need fewer hospital admissions and anaesthetics. Lasers can be used to remove small cancerous nodules from the mouth or larynx. The appearance following laser surgery is that of a small crater.

The term 'laser' may be quite frightening to the patient, so reassurance should be given by explaining that it is merely a fine beam that can be directed to the area concerned.

Pre-operative care

The procedure is more commonly performed as a day case, depending on the investigations required.

The procedure

Following general anaesthesia, a special flexible or PVC tube is introduced into the respiratory tract, and air is administered. This minimizes the possible risk of ignition of gases in the respiratory tract owing to the beam intensity and protects the surrounding area. The laser is directed very accurately at the area to be treated.

Post-operative care

There is little operative swelling, so pain should be minimal. Mild analgesics may be required if there is throat discomfort caused by the anaesthetic tube. Eating and drinking may be resumed as soon as the patient is fully awake. Patients may go home on the day of operation if the surgeon allows.

Discharge advice

Voice rest may be advised for a few days if laser treatment has been given to the larynx. This helps to minimize damage to the vocal cords. An outpatient appointment is usually planned for 2–8 weeks later.

The ear

- Hearing and balance are affected by damage or obstruction to the outer, middle and inner ear

The function of the outer and middle ear is to transmit sound waves to the inner ear, where they are converted to nerve impulses and sent to the brain for interpretation. The sound waves hit the tympanic membrane and ossicles – the malleus, incus and stapes within the middle ear (Fig. 5.1) – which, by their movement, carry the sound to the inner ear. Interruption of or blockage to this passage of sound waves will cause deafness. The eustachian tube leads from the middle ear to the nasopharynx. Blockage of this can affect hearing by altering the pressure in the middle ear and causing fluid accumulation, which is why people with colds often complain of deafness.

Myringotomy and grommet insertion

Myringotomy is a small surgical incision made in the tympanic membrane (Fig. 5.2). A small tube inserted into this incision – a grommet – ventilates the middle ear and prevents pressure and fluid accumulation (Dingle et al., 1995).

Grommets normally fall out 6–18 months after insertion. The procedure is most commonly undertaken in childhood, parents usually having noticed that the child is having difficulty hearing or the problem having been picked up by school screening. In adults, it is undertaken for malfunction of the eustachian tube as a result of malignancy or for functional reasons.

- Poor hearing is detrimental to child development
- Effective screening will facilitate the early diagnosis and treatment of hearing problems

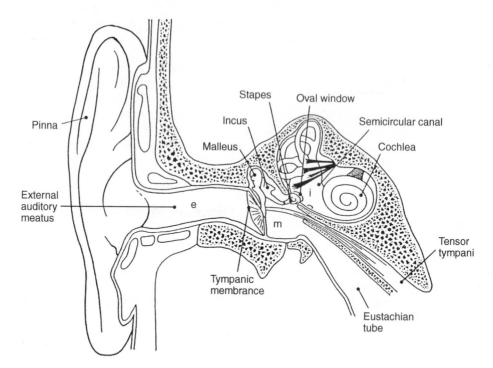

Figure 5.1 The middle ear

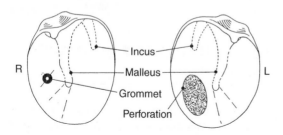

Figure 5.2 The tympanic membrane (eardrum)

PRE-OPERATIVE CARE

The operation is performed under general anaesthetic as a day case. Since it is mainly children who require the procedure, parents should, whenever possible, be encouraged to be present beforehand. The level of the child's hearing is assessed pre-operatively by undertaking an audiogram and an ear pressure (impedance) test. This painless procedure is required as a baseline for comparison with any subsequent post-operative audiograms.

The child is fasted for 6 hours before operation. It is usually cancelled if the child has a cold or a sore throat. A mild oral premedication syrup is given 2 hours pre-operatively to induce sleepiness.

POST-OPERATIVE CARE

After the anaesthetic, the child is encouraged to lie in a semiprone position. There may be clear or slightly bloodstained discharge from the ear; this is normal and parents should be forewarned. Eating and drinking can resume when the child is fully awake. Reports of pain after this procedure are rare, and there is usually an immediate improvement in hearing.

DISCHARGE ADVICE

Children can return to school after 1 week, and an outpatient appointment is made for 6 weeks post-surgery. Parents are advised to contact the hospital or their GP if severe earache occurs, as this abnormal finding may indicate infection.

Ears should be kept dry. Some surgeons allow swimming but not diving, swimming underwater or getting bath water in the ears. A little petroleum jelly on cotton wool will keep ears dry during hair washing and bathing but must be removed afterwards. Parents should be advised not to attempt to clean the ears with cotton buds.

It is helpful if the parents are shown a grommet so that they know what to look for should one fall out prematurely, which occasionally happens. It may need to be reinserted.

Mastoidectomy

Mastoidectomy is the surgical removal of infected or diseased tissue from the mastoid cavity, which may have caused a perforation of the eardrum. It is often associated with an expanding keratin-containing epithelial cyst, a cholesteatoma, which, if not removed, can cause destruction of bone and other structures surrounding the mastoid cavity. Untreated infection can erode bone and lead to nerve damage or meningitis. The operation is performed under general anaesthetic and may be a simple or cortical, modified radical or radical procedure, depending on the extent of disease. The operation will not usually improve the patient's hearing in that ear.

PRE-OPERATIVE CARE

The patient is admitted the day before surgery, and mastoid X-rays and hearing tests are undertaken. A small area behind the ear is sometimes shaved in theatre immediately prior to surgery. The patient should be informed that there will be a few post-auricular sutures and, in some cases, a small drain. There is a minimal risk of damage to the facial nerve, but this should be explained by the doctor obtaining consent. Some patients express anxiety about packs or dressings. Reassurance can be given, explaining that analgesics will be given for discomfort.

THE OPERATION

The operation is performed under a general anaesthetic using hypotensive anaesthesia to minimize bleeding during surgery. The surgeon cleans the ear and makes a pre- or post-auricular incision depending on the type of mastoidectomy required. All infected tissue and bone are then removed, leaving a smooth clean cavity. An antiseptic pack such as bismuth iodoform paraffin paste (BIPP) is placed in the ear cavity, and the wound is sutured. A small drainage tube may be placed at the lower part of the wound to allow drainage of blood and thus reduce the risk of infection. A pressure dressing is applied over the wound to prevent haematoma formation. The operation lasts for 1–2 hours.

POST-OPERATIVE CARE

The patient can be positioned in the most comfortable way but should avoid lying on the operated side. Damage to the facial nerve which passes close to the mastoid process and through the middle ear, is a rare complication. It causes weakness on one side of the face, which can be detected by asking the patient to show his teeth or smile. Blood pressure, pulse and facial nerve recordings should be made regularly for 4–6 hours after surgery.

The patient should be advised not to make sudden head movements as this may result in dizziness or vomiting; an anti-emetic should be given to alleviate these symptoms. The patient will often experience moderate pain around the operated ear and side of the head and will require regular analgesia. After 4 hours, eating and drinking may be resumed if there is no sickness.

Mobilization begins the day after surgery. The dressing and drain are removed 1–2 days post-surgery. The patient should initially be helped to get out of bed in case there is dizziness or unsteadiness. Owing to the packing in the ear, temporary deafness may be a problem. The patient sometimes complains of a feeling of 'squelching and muzziness in the ear'. It is important to ensure the patient understands what they are told. The patient is normally allowed home 1–3 days after operation.

DISCHARGE ADVICE

Sutures will be removed after 1 week by the patient's GP or clinic nurse. The patient is advised to keep the ear dry, and a small plug of cotton wool, which can be changed if it becomes soiled, is inserted into the ear canal. Care must be taken not to disturb the underlying pack, which is removed by the surgeon in the OPD 2–3 weeks later. The patient should be advised that a small amount of leakage into the ear canal is normal, but if this becomes excessive or smells offensive, or if there is pain, the GP or hospital staff should be contacted. The patient can return to work after 10 days.

- Middle ear disease can cause serious complications if left untreated
- Most mastoidectomy procedures will remove disease but not improve hearing

Myringoplasty

This operation repairs a perforation of the tympanic membrane using a small graft, and is performed under general anaesthetic.

PRE-OPERATIVE CARE

The patient is admitted to hospital the day before operation. An audiogram is required. The operation is always cancelled if the patient has had a recent cold or infection, because the graft is then more likely to become displaced.

THE OPERATION

Following induction of general anaesthesia, the patient is placed in a semiprone position with the affected ear uppermost. The surgeon cleans the ear and makes a pre-auricular incision; then, with the aid of a microscope, she places the graft over the hole in the tympanic membrane. This graft is usually harvested from the temporal region of the patient's affected ear. A small pack is placed in the ear to keep the graft in place, and a pressure dressing may be applied.

POST-OPERATIVE CARE

Post-operative care is as for mastoidectomy. The patient should be reminded to avoid 'fierce' nose blowing, and the mouth should be kept open during sneezing. This will reduce pressure in the middle ear and thus prevent graft displacement. The patient is usually allowed home 1–2 days after the operation.

DISCHARGE ADVICE

This is as for mastoidectomy. The surgeon will remove the ear pack in the OPD 1–2 weeks after discharge. Advice is given to avoid situations causing pressure changes in the middle ear, for example flying, for at least 2 weeks post-operation. The patient can be advised to return to work after the first outpatient appointment.

- A perforated tympanic membrane may compromise hearing and result in infection

Stapedectomy

The stapes is the third ossicle in the middle ear. It is stirrup shaped and rests against the oval window of the inner ear. Sound waves cause the ossicles to vibrate, and, by their tapping the oval window, the sound waves are transmitted to the inner ear and then via the auditory nerve to the brain. If the stapes becomes fixed to the oval window, no transmission occurs, resulting in deafness. Stapedectomy is the removal of the stapes and its replacement with a prosthesis – a plug resting against the oval window and hooked over the incus.

PRE-OPERATIVE CARE

The patient is admitted to hospital the day before operation so that an audiogram and impedance test can be carried out. One major complication is that complete deafness in the ear can occur if the operation is unsuccessful; this will be explained beforehand by the doctor.

THE OPERATION

Once anaesthetized, the patient is placed in a semiprone position, and the surgeon cleans the ear. A microscope is used during the procedure, which involves lifting the eardrum and looking into the middle ear. The stapes is partly removed, and the surgeon then joins the incus bone to the stapes using a tiny connection, usually made of teflon or wire. A small pack is sometimes placed in the ear canal. The operation takes 1–2 hours.

POST-OPERATIVE CARE

This is as for mastoidectomy. The patient is normally allowed home 1–3 days post-operatively if there is no persistent dizziness.

DISCHARGE ADVICE

Discharge advice is also as for mastoidectomy. Strenous exercise, heavy lifting and straining

must be avoided before the OPD appointment. Packing in the ear will be removed by the surgeon 1–2 weeks post-operation. There is often a significant improvement in hearing after surgery, which will be further improved following removal of the ear packing.

The patient should be asked to contact the hospital if vomiting or dizziness occurs as it may indicate an inner ear infection. Patients may return to work after the first outpatient appointment.

- Ossicular damage significantly affects sound transmission and may affect balance if the inner ear becomes involved

The nose

- Nasal blockage affects breathing and appetite, and may result in frequent headaches, snoring and reduction in the ability to smell
- Owing to the vascularity of the nose, any bleeding should be treated promptly as it can be fatal

The nose and nasal passages, the first part of the respiratory tract, warm, moisten and filter the air before it passes into the lungs. The sinuses (Fig. 5.3) are air-filled cavities lined with mucous membrane, lying in the front of the skull, which open into the nasal passages. Olfactory nerves in the nasal mucosa enable us to detect smells. Deviation of the nasal septum or blockage within the nasal cavity will result in difficulty in breathing and loss or reduction in the ability to smell.

Nasal polypectomy

Nasal polyps, grape-like swellings hanging in the nasal fossa, are caused by local oedema of the nasal mucosa. They are usually bilateral and associated with allergies. When polyps occur singly, they are often malignant. Polyps can be removed

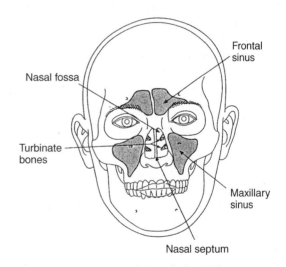

Figure 5.3 The nasal cavity and sinuses

under general or local anaesthetic in a procedure lasting about 20 minutes. All polyps are sent for histology.

PRE-OPERATIVE CARE

The patient is admitted to hospital either the day before or on the day of the operation. Blood tests,

X-rays and skin tests (to indicate allergies; Scadding, 1995) are usually carried out prior to surgery. The admitting nurse should check whether the patient is using nasal sprays or taking medication, for example steroids. The patient is also advised that packs may be in place post-operatively.

THE OPERATION

Once the patient, or the area, is fully anaesthetized, the polyps are snared off. To ensure that no bleeding occurs, nasal packs may be inserted into the nasal passages. These are often made of ribbon gauze and may be impregnated with an antiseptic such as BIPP.

POST-OPERATIVE CARE

The patient should be nursed in the most comfortable position, but nasal congestion is reduced and breathing is easier in an upright position. Watering of the eyes occurs owing to the packs pressing on and blocking the nasolacrimal (tear) ducts. Some patients experience headache and some discomfort, often saying, 'I can't breathe'. Analgesics and an ice pack applied to the forehead help to relieve this. Some blood may ooze through the pack, in which case a small pad is placed under the nose and changed as necessary. Dryness from mouth breathing can cause discomfort, mouthwashes helping to maintain moistness and freshness. Any nasal packs are removed 6–24 hours after operation by a nurse or the surgeon. The patient should be encouraged to remain on his bed for an hour afterwards. Very hot drinks should be avoided for at least 2 hours as vasodilatation may cause the nose to bleed. If BIPP packing is used, patients often liken its removal to the Indian rope trick (as much as 2 m can be used).

DISCHARGE ADVICE

The patient should be able to go home later that day or the next. There may be some swelling, nasal discharge, nasal obstruction and reduction in sense of smell for about 2 weeks post-operatively. A nasal spray or inhaler is sometimes prescribed to relieve this (El-Nagger et al., 1995). Alcohol should be avoided in the first week as it will cause vasodilatation.

Patients are usually advised to take a week off work, and an outpatient appointment is given for 6 weeks post-discharge. Patients with a unilateral polyp may be seen sooner than this so that further treatment can be planned. The patient should be advised to contact his GP or the hospital staff if persistent headache or nasal discharge occurs. Polyps tend to recur.

STUDENT ACTIVITY

Eat a meal with nose plugs in place. How does it affect your sense of taste and appetite?

Submucous resection

The septum is the cartilaginous partition between the nostrils; it may become damaged after trauma. Submucous resection involves lifting the mucous membrane, trimming the cartilage and replacing the mucous membrane. Splints are sometimes inserted into the nose to prevent adhesions, and nasal packs are inserted to prevent bleeding.

PRE- AND POST-OPERATIVE CARE

These are as for nasal polypectomy. Nasal packs are removed the day after operation. The splints are removed by the surgeon 1 week post-operatively. Antibiotics are often prescribed while the splints are in the nose. Nasal obstruction may continue for 3–4 weeks. The patient can return to work 2 weeks after the operation.

Sinus washout

This procedure involves introducing water into the maxillary sinuses to remove any infected material. It can be done under local or general anaesthetic, as a day case or as an outpatient procedure. The nurse should remain with the patient throughout as it may be unpleasant. Patients are often aware of 'pressure as the trocar is pushed in and the horrible noise of the bone cracking'. Sinus X-rays will be performed before the washout. When the procedure is carried out under local anaesthetic, cocaine paste or solution on small wires is used to numb the lining of the nose. The nurse should be aware that a reaction to cocaine may occur and should be dealt with promptly by immediate removal of the cocaine wires.

Cocaine reaction

- Raised blood pressure
- Tachycardia
- Restlessness
- Pallor and shock
- Convulsions in extreme cases
- If a reaction is noted, remove the cocaine wires immediately and contact a doctor

When the patient is anaesthetized, a small trocar and cannula are inserted into the maxillary sinus via the nose, a cracking sound being heard as the cannula enters the sinuses. The sinus is then washed out with a warmed saline solution. A small pack may be inserted.

DISCHARGE ADVICE

The patient can be allowed home in the evening after removal of the pack if no bleeding occurs, and is seen in the OPD by the surgeon after 4–6 weeks. Some initial swelling may occur, which may cause obstruction of the nose and discomfort. The patient can return to work when he feels fit.

The throat

Tonsillectomy

Tonsillectomy is removal of the tonsils, which are situated on each side at the back of the mouth and oropharynx. They are vascular pads of lymphoid tissue that help to 'fight' infection. Enlargement of the tonsils occurs from repeated infection and causes halitosis and difficulty in breathing and swallowing. Recurrent tonsillitis leads to absence from school and work, affecting mostly children and young adults (McKenzie, 1986).

PRE-OPERATIVE CARE

The patient may be admitted to hospital on the day of surgery or the previous day. Parents should be encouraged to stay with their child to provide reassurance. Pre-operative blood tests check the haemoglobin level and provide a cross-match sample in case transfusion is required. The operation may be cancelled if a recent cold has occurred or if signs of infection are present as these may increase the risk of post-operative bleeding.

THE OPERATION

The tonsils are dissected out and removed through the mouth. Small bleeding vessels are sealed off with diathermy or sutures that dissolve after a few days. The operation takes about half an hour.

POST-OPERATIVE CARE

The patient should be nursed in a semiprone position, allowing any blood to drain from the mouth and preventing its being swallowed. Observations of blood pressure and pulse are initially recorded half-hourly, then less often as the patient's condition stabilizes, to note any signs of bleeding, indicated by frequent swallowing, bleeding from the mouth and a rise in pulse rate. The doctor must be called if this occurs. Once awake, the patient should regularly be given analgesics in the form of an injection or soluble tablets as the throat will be very painful. Patients often will say 'It is like swallowing razor blades'.

Cold drinks can be offered after 2 hours and eating after 6 hours if there is no nausea or vomiting. Diet should include crisp foods and plenty of fluids to help the flow of saliva, which will keep the tonsil bed clean and encourage healing. Regular analgesia, particularly before mealtimes, is required for the first few days. Patients often complain of earache, which is referred pain from the glossopharyngeal nerve; this is relieved by the analgesia (Toma *et al.*, 1995).

Good mouth care is important to prevent collection of debris on the tonsil beds, which may lead to infection. A mouthwash should thus be encouraged after food and milky drinks. The teeth should be brushed as normal.

DISCHARGE ADVICE

Patients are allowed home 1–2 days after operation and need to have 2 weeks off work or school. They should avoid smoky, crowded places for the first week to decrease the risk of infection. Mouthcare advice should be followed at home. Drinking water or taking a mouthwash after food is important to keep the area clean. Gargles can cause discomfort and are not necessary.

If a temperature or bleeding from the mouth develops, the GP or hospital should be contacted. It will not be necessary for patients to be seen again at the hospital unless they have further problems.

- Post-operative bleeding, particularly in children, can be fatal if not dealt with immediately

- The resumption of a normal diet will aid recovery and help to prevent complications

- Effective analgesia is paramount to aid a swift recovery

Tracheostomy

- Temporary/permanent stoma
- Can speak with the aid of special valves/tubes or by placing a finger over tracheostomy tube

NB *Tracheotomy* is the surgical incision through the skin, muscle and trachea. *Tracheostomy* is the stoma itself.

Adenoidectomy

The adenoids are pads of lymphoid tissue situated on the posterior wall of the nasopharynx. By 14–15 years of age, adenoid tissue usually completely atrophies. In some children, enlarged adenoids can cause nasal obstruction, resulting in mouth breathing and recurrent pharyngeal infections. The eustachian tube becomes blocked, causing glue ear (McKenzie, 1986).

PRE-OPERATIVE CARE

Pre- and post-operative care are as for tonsillectomy, the main post-operative complication being haemorrhage, usually from the nose. The adenoids and tonsils are sometimes removed simultaneously, or a grommet may be inserted when removing the adenoids.

Tracheostomy

A tracheostomy is an artificial opening made into the trachea, which is then kept open by a tracheostomy tube (Figs 5.4 and 5.5). Surgery may be planned or emergency. Patients undergoing oropharyngeal surgery are susceptible to swelling that may result in airway obstruction. In these cases, a planned tracheostomy may be undertaken at the time of surgery.

Where there is airway obstruction resulting in severe breathing difficulties, for example from tumours of the larynx or thyroid, trauma or acute inflammation of trachea or larynx, or congenital abnormality, an emergency tracheostomy may be required. The patient will present with breathlessness, stridor and tachycardia. The procedure

Laryngectomy

- Permanent stoma
- Can speak using oesophageal speech

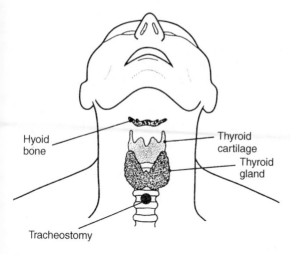

Figure 5.4 Front view of neck and tracheostomy tube

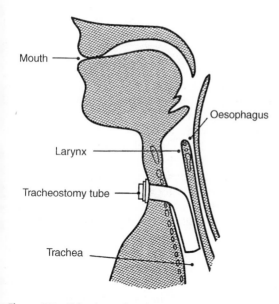

Figure 5.5 Side view of neck and tracheostomy tube

is usually carried out under a general anaesthetic but may be undertaken using local anaesthesia.

PLANNED TRACHEOSTOMY

Pre-operative care

The patient will be admitted 1–2 days before operation for investigations and assessment, including blood tests, chest X-ray and ECG.

Psychological support is very important as the patient is likely to be highly anxious about both surgery and the inability to talk because of the tracheostomy, the escape of air through the tracheostomy preventing air passing through the vocal cords (larynx). Seeing booklets and equipment will help to allay some fears. The patient will need reassurance that he will be able to make his needs understood. Picture cards, pen and paper can be used effectively as communication tools. It is important to involve the family as much as possible.

The physiotherapist and cancer care counsellor (where appropriate) will see the patient pre-operatively as they will be involved in his post-operative management (Royal National Throat, Nose and Ear Hospital, 1993).

The operation

Once the patient has been anaesthetized, the surgeon will make a small transverse incision between the second and third tracheal rings at the front of the neck. A tracheostomy tube, its size determined by the surgeon, is then inserted into the hole and held in place with sutures or tapes tied securely in a knot. A small dressing is applied around the tube to prevent it rubbing or pressing on the skin. The tracheostomy may be performed before or after the main surgical procedure.

Post-operative care

Equipment at bedside

- Suction equipment – suction catheters and gloves
- Tracheal dilators
- A spare tracheostomy tube with introducer
- Humidification equipment
- Oxygen
- Communication materials, e.g. pen, paper and picture board

The patient is returned to the ward or ITU when the anaesthetist is satisfied with his condition. When awake, the patient is nursed in an upright position, well supported with pillows, to allow better chest expansion and make breathing easier. A nurse will remain with him for the first 6–12 hours post-operatively, to monitor him, particularly his airway, closely. Blood pressure, pulse and respiration should be checked 0.5–2 hourly during this time.

The tracheostomy tube often used has a small inflatable cuff at its lower end to prevent blood and secretions passing down the trachea into the lungs. The cuff should be inflated for as short a time as possible, or a low-pressure type of cuffed tube used, as pressure on the tracheal wall can lead to mucosal damage and narrowing of the trachea.

Tracheal suction should be performed when the chest secretions sound wet or 'bubbly'. A sterile suction catheter and gloves must be used and discarded after each insertion. The diameter of the suction catheter should be no more than half the diameter of the inner lumen of the tracheostomy tube to ensure that air can still pass around the catheter during suctioning (Florentini, 1992).

Correct size of suction catheter (Serra *et al.*, 1986)

(Diameter of tracheostomy tube ÷ 2) × 3 = Catheter size

e.g. If tracheostomy tube size is 8:

8 ÷ 2 = 4

4 × 3 = 12 FG catheter

Suctioning

- Suction apparatus for adults is kept at a pressure of 100–120 mmHg to prevent mucosal damage
- Sterile technique is used
- Gloves are used at all times
- A fresh catheter is employed each time
- The catheter internal diameter should be no more than half the diameter of the tracheostomy tube
- The time from insertion to removal of the catheter should not exceed 10–15 seconds
- Allow the patient to rest between each suction application
- Only apply suction on removal of the suction catheter and not on insertion

---

Humidified oxygen as prescribed is administered immediately post-operatively through the tracheostomy stoma. When oxygen is no longer required, the air is humidified using a moistened bib positioned over the stoma, together with regular normal saline nebulizers. This is very important as the air is no longer being humidified through the nose. Dry air will cause the secretions in the lungs to become thick and difficult to remove by either coughing or suctioning, which will in turn lead to obstruction or infection. The physiotherapist will encourage the patient to expand his lungs and cough up any secretions. The patient often states how strange it feels trying to cough and finding the noise coming from an unusual place.

- Effective humidification and tracheal suction is essential to maintain a patent airway
- It is important that the tracheostomy tube does not become displaced or blocked

---

Pain is relieved by regular analgesia, either intramuscularly or intravenously through a syringe pump in the first 24–48 hours. After this, milder analgesia should be sufficient.

If oropharyngeal surgery has been performed, the patient may remain nil by mouth for several days. Hydration will be maintained with an intravenous infusion or feeding through a nasogastric tube, as instructed by the surgeon.

Mobilization should be encouraged from the first post-operative day to prevent complications.

The tracheostomy tube is usually changed after 2–3 days to a non-cuffed tube by an experienced registered nurse or doctor. The new tube should be inserted immediately after the dirty tube is removed. In the first few days, the stoma may close rapidly, blocking the tracheostomy opening. Tracheal dilators to keep the stoma open and suction equipment should be available. Where possible, it is advisable for two people to carry out this procedure.

Tracheostomy tapes and dressings are changed as necessary, taking care to hold the tube in position as this is done. The skin around the tracheostomy tube is cleaned with normal saline every 4–6 hours to prevent collection of secretions and soreness of the skin.

EMERGENCY TRACHEOSTOMY

Pre-operative care

Owing to the acute condition of the patient, there is often little time for preparation, but as much information as possible should be given. The operation is performed as soon as it can be arranged.

The operation

This can be performed under general or local anaesthesia, depending on the patient's condition. It proceeds as for planned tracheostomy. The surgeon will often, following the tracheostomy, examine the patient to assess the cause and extent of the obstruction.

Post-operative care

This is as for planned tracheostomy. Eating and drinking can resume as soon as the patient is awake and able to swallow.

TEMPORARY TRACHEOSTOMY

The tracheostomy tube can be withdrawn when the surgeon has confirmed that the cause of obstruction has been removed. An airtight dressing is applied over the site. The wound will heal naturally over the next 2–3 weeks and rarely needs suturing, leaving only a small scar. Patients will be seen in the OPD 1–2 weeks after discharge. They should be able to return to work and normal activities as soon as they feel well enough.

PERMANENT TRACHEOSTOMY

Where the patient requires a tracheostomy on a long-term or permanent basis, he needs support and teaching to enable him to look after the tube and the equipment he will receive (Mason *et al.*, 1992). The tracheostomy tube may be replaced by a silver or polyurethane type with an inner tube. This is easier as the patient can remove the inner tube for regular cleaning without having to disturb the main one. A valved inner tube or attachment may be used, allowing the patient to speak without using his fingers to block the tube.

The patient and family need to be aware of the importance of humidifying the air breathed by using moistened bibs or specially produced protectors over the tube. This will also prevent dust going into the tube, which would make the patient cough and might cause a chest infection. Patients also need to be taught how to care for equipment, for example suction machines, that they will need to take home.

Before the patient returns home, it is important that his GP and community nurse are informed, so regular visits can be arranged until he feels confident managing alone. The complete tracheostomy tube will need to be changed every 2–4 weeks. This can be done by the community nurse or hospital staff, and when he feels confident, by the patient himself.

Regular outpatient visits will be arranged to monitor progress. The patient can return to work and normal activities when he feels able.

Specific discharge guidelines
- District nurse informed
- Suction equipment
- Dressings, suction catheters
- Spare tracheostomy tubes
- Contact telephone number for ward staff

STUDENT ACTIVITY

Order a drink without using speech.

Total laryngectomy

The larynx is situated between the hypopharynx and the trachea, with the oesophagus posteriorly. One of the functions of it is the production of sound for speech.

Laryngectomy means removal of the larynx; it is usually carried out because of malignancy or, occasionally, severe trauma. Patients will not be able to speak as before but will eventually be taught a new method of communication.

PRE-OPERATIVE CARE

The patient is admitted to hospital 1–2 days pre-operatively for the necessary investigations, such as blood tests, chest X-ray and ECG.

The patient and family will naturally be anxious about the operation and the subsequent loss of voice. They may express concerns about the prognosis, particularly if referral for surgery has been made urgently. Staff should be sensitive to this, and discussion between doctors, nurses, other health-care members, patients and family should be arranged. Key health-care staff such as the speech therapist, physiotherapist and cancer care counsellor will introduce themselves to the patient before the operation. A person who has had a laryngectomy and is leading a full and active life can also be introduced if this is felt to be appropriate.

There must be a full explanation of the permanent changes caused by the operation, for example the hole in the neck, coughing, breathing through the hole, communicating and the equipment that may be used post-operatively. Booklets will enable patients and their family to refer back to written information. Also useful is information about the Laryngectomy Club (NALC) (*see* end of chapter).

THE OPERATION

This is performed under a general anaesthetic and lasts 3–4 hours. The larynx is removed through a transverse neck incision. The top of the trachea is brought out onto the skin and sutured in place, forming a permanent stoma through which the patient breathes. A tube may be inserted into the stoma and secured around the neck with tapes.

Tubes are placed in the neck wound site to allow drainage of blood and serous fluid. A pressure dressing is sometimes applied to the neck to aid drainage of fluid and prevent its collection in the wound.

A fine-bore naso-gastric feeding tube is inserted and secured in place.

POST-OPERATIVE CARE

The immediate post-operative care is as for a tracheostomy. Humidification, initially using humidified oxygen, is extremely important. When the patient no longer requires oxygen, moistened bibs and normal saline nebulizers are used for humidification.

Any pressure dressing used will remain in place for 2–3 days.

Drainage tubes are removed when there is minimal drainage, usually 2–3 days after the operation. If a tube has been used, this is removed completely after 2–3 days, unless swelling around the stoma might cause obstruction to the airway. Patients are often afraid to move or touch their neck in case they cause damage.

Hydration is maintained by intravenous fluids until nasogastric feeding is established. The enteral feeding will continue for 10–14 days to ensure healing of the wounds (Millinson, 1991). A dietitian will assess nutritional requirements and prescribe an appropriate feeding regimen. A barium swallow X-ray may be performed to confirm that the wound has healed prior to re-establishing diet and fluids. The patient will commence with a soft diet and then move to a more substantial one when discomfort subsides.

Sutures in the neck and stoma are removed 7–10 days post-operatively.

Once the tubes and drains have been removed, the patient is taught how to care for the stoma. Patients often feel very depressed when the realization of loss of voice and permanence of stoma becomes apparent.

Understanding, patience and sensitivity from the staff and family help the patient to overcome these feelings. He must be allowed to learn new tasks at his own pace. Patients find it 'very frustrating not being able to communicate by voice'.

The patient is allowed to go home approximately 2 weeks after the operation, when he is confident and competent in managing his care.

DISCHARGE ADVICE

Booklets given on admission will answer many of the patient's queries on returning home. Again, the importance of humidification is stressed, as is avoiding overexertion and crowded places in the first few weeks when he is more susceptible to infection. All operation scars should be protected from the sun with sunblock, scarves, etc.

In special circumstances but not for most patients, swimming is possible. No water must be allowed to go into the stoma, so care must be taken when showering or hair-washing (Keith, 1991).

Arrangements should be made for the GP and/or district nurse to visit regularly for 2–3 weeks to ensure that the patient is coping (Thurston-Hookway and Seddon, 1989).

An outpatient appointment for 2 weeks after discharge and speech therapy appointment, as timed by the surgeon, to commence speech training are arranged. Hospital contact telephone numbers are given to provide advice or support.

Some patients find it helpful to join a support group. There is usually one attached to the hospital, but the National Association of Laryngectomy Clubs will be able to help and advise both patient and family (Stokes, 1983).

- The stoma is permanent
- Humidification and suction are essential
- Patients and relatives will need support to accept the changes to their lives
- Stoma occlusion is life-threatening

Glossectomy

This operation involves removal of all (total) or part (hemi) of the tongue when cancer is present. It is sometimes necessary to resect the mandible and floor of the mouth using skin grafts or flaps to repair the defect (Biller *et al.*, 1983).

PRE-OPERATIVE CARE

The patient is admitted 1–2 days pre-operatively for preparation, for example blood tests and X-rays. He will need a full explantation, support and reassurance from all involved staff. A temporary planned tracheostomy may be required; the patient will need help to understand the reasons for this and what it involves.

Removal of all or part of the tongue creates difficulty in eating, drinking, swallowing and speech, so the patient needs to be aware that recovery will take weeks and possibly months.

The speech therapist, physiotherapist and cancer care counsellor will be actively involved and see the patient before the operation.

THE OPERATION

The operation is performed under a general anaesthetic and lasts 4–6 hours depending on its extent. The tongue is brought forward and secured with a traction suture. The affected part of the tongue is excised by resecting towards the floor of the mouth. Any structures or tissue involved in the tumour are then removed. Reconstruction will be achieved by suturing, skin grafting or skin flaps, depending on the extent of the defect. The type of skin flap used will be decided by the surgeon.

Tubes are inserted into the wound to allow drainage of blood or serous fluid. A nasogastric or gastrostomy feeding tube is inserted, and a pressure dressing may be applied to aid drainage of blood and prevent any haematoma.

POST OPERATIVE CARE

The patient is nursed upright, supported with pillows when awake. A nurse will be in constant attendance for 6–12 hours.

If a tracheostomy has not been performed, the nurse must monitor the airway closely as acute swelling can cause obstruction of the airway, the doctor must then be informed immediately.

Monitoring of airway for:

- respiratory distress
- stridor
- agitation
- dyspnoea

Mouth care is of paramount importance, since the collection of debris and secretions may cause infection and break-down of the mouth wound (Buglass, 1995). It is necessary to liaise with the surgeon about the permitted degree of mouth

Requirements

- Good light
- A gentle procedure
- Swabs/syringe with a quill
- A soft toothbrush for teeth only
- A solution of e.g. warm saline, Chlorhexidine or sodium bicarbonate

care, as some areas, for example, the area of a skin graft, which will be very delicate until healed properly, may need to be avoided.

Hydration is maintained by intravenous infusion until nasogastric or gastrostomy feeding is established. This is required for at least 1 week, but may be necessary for several, depending on the extent of surgery.

The tracheostomy is removed once surgical swelling subsides. The drains are removed after 3–4 days and the sutures after 7–10 days; sutures in the mouth usually dissolve by themselves.

The patient will initially have difficulty in articulating and will need much support. Articulation will improve as the swelling subsides, but there may be long-term speech problems. When swallowing is recommenced, the patient may have some difficulties, and the speech therapist will be able to help in swallowing and speech rehabilitation (LaBlance *et al.*, 1991). Many patients feel embarrassed at eating in company because of dribbling of food and drink. The action taught can be likened to that of a baby bird swallowing.

Most patients are ready for discharge 2–3 weeks after surgery, but some may need to continue enteral feeding support at home. They will need regular attendance by their GP and district nurse over this period.

An outpatient appointment is usually made for 1–2 weeks after discharge. The decision to resume work will be made by the surgeon in consultation with the patient.

Summary

1 The specialty extends from simple tonsillectomy, performed as a day case, to complex surgery for malignancy, requiring an extended stay and prolonged multidisciplinary support.

2 Developments in techniques for sleep apnoea are outlined.

3 Suggestions for communication with the deaf person and the speech-deprived patient are reviewed.

4 Peri-operative care for patients undergoing endoscopy and laser surgery are summarized.

5 A simple outline of the structure and function of the ear, nose and throat is given before the principles of peri-operative care of the most frequently performed operations in each area.

6 Precise advice on discharge is given for each operation described.

CASE HISTORY

Mr Joseph, aged 61, works as an engineering lecturer and is a keen swimmer. He has complained of hoarseness with earache for 3 months. On initial microlaryngoscopy and biopsy, he was found to have carcinoma of the supraglottic region, extending to the vocal cords. He has been admitted for laryngectomy and anticipates loss of speech and change of body image, as well as expecting to lose his job. How will the nurse and multidisciplinary team help Mr Joseph to prepare and come to terms with these major changes in his life?

Review Questions

1 Describe the chain of ossicles in the middle ear. How do they transmit sound?

2 How can the ears be kept dry during bathing?

3 Why is the consumption of alcohol discouraged after nasal surgery?

4 What is the difference between conductive and sensorineural deafness?

5 Why do polyps occur, and what is the treatment for nasal polyps?

6 Explain to a patient why you go deaf when your nose is blocked.

7 Why should a patient sneeze with his mouth open after ear surgery?

References

Biller, H., Lawson, W. and Baek-Se-Min 1983 Total glossectomy. *Archives of Otolaryngology* **109**(2), 69–73.

Buglass, E. 1995 Oral hygiene. *British Journal of Nursing* **4**(9), 516–19.

Camillieri, A.E., Ramamurthy, L. and Jones, P.H. 1995 Sleep nasendoscopy: what benefit to the management of snorers? *Journal of Laryngology and Otology* **109**(12), 1163–5.

Dingle, A., Flood, L.M., Kumar B.U. and Newcombe, R.C. 1995 Tympanosclerosis and mini-grommets: the relevance of grommet design. *Journal of Laryngology and Otology* **109**(10), 922–5.

El-Nagger, M., Kale, S., Aldrew, C. and Martin, F. 1995 Effect of Beconase nasal spray on olfactory function in post nasal polypectomy patients: a prospective controlled trial. *Journal of Laryngology and Otology* **109**(10), 941–4.

Florentini, A. 1992 Potential hazards of tracheobronchial suctioning. *Intensive and Critical Care Nursing* **8**(4), 217–26.

LaBlance, G., Kraus, K. and Steckol, K. 1991 Rehabilitation of swallowing and communication following glossectomy. *Rehabilitation Nursing* **16**(5), 266–70.

McKenzie 1986 *The special senses*, 2nd edn. Edinburgh: Churchill Livingstone.

Mason, J., Murty, G.E., Foster, H. and Bradley, P.J. 1992 Tracheostomy self care – the Nottingham system. *Journal of Laryngology and Otology* **106**(8), 723–4.

Millinson, K. 1991 Taking care of John's mouth. *Nursing Times* **87**(21), 34–5.

Moralee, S.J. and Murray, J.A. 1995 Would day-case adult tonsillectomy be safe? *Journal of Laryngology and Otology* **109**(12), 1166–7.

Royal National Throat, Nose and Ear Hospital NHS Trust 1993 *Tracheostomy care* Patient Care Series. London: RNTNE.

Scadding, G. 1995 The perennial problem. Clinical Focus – Otorhinolaryngology. *Head and Neck Surgery* **1**(1).

Spraggs, P.D. and Harries, M. 1995 The modified Valsalva manoeuvre to improve visualisation of the hypopharynx during flexible nasopharyngoscopy. *Journal of Laryngoscopy and Otology* **109**(9), 863–4.

Stokes, D. 1983 Laryngectomy: nursing care; a patient's view. *Nursing* (London) **2**(18), 520–1.

Thurston-Hookway, F. and Seddon, S. 1989 Care after laryngectomy. *Nursing* **3**(35), 5–10.

Toma, A.G., Blanchard, J., Eynon-Lewis, N. and Bridger, M.W. 1995 Post-tonsillectomy pain: the first ten days. *Journal of Laryngology and Otology* **109**(10), 963–4.

Whinney, D.J., Williamson, P.A. and Bicknell, P.G. 1995 Punctalate diathermy of the soft palate, a new approach in the management of snoring. *Journal of Laryngology and Otology* **109**(9) 849–52.

Further reading

Keith, R.L. 1991 Looking forward: a guide book for the laryngectomee, 2nd ed. New York: Theime Medical.

Kendrick, A. and Wiltshire, N. 1995 Sleep apnoea. *Professional Nurse* **10**(10), 624–8.

Rosenfeld, R.M. 1995 Non-surgical management of surgical otitis media with effusion. *Journal of Laryngology and Otology* **109**(9), 811–16.

Serra, A., Bailey, C.M. and Jackson, P. 1986 *Ear nose and throat nursing*. Oxford: Blackwell Scientific.

Useful contacts

BACUP	
Cancer Information Service	
Freeline	(0800) 181199
Cancer Counselling Service	0171–696 9000
British Association for Counselling	(01788) 578328
Cancer Link	0171–833 2451
Cancer Relief Macmillan Fund	0171–351 7811
Let's Face It	(01344) 774405
National Association of Laryngectomee Clubs	0171–381 9993
Oesophageal Patients' Association	0121–704 9860

Breast surgery

6

Penelope Simpson

Introduction

The care of the patient needing removal of the breast or part of the breast for benign disease, carcinoma or cosmetic reasons is best performed by a specialized team, including a breast care nurse.

The majority of breast lumps are found by women themselves or their partners. It is therefore of vital importance that women are taught to be breast aware and responsible for noting changes in their breasts (Burton, 1995).

One in ten women develops breast cancer, between 5% and 10% of cases being linked with gene defects (Eeles, 1995). Some women take the difficult decision to have both breasts removed when it is discovered that they are carrying faulty genes *BRCA1* or *BRCA2*, responsible for about two-thirds of inherited cases of breast cancer.

Most breast lumps prove to be benign, but the patient will believe that she has cancer until proven otherwise.

Patient comment

'My first thought was, "Oh no, I'm going to die".'

Men also suffer from breast cancer, but it is rarer, estimated at 1 in 200 (Chaplin, 1996).

If a diagnosis of carcinoma is confirmed, breast surgery will be combined with adjuvant treatment, radiotherapy, chemotherapy or tamoxifen. These may be given pre- and/or post-operatively. Adjuvant therapy can significantly improve both survival and risk of relapse in patients who have a mastectomy (Bonadonna *et al.*, 1995) or lumpectomy (Jacobson *et al.*, 1995). The patient should be involved in deciding which is the most appropriate treatment (Hollinworth, 1992; Whitman, 1994), and this opportunity is usually welcomed. Immediate and long-term options need to be discussed.

At some point in the treatment programme, it is possible to refashion a post-mastectomy breast by one of the following reconstruction methods:

- *subpectoral*, in which a breast implant is placed beneath the pectoralis major or serratus anterior muscle;
- *subcutaneous* placing of the implant beneath the skin of the breast following subcutaneous mastectomy;
- *myocutaneous flap*, the two most common sites being the latissimus dorsi in the back or the rectus abdominis in the abdomen;
- *tissue expansion techniques.*

For these, the patient may be referred to a plastic surgery team. Other centres offer a total service, including reconstruction immediately or at an appropriate time later. Sanchez-Guerro *et al.* (1995) conclude that there is no evidence that silicone breast implants are associated with a greater risk of connective tissue disease.

The timing of breast surgery in relation to the menstrual cycle can have an impact on the 5-year survival rates of those with carcinoma. Women appear to do better if operated on in the second half of their cycle, i.e. the 14 days or so before their period (Hrushesky *et al.*, 1989). Surgery, including lumpectomy, should therefore be offered to women on their 'best' days (Badwe *et al.*, 1991).

Investigations

Careful examination of both breasts is essential, and various investigations may be performed to aid diagnosis (*see* a handbook of investigations, e.g. Booth, 1983, for further details).

1 Mammography will have been performed before admission and may have been the point at which the mass was detected.

2 Needle aspiration (Hindle *et al.*, 1993) will check for cysts and gain material for cytology. It can be very painful (Millward, 1994). The tumour can be graded by cytology, allowing

'assessment of the biological aggressiveness of the cancer without removing it' (Robinson *et al.*, 1994).

3 Ultrasonography may be used to visualize the mass.

4 Bone scan, liver ultrasonography and chest X-ray may be employed to detect metastatic spread in the event of malignancy. This will help in choosing surgery and follow-up treatment.

Pre-operative care

Admission will take place anything from 2 days to a few hours before surgery, depending on the number of investigations needed. Many of these will have been performed in the OPD, and the patient may have been seen in a pre-admission clinic.

Consideration must be given to age, menstrual status and the presence of other debilitating conditions before the therapeutic programme

is decided. Leaflets, audiocassettes and videocassettes on surgical options should be available to reinforce discussions with the multidisciplinary team. The patient should be offered time with the breast care nurse and the option of having her partner present (Taylor, 1991) to enable them both to discuss surgery and future implications. Crockford *et al.* (1993) and the Health Committee (1995) support the appointment of a breast care nurse for every hospital dealing with breast surgery patients, and Hammond *et al.* (1995) describe the role of a breast care nurse practitioner who works interchangeably with a senior house officer in outpatient clinics.

Once the type of surgery has been decided on, the nurse must make sure that the patient understands what she will experience. Sensory information is as important as process information in trying to reduce unpleasant surprises. The patient needs to know what to expect post-operatively in terms of pain and its relief, dressings, intravenous infusions and drains.

Patient comment

'It was helpful to know that the wound was going to feel painful, hot and tight. It made it less frightening.'

The patient needs to know what is expected of her and will be taught (and regularly perform post-operatively) deep breathing, arm, leg and mobility exercises. She may be asked to shave her axilla.

Breast cancer patients (even those whose lumps turn out to be benign) suffer both emotionally and psychologically (Shrotria 1992; Crockford *et al.*, 1993). The patient will need psychological support throughout her stay as possibly having cancer will be a major shock. She may benefit from relaxation training to reduce anxiety and depression to reasonable levels, and may be tearful, withdrawn or very optimistic. The nurse must be there for the patient even if she is seen as 'self-caring' in the physical sense. Some patients benefit from meeting a former breast cancer patient trained to offer support.

Types of operation

This varies according to the size and position of the mass, the reason for surgery, the skill and preference of the surgeon, the patient's choice and the decision about any further reconstruction.

- *Lumpectomy* – the removal of all clinically suspicious tissue.

- *Partial mastectomy/wide local excision/wedge resection* – removal of the tumour together with a margin of microscopically normal tissue, with sampling/dissection of the lymph nodes.

- *Quadrantectomy* – removal of the quadrant of the breast containing the malignant mass, leaving the rest intact.

- *Simple mastectomy* – removal of the entire breast with the overlying skin down to the muscle, the pectoralis muscles being left intact. The axillary nodes may be sampled or cleared.

- *Subcutaneous mastectomy* – the incision is made in a relatively unobtrusive place to remove all tissue down to the muscle, conserving the skin, areola and nipple for immediate or future reconstruction with a silicone or other prosthesis.

- *Extended simple mastectomy* – removal of the entire breast along with the overlying skin down to the muscle, the axillary tail and the accessible nodes in the lower axilla, dividing the pectoralis minor muscle to gain access.

- *Modified radical (Patey) mastectomy* – removal of all breast tissue with the overlying skin down to the muscle, and removal of the pectoralis minor muscle to expose the whole axilla, which is cleared of nodes. The pectoralis major muscle remains intact.

- *Frozen section* – may be offered to some patients. The lump is removed under general anaesthetic, send to pathology, frozen, sliced with a microtome and examined under a microscope. If it proves to be malignant, the team can proceed to mastectomy or a previously agreed excision. This saves the awful wait for the results and the need for a second anaesthetic.

The patient is usually positioned supine on the operating table, with the arm of the affected side extended and supported at right angles to the body. The length of surgery depends on its complexity. Performing a 'keyhole' excision of breast tissue from a circumareolar (around the nipple) incision takes more time than does a straight-forward removal of breast tissue including skin. As breast tissue is highly vascular, a drain may need to be inserted through a separate stab incision and stitched into place.

Insertion of a subcuticular suture takes longer than using simple skin sutures or clips. A dressing will be applied, which may include a certain amount of padding or even a pressure bandage.

Patient comment

'When I woke up, there was so much padding on my chest that I didn't know if they had taken my breast off or not. I felt curiously detached about it.'

Post-operative care

Post-operative care is aimed immediately at preventing complications such as pain and, in the long term, at supporting patients through changes in body image and fear of return of the cancer.

When transferring the patient to the ward, great care must be taken to ensure that the affected arm is not abducted. The wound and drains will be monitored for excessive blood loss. If necessary, an intravenous infusion will be maintained until the patient is drinking freely. Regular analgesics will be given to enable her to sit up and perform deep breathing exercises. Providing her blood pressure is reasonable, she should get out of bed to pass urine within hours of surgery.

If a pressure bandage has been applied, it will be removed after 24 hours.

Patient comment

'I woke up with a dry mouth, a tight band around my chest, tubes and wires sticking out, feeling as if I had been run over.'

Drains will be removed when drainage is minimal, which may be 24–72 hours post-surgery. The patient may appreciate analgesic cover for this procedure, as pain may ensue. If there is no need for intravenous access for drugs or blood transfusion, intravenous infusions can be removed once the patient is tolerating adequate amounts of oral fluids.

The patient will need physiotherapy support, particularly after axillary surgery and mastectomy, to prevent the complications of reduced mobility. She will be taught how to exercise the arm and shoulder on the affected side to regain and maintain the full range of movement. Exercises, at first gentle, will become progressively harder.

STUDENT ACTIVITY

In privacy, stripped to the waist, sit in front of a full-length mirror. Put the shoulder joint through its full range of movement and note how it pulls on the skin of the axilla, chest and breast. Compare both sides. Get used to how your breasts look and feel.

The breast care nurse will visit the patient and will, along with the nursing staff, encourage the patient to express and discuss her worries and questions before leaving hospital. It is important to prepare the patient, with support and reassurance, to view her wound either in hospital or at home. It may be helpful to have her partner present.

Patient comment

'My feller took a swift look, gripping my hand tightly, and said "I'm a leg man myself".'

Discharge advice

How soon the patient goes home depends on the extent of surgery and the support available to her. A patient who has undergone a simple, uncomplicated lumpectomy may be allowed home the same day. She will be given an outpatient appointment for approximately 2 weeks later to receive the pathology results and discuss progress.

Patient comment

'It was the longest ten days of my life, like waiting for a death sentence. I couldn't think about anything else at all.'

All patients who have retained any breast tissue will be advised to wear a supporting (boneless) bra to sleep in as well as one to be worn all day.

Patient comments

'I wanted to resume our sex life as soon as possible, so I bought a frilly peephole bra that showed my nipples but not the scars or bruises. It felt naughty, but feminine, which was just what I needed.'

'It took me about 4 days to recover from the [lumpectomy] surgery.'

The patient should be advised to avoid lifting any heavy objects using the affected side until about a week after suture removal.

For more comprehensive surgery, a stay of 3–5 days may be indicated. If the sutures can be removed by the district or practice nurse, the patient can go home as soon as she is fit.

Once the dressing has been removed, the patient can wash her wound using soap and water. Once the sutures have been removed, daily application to the scar of a moisturizing lotion, using a gentle stroking action, is needed, although this is contraindicated if radiotherapy is anticipated. Moisturizing helps the scar to stay supple and enables the patient to incorporate the new sensations into her altered body image. She might also ask her partner to apply the moisturizer. After 6 weeks, a slightly more energetic massage technique is advisable, possibly using a thicker cream. If there is any possibility of exposure of the scar to sunlight, total sunblock must be applied for at least 2 years – for life if radiotherapy has been used on the area.

Patients who have undergone a mastectomy will be provided with a soft temporary prosthesis to wear for the first few weeks until wound healing is well advanced. The physiotherapy exercises should be continued to ensure full movement of the arm and shoulder; lifting heavy shopping or a vacuum cleaner with the operated side should be avoided for the first few weeks. Wearing a seatbelt may be painful; a device to relieve the pressure can be bought in car accessory outlets.

To reduce the possibility of lymphoedema in the affected arm, the patient should:

- use her arm as naturally as possible;
- do her exercises;
- avoid cuts, bruises and insect bites by using a thimble when sewing, appropriate gloves for gardening, housework, DIY and cooking, and an electric razor or hair-removing cream, as well as taking great care when cutting her nails;
- avoid tight clothing around the arms and shoulders;
- ensure that any blood samples or blood pressure measurements are taken on the other arm.

The patient may find it helpful to see or telephone the breast care nurse again, or have the addresses and telephone numbers of breast cancer care and support groups. She may need help to go through the grieving process and come to terms with her loss. Once at home, many questions occur, for example on nutritional advice (Monnin et al., 1993; Clayton and Jones, 1994).

A more permanent prosthesis (Horsfield, 1994) will be fitted 6 weeks after surgery or soon after the completion of radiotherapy when the skin is well healed. Driving can be resumed when the full range of movement has been regained. Most patients can return to work after 6–8 weeks unless they are receiving chemotherapy or radiotherapy. In this case, they are advised to conserve their energy, as these treatments can make them very tired (Millward, 1994), an effect that increases over time (Graydon, 1994). Some patients, however, choose to work during their treatment.

The patient will be followed up regularly for 10 years. Ideally, she should wait for at least 2 years after completion of treatment before becoming pregnant.

Complications

Should any immediate problems arise, the patient is advised to telephone her ward, breast care nurse or GP. She will be advised to look out for and report the signs of infection:

- pain;
- tenderness;
- redness;
- swelling;

Some breast scars undergo keloid changes, becoming raised, red (black in those with pigmented skin), lumpy and itchy. The GP should refer the patient to a plastic surgeon. Steroid injections may be needed.

A high proportion of women who have undergone surgery for breast cancer develop psychological problems warranting psychiatric treatment. Wilkinson *et al.* (1988) and Taylor (1991) have identified limited counselling by specialist nurses as being the most successful intervention to reduce depression and anxiety.

Some patients develop post-mastectomy pain days or weeks after surgery. The pain becomes chronic, stable and of long duration (Stevens *et al.*, 1995), typically localized to more than one area. The patient may need referral to a pain clinic.

If the affected arm swells, the patient should contact the GP or the breast care/lymphoedema nurse. Lymphoedema treatment may include external support, massage, exercise, care of the skin and, very rarely, surgery.

With breast cancer, there is the possibility of recurrence and/or distant spread, and the patient will be monitored by the oncology team at increasingly longer intervals. If the cancer is of an inherited type, the family can be screened in a family cancer clinic, where a geneticist will estimate the risk. The woman faces 'the lifelong threat of recurrence, a fear which is never truly absent, acting as a lingering ghost in the background' (Kramer, 1988). She may well wish to use complementary therapies to boost her defences and coping mechanisms.

Summary

1 Surgery ranges from simple lumpectomy, performed as a day case, to more extensive surgery for malignancy, requiring an extended stay and multidisciplinary support over time.

2 Investigations and incidence are outlined.

3 Options for reconstructive surgery to the breast are briefly reviewed.

4 Peri-operative care for patients undergoing breast surgery is summarized and the range of options defined.

5 Advice on discharge is given for each operation described, with indications for follow-up.

CASE HISTORY

Ms Doran, aged 52, works part time as a fitness instructor at a leisure centre. She has found a breast lump, shown on needle aspiration to be a fairly aggressive malignant growth. How can the nurse help her to review her options in deciding the best treatment for her?

Review Questions

1 Are both breasts the same size in most people?

2 What is the name for male breast enlargement?

3 Why is the lifetime use of sunblock necessary on skin that has had radiotherapy?

4 Why does removal of lymph nodes increase the risk of infection in the affected arm?

5 What nutritional advice is relevant to the needs of the patient who has had breast surgery for malignancy and faces adjuvant therapy?

ACKNOWLEDGEMENTS

In memory of Liz Kenny, and with many thanks to Ruth Markby, breast care nurse and reviewer, and Clare Beattie, the original author.

References

Badwe, R.A., Gregory, W.M. and Chandry, M.A. 1991 Timing of surgery during the menstrual cycle and survival of pre-menopausal women with operable breast cancer. *Lancet* **337**, 1261.

Bonadonna, G., Valagussa, P. and Moliterni, A. 1995 Adjuvant cyclophosphamide, methotrexate and fluorouracil in non-positive breast cancer. *New England Journal of Medicine* **332**(14), 901–6.

Booth, J.A. (ed.) 1983 *Handbook of investigations*. Lippincott Nursing Series. London: Harper & Row.

Burton, M. 1995 Guidelines for promoting breast care awareness. *Nursing Times* **91**(24), 33–4.

Chaplin, B. 1996 Breast cancer: knowledge for practice. *Nursing Times*/Professional Development Unit 26 **92**(10), 1–4.

Clayton, P. and Jones, J. 1994 Vitamin diet lifts breast cancer hope. *Observer* April 24, 7.

Crockford, E.A., Holloway, I.M. and Walker, J.M. 1993 Nurses' perceptions of patients' feelings about breast surgery. *Journal of Advanced Nursing* **18**, 1710–18.

Eeles, R. 1995 Developments in the study of familial breast cancer. *Nursing Times* **91**(5), 29–33.

Graydon, J.E. 1994 Women with breast cancer: their quality of life following a course of radiation therapy. *Journal of Advanced Nursing* **19**, 617–22.

Hammond, C., Chase, J. and Hogbin, B. 1995 A unique service? *Nursing Times* **91**(30), 28–9.

Health Committee 1995 *Third report on breast cancer services*. London: HMSO.

Hindle, W.H., Payne, P.A. and Pan, E.Y. 1993 The use of fine needle aspiration in the evaluation of persistent palpable dominant breast masses. *American Journal of Obstetrics and Gynaecology* **168**(6:1), 1814–18.

Hollinworth, H. 1992 Choice without fear. *Nursing Times* **88**(50), 27–9.

Horsfield, S. 1994 Adhesive prosthesis. *Nursing Times* **90**(8), 44–5.

Hrushesky, W.J.M., Bluming, A.Z., Gruber, S.A. et al. 1989 Menstrual influence on surgical care of breast cancer. *Lancet* **2**, 949–52.

Jacobson, J., Danforth, D. and Cowen, K. 1995

Ten year results of a comparison of conservation with mastectomy in the treatment of stage I and II breast cancer. *New England Journal of Medicine* **332**(14), 877–911.

Kramer, A.S. 1988 Immediate breast reconstruction. *Plastic Surgical Nursing* **8**(4), 150–4.

Millward, J. 1994 On the receiving end of breast cancer. *Journal of Clinical Nursing* **3**(3), 134–7.

Monnin, S., Schiller, M.R., Sachs, L. and Smith, A.M. 1993 Nutritional concerns of women with breast cancer. *Journal of Cancer Education* **8**(1), 63–9.

Robinson, I.A., McKee, G., Nicholson, A. *et al.* 1994 Prognostic value of cytological grading of fine-needle aspirates from breast carcinoma. *Lancet* **271**(8903), 947–9.

Sanchez-Guerro, J., Coldita, G.A. and Karlson, E.W. 1995 Silicone breast implants and the risk of connective-tissue diseases and symptoms. *New England Journal of Medicine* **382**(25), 1666–70.

Shrotria, S. 1992 Knowing the facts. *Nursing Times* **88**(50), 24–6.

Stevens, P.E., Dibble, S.L. and Miaskowski, C. 1995 Prevalance, characteristics, and impact of postmastectomy pain syndrome: an investigation of women's experiences. *Pain* **61**(1), 61–8.

Taylor, J. 1991 A place for women. *Nursing Times* **87**(35), 54–5.

Whitman, M. 1994 Breast surgery: helping patients choose. *Nursing* **24**(8), 25.

Wilkinson, S., Maguire, P. and Tait, A. 1988 Life after breast cancer. *Nursing Times* **84**(40), 34–7.

Further reading

Bennicke, K. Conrad, C., Sabroe, S. and Sorensen, H.T. 1995 Cigarette smoking and breast cancer. *British Medical Journal* **310**(6992), 1431–3.

D'Angelo, T.M. and Gorrell, C.R. 1989 Breast reconstruction using tissue expanders. *Oncology Nursing Forum* **16**(1), 23–7.

Hunter, D.J., Speigelman, D., Adami, H-O. *et al.* 1996 Cohort studies of fat intake and the risk of breast cancer – a pooled analysis. *New England Journal of Medicine* Feb 8, 356–61.

Lynn, J. 1993 The waiting game. *Nursing Standard* **10**(8), 22–3.

Noblet, M. 1994 Discrene, an alternative to conventional breast prosthesis. *Journal of Cancer Care* **4**, 203–7.

Slattery, M.L. and Kerber R.L. 1993 A comprehensive evaluation of family history and breast cancer risk: the Utah population database. *Journal of the American Medical Association* **270**(13), 1563–8.

Webb, C. 1985 *Sexuality nursing and health*. Chichester: John Wiley & Sons.

Useful addresses

Breast Cancer Campaign   High Street, Marlow, Buckinghamshire SL7 1AQ. Provides information, patient leaflets, breast bulletins, patient videos and lecture kits.

Breast Cancer Care   Kiln House, 210 New Kings Road, London SW6 4NZ. Tel administration: 0171–384 2984; helpline: 0171–384 2347; freeline: (0500) 245345

Suite 2/8, 65 Bath Street, Glasgow G2 2BX. Tel: 0141–353 1050

Bristol Cancer Help Centre   Grove House, Cornwallis Grove, Bristol BS8 4PG. Tel: 0117–974 3216.

British Association of Cancer United Patients (BACUP)   3 Bath Place, Rivington Street, London

EC2A 3JR. Information line: (0800) 181199, administration: 0171–696 9003.

CancerLink   17 Britannia Street, London WC1X 9JN. Tel: 0171–833 2451.

9 Castle Terrace, Edinburgh EH1 2DP. Tel: 0131–228 5557.

Women's Health   52 Featherstone Street, London EC1Y 8RT. Helpline: 0171–251 6580; administration: 0171–251 6333.

Women's Nationwide Cancer Control Campaign South Audley Street, London W1Y 5DQ. Administration: 0171–729 1735, helpline: 0171–729 2229.

Cardiac and non-cardiac thoracic surgery

7

Jennifer S. Wesson and Helen R. Neary

CARDIAC SURGERY

Introduction

Cardiac surgery can be broadly divided into procedures for congenital and acquired disorders. This chapter focuses on surgery for acquired cardiac disorders, the main indications being:

- coronary artery disease;
- valve disease (stenosis or regurgitation);
- thoracic aortic aneurysm or dissection;
- post-infarction ventricular septal defect;
- endocarditis;
- dysrrythmias resistant to medical treatment (ablative dysrrhythmia surgery).

Coronary heart disease

Coronary heart disease (CHD) accounts for the highest incidence of acquired heart disorders and will be the main focus of this chapter. It is the biggest single cause of death in the UK, accounting for 26% of all deaths in England in 1992 (Department of Health, 1994). Its manifestations are multiple, including sudden death, angina pectoris, myocardial infarction and heart failure. At its most extreme, a patient may be considerably handicapped, suffering stringent restrictions on his activities.

CHD results from progressive blockage of the coronary arteries (Fig. 7.1) by atherosclerosis – the accumulation and proliferation of lipid substance and fibrous tissue in the vessel wall (atheroma).

This leads to a reduced blood flow through the lumen, inadequate myocardial perfusion and oxygenation and, ultimately, ischaemia (Shuttleworth, 1996).

> **STUDENT ACTIVITY**
>
> Look up the pathogenesis of atheroma. What factors predispose to this condition?

Unlike other vital organs, the heart, even at rest, extracts a high percentage of the oxygen available to it via the coronary arteries. Thus it has no safety margin as oxygen extraction is already nearly maximal. Myocardial ischaemia becomes clinically significant when supply fails

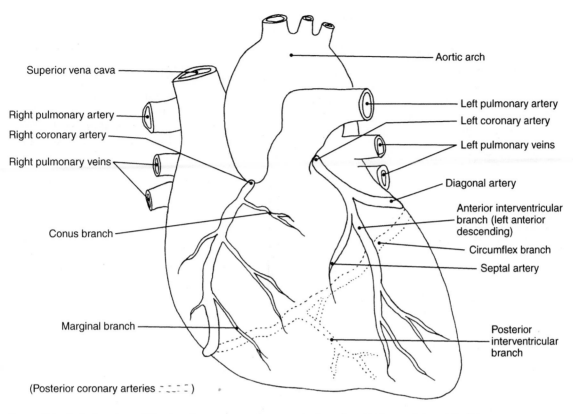

Figure 7.1 Anterior view of the heart: coronary artery supply. (===), posterior coronary arteries

to meet demand, usually when 60% or more of the vessel lumen is occluded (Possanza, 1996).

Causes of coronary heart disease

The cause of CHD is multifactorial, and extensive epidemiological investigation over many years has led to the identification of well-recognized risk factors (Donaldson and Donaldson, 1993; Tortora and Grabowski 1993):

1 *Cigarette smoking.*

2 *Raised blood pressure.* A systolic blood pressure of 160 mmHg carries nearly three times the risk of a major coronary event of one of 130 mmHg (Fox, 1996).

3 *Raised blood cholesterol and dietary considerations.* When plasma cholesterol rises above 4.1 mmol/L, the risk of clinical coronary artery disease increases (Witztum, 1994).

4 *Physical inactivity.* A lifestyle lacking in exercise can contribute to the development of heart disease (Jones, 1996).

5 *Obesity and weight fluctuations.* Being greater than 30% overweight predisposes a person to heart disease. Predictors of obesity are body mass index and waist hip ratio (Department of Health, 1994).

6 *Genetic predisposition.* A parental or sibling history of myocardial infarction is strongly associated with an excess risk of cardiovascular disease, especially when associated with other risk factors (Underhill *et al.*, 1989).

7 *Diabetes mellitus.* A high glucose level may irritate the endothelial layer of the vessel, leading to atherosclerosis (Department of Health, 1994).

8 *Stress*. Certain behaviour and personality types have also been identified as predictors for the development of CHD (Underhill *et al.*, 1989).

9 *Oxygen free radical damage*. Oxygen free radicals attack polyunsaturated fatty acids, causing cellular damage (Parkinson, 1995), which affects the arterial endothelium and accelerates atherogenesis (Hoffman and Garewal, 1995).

Owing to the protective effects of oestrogen, the incidence of heart disease tends to remain lower in women until after the menopause; consequently, men have received more attention and treatment for CHD (Penkofer, 1993). It should be remembered, however, that both sexes share the same risk factors, and it is the reduction of these risk factors that is paramount, as identified in *The Health of the Nation* (Department of Health, 1992), whose aim is to reduce the death rate from CHD by 30–40% by the year 2000.

Valvular heart disease

Valve disease is mainly attributed to rheumatic heart disease. Any of the valves can be affected, but the mitral or aortic valves (Fig. 7.2) are most commonly left with impaired function owing to the formation of scar tissue. Valve leaflets may be thickened, calcified or fused together. This may result in a narrowed valve orifice causing stenosis and obstruction to flow, or a regurgitant or leaky valve incapable of preventing retrograde blood flow through its orifice. Bacterial invasion of the deformed heart valve can subsequently lead to bacterial endocarditis.

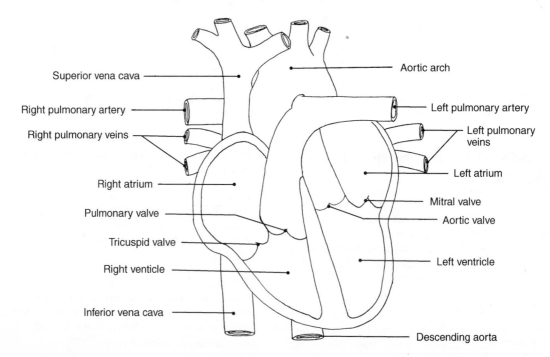

Figure 7.2 Anterior view of the heart: heart valves

Treatment of coronary heart disease

The number of patients undergoing heart surgery for acquired disease has risen dramatically over the past 20 years. The profile of patients being admitted for cardiac surgery is changing, those previously suitable for surgery being successfully treated with new techniques coming under the auspices of the cardiologist.

Patients are usually referred to a major cardiac centre for investigation, although mobile cardiac catheterization units now offer services to hospitals where fixed facilities are not available (Owen, 1994).

Diagnostic techniques

ELECTROCARDIOGRAPHY (ECG)

This is non-invasive study of the electrical activity occuring during each heart contraction. It will reveal heart rate and rhythm, ventricular hypertrophy and any areas of ischaemia (Quinn and Jones, 1996).

EXERCISE STRESS TESTING

The monitoring of ECG and blood pressure under conditions of controlled exercise. This usually takes the form of a treadmill or exercise bike. The test becomes positive if ischaemic ECG changes are seen (with or without chest pain). The point when the test becomes positive is relevant to the diagnosis.

> ### Patient comment
>
> 'I was very anxious before going for the stress test. I thought that I would have chest pain and something dreadful would happen. The staff were great. I was told exactly what to do and what would happen, and they watched me closely all the time.'

ECHOCARDIOGRAPHY

This is a transthoracic or transoesophageal ultrasound scan of the heart that can assess blood flow in different parts of the heart, ventricular function and any abnormalities of the heart valves or septum. Pericardial effusion and cardiac tamponade can also be diagnosed.

CORONARY CARDIAC CATHETERIZATION

A catheter is inserted percutaneously, usually via a femoral artery, and advanced into the aorta, coronary vessels and heart. Contrast medium is injected into the coronary arteries. Cardiac anatomy and the efficacy of the ventricles and valves can be demonstrated, and the pressure and oxygen saturation in each heart chamber measured. Coronary artery anatomy, and the extent and location of partially or completely occluded coronary arteries, can be visualized (Thomas, 1994).

Medical management

Many patients with CHD can be managed medically with success. Medication is usually a combination of nitrates, angiotensin-converting enzyme (ACE) inhibitors, beta-adrenergic blockers and calcium-channel blockers.

Minimal invasive therapy

Many patients with CHD are treated successfully with non-surgical interventions such as percutaneous transluminal coronary angioplasty (PTCA), percutaneous balloon mitral valvuloplasty or implantation of a coronary stent (a wire mesh tube positioned at the site of the obstruction to hold the blocked artery segment open). New techniques are being developed and researched, for example 'angel wings', a nickel and titanium alloy disc covered in a polyester gauze that is inserted via a cardiac catheter to close an atrial septal defect.

Surgical management

Approximately one-third of patients with angina who are referred for cardiac catheterization are suitable for treatment by PTCA (British Heart Foundation, 1995), the remainder being referred for surgery. Consequently, the patient admitted for cardiac surgery is likely to have more advanced disease and left ventricular dysfunction (Bojar, 1994), and often tends to be older. Even though increasing age is recognized as a risk factor for mortality, it has not been demonstrated as an absolute contraindication, so surgery in the octogenarian is a therapeutic option (Vaca and Moskoff, 1994). This patient group often tends to have other co-morbidities, such as cerebrovascular disease, hypertension and peripheral vascular disease, increasing the operative risk and the incidence of complications.

Indications for coronary artery bypass surgery

- Chronic stable angina unrelieved by drugs (especially if the left main coronary artery is obstructed);
- Unstable angina;
- Acute ischaemia or haemodynamic instability following attempted PTCA;
- Left main vessel stenosis greater than 50%;
- Triple vessel disease with an ejection fraction of less than 50%;
- Patients whose disease is not suitable for PTCA.

Selection for surgery also depends on the severity of symptoms, left ventricular function, the size of the coronary arteries, the location of the obstruction and the suitability of donor vessels.

The aim of coronary artery bypass graft surgery (CABG) is to improve perfusion to a region of ischaemic myocardium by bypassing the oc-

Table 7.1 Commonly used types of graft

- Left or right internal mammary artery (IMA)
- Saphenous vein
- Radial artery
- Gastroepiploic artery
- Inferior epigastric artery

cluded area. Occlusion by atherosclerosis tends to be confined to the proximal sections of the large coronary arteries, so bypass grafting is to the more distal section of the vessels (Sanderson and Kurth, 1983; Shuttleworth, 1996).

This is achieved using a variety of conduits fashioned from the patient's own tissue to divert the blood from the aorta to the vessel distal to the occlusion (Table 7.1), using cardiopulmonary bypass, described below. The type of graft depends on the site of occlusion and the availability of suitable donor vessels.

Patient comment

'I had read that the vein in the leg is used for the operation and I did wonder whether my varicose vein would cause a problem. The surgeon tells me that other grafts will be used because the varicose vein won't be suitable.'

Preparation for surgery

Unless surgery is required urgently or as an emergency, the patient will join the routine waiting list. The wait for cardiac surgery has been identified as a very stressful period for both the patient and family (Gillis, 1984) and a pre-admission programme has been found to reduce fears and anxieties (Nelson, 1996).

During this time, the patient will have access to health education and support from his own GP surgery. Advice is given on a healthier lifestyle, including the cessation of smoking at least 2 months prior to surgery to reduce the risk of post-operative pulmonary complications.

The patient may be seen by a rehabilitation nurse approximately 1–2 weeks prior to surgery, to begin to prepare the patient and his family for the hospitalization, surgery, post-operative recovery and rehabilitation period that lies ahead by anticipating the need for information and the issues that are likely to heighten anxiety. The patient will be informed that the hospital stay is likely to be 5–8 days and that he will be unable to drive immediately after surgery; thus discharge planning can already begin. The patient may also be advised to contact the ward the evening prior to admission to confirm availability of a bed.

Patient comments

'It was reassuring to hear what was expected of me and what was likely to happen during my hospital stay. Having my wife with me was comforting too – I think that she is almost as apprehensive as I am.'

'At first I didn't like the idea of the possibility that the ward would not being able to accommodate me and my surgery could be cancelled at the last minute, but then I thought that if I needed surgery urgently, I'd expect to jump the queue too.'

Admission

The patient is usually admitted to hospital the day before surgery. The admission procedure varies depending on the admitting cardiac centre, but pre-operative medical investigations are usually already complete.

Basic clerking and general pre-operative procedures are carried out as discussed in Part One of this book. An ECG and chest X-ray are performed to provide a baseline for post-operative comparison. Blood samples are taken for group and cross-matching, full blood count, blood chemistry and fasting lipid level. Liver function tests and coagulation screening are particularly relevant if the patient is already taking anti-coagulants, for example in valve disease or atrial fibrillation. Lung function tests may also be required, especially if the patient has continued to smoke. Drug therapy during the pre-operative period will vary between cardiac centres; examples can be seen in Table 7.2. Most medications, for example diuretics, anti-arrythmics and anti-angina treatments, will continue as normal.

Table 7.2 Pre-operative medical management

Drug	Administration	Rationale
Warfarin/aspirin	Stop 2 days prior to surgery	To reduce the risk of excessive post-operative bleeding
Dipyridamole	Pre-operatively	To reduce platelet dysfunction during cardiopulmonary bypass and improve graft patency
Propanolol	If already taking long-acting beta-blockers	To replace a long-acting with a shorter-acting beta-blocker
Digoxin	Omit on morning of surgery	Is a risk of increased sensitivity to digoxin as a result of fluid and electrolyte shifts during surgery
Heparin	Stop 4 hours prior to surgery and check coagulation screen	Is a risk of prolonged clotting times or heparin-induced thrombocytopenia

Nursing assessment

(*See* Part One)

Patient comment

'It was nice to have my own named nurse. She greeted me on my arrival to the ward and will be with me when I go to theatre tomorrow. I understand that she will look after me when I come back from intensive care too.'

Religious or cultural needs must be addressed. A past medical and nursing history is taken, which may reveal previous ill-health or disability affecting subsequent care, for example diabetes mellitus increasing the risk of a mediastinal wound infection. The nurse will also begin to anticipate the patient's discharge status: Is there a carer at home? Are there any dependents who rely on the patient?

Patient comment

'It was reassuring that the nurse realized that the arthritis in my hip means that I have great difficulty and suffer extreme pain when lying on my left hand side.'

Emotional needs

Fear, anxiety and knowledge deficit are the most commonly identified pre-operative problems (Underhill *et al.*, 1989). Reducing anxiety at this stage lessens the risk of pre-operative angina or infarction and enhances the patient's involvement in post-operative care and recovery. Fear may be related to the fear of the unknown, the experience of pain, a change in body image or the possibility of death. Usual family roles and support systems should be assessed, and education and support be provided to sustain these roles.

Patient comment

'I told the nurse that I was frightened about the amount of pain I was going to experience, and how this worry had kept me awake at night. She talked to me for a while about the night sedation I could have, about the pre-medication before going to theatre, the anesthetic and the amount of sedation and painkillers I would receive in intensive care. She showed me some relaxation techniques and talked about how I could ask the nurses to change my position in bed to make me more comfortable. I felt better afterwards.'

A high degree of anxiety may prevent the understanding and retention of any information presented (Gilliss, 1984). Much of the information may have to be repeated several times if communication is to be effective. Patients who are anxious retain only 30–40% of any verbal information given to them (Cheetham, 1993), so many cardiac centres provide written information to supplement that given verbally, as highlighted by the Government's White Paper *Working for Patients* (Department of Health, 1989). The British Heart Foundation also provides a useful series of leaflets.

Some patients find it helpful to talk to other patients already recovering from cardiac surgery. For some patients, the main cause of anxiety may be unrelated to their actual treatment in hospital.

Patient comment

'The nurse understood my concern about walking the dog each day. My neighbour will help out if I ask, but they are always so busy, and I don't like to rely on them too much. Plus the fact, I actually enjoy our daily walks.'

Physical needs

When cardiac dysfunction reduces cardiac output, other vital organs may also be adversely affected, which should be detected in the nursing assessment. For example, the kidneys receive 25% of cardiac output, so any significant reduction in this may affect glomerular filtration rate, which depends on renal artery perfusion.

As the size of the older population increases, nurses need to become familiar with the normal physiological changes associated with advancing age and anticipate the likelihood of post-operative complications (*see* Chapter 2). Baseline observations of vital signs must be made, a change in the trend of observations rather than a one-off recording usually being more significant (Endacott, 1993).

A weak pulse may indicate a reduced stroke volume or increased vasoconstriction. If a dysrrythmia is present and the heart rate is less than 60 or more than 100 per minute, impaired tissue perfusion should be suspected (Endacott, 1993).

Blood pressure is an indicator of cardiac output and depends on contractility, blood volume, vessel elasticity and resistance to blood flow. The difference between the systolic and diastolic blood pressures is known as the pulse pressure; the level of this provides information about the condition of the arteries. For example, in atherosclerosis, the pulse pressure is increased (Tortora and Grabowski, 1993).

An elevated temperature may be indicative of infection. The prevention or detection of infection is essential because of the use of prosthetic devices in some valve replacement surgery. Any pre-operative infection can increase the risk of post-operative sternal wound infection, sepsis or pneumonia (Possanza, 1996). Patients admitted for valve surgery should undergo a dental assessment to identify any gum infection or severe dental decay, and relevant treatment should be carried out prior to surgery. Any chronic infection, for example sinusitis, must be treated pre-operatively, as must any respiratory infections predisposing to post-operative pulmonary complications. The skin is observed for any signs of local infection that could increase the risk of a sternal wound infection.

The temperature of extremities should also be noted as an indicator of cardiac output and the presence of pulses observed. A capillary refill time of greater than 3 seconds may indicate inadequate tissue perfusion.

Respiratory function is assessed by respiratory rate, depth, pattern, use of accessory muscles and presence of any wheeze or shortness of breath. Arterial oxygen saturation (Sao_2) may prove useful but can be unreliable due to patient movement, reduced perfusion or anaemia (Endacott, 1993). Causes of an increased respiratory rate, such as pain, anxiety and pyrexia, should be excluded prior to further investigation. A cough may be indicative of a respiratory infection, pulmonary oedema or congestion. Those patients who smoke may need further assessment, as the irritant effects of smoking on the tracheobronchial tree predispose the patient to post-operative pulmonary complications. These patients tend to be sensitive to the irritant effects of inhalational anaesthetics, and have thick, tenacious secretions

(Sanderson and Kurth, 1983). Those who have recently given up smoking may require additional understanding and diversional support. Nicotine patches also appear to be helpful.

Skin colour is a good indication of respiratory and cardiac function. Central cyanosis indicates impaired gas exchange, and peripheral cyanosis reduced blood flow. Pallor may suggest poor perfusion owing to catecholamine release and vasoconstriction, or anaemia that may need correcting prior to surgery. In the elderly, pre-operative anaemia or hypovolaemia can increase the risk of post-operative complications (Ferraris and Ferraris, 1996).

Distended jugular veins or raised jugular venous pressure (JVP) reflects increased pressures in the right side of the heart. The veins are usually visible when the patient lies flat but disappear when he sits at 45°. A raised JVP may indicate hypervolaemia, vena cava obstruction or right ventricular failure.

STUDENT ACTIVITY

Observe a colleague lying flat and try to identify the jugular veins. Get the person to sit up and see if the veins disappear.

Generalized oedema is the abnormal accumulation of fluid in the interstitial spaces, becoming visible following the retention of approximately 5 L of extracellular fluid (Coombs, 1995). It may suggest right-sided heart failure, but other causes, for example hypoalbuminaemia, should be excluded.

Orientation and information needs

A visit from an ITU nurse the day before surgery has been associated with a significant decrease in anxiety in the 24–72 hour post-operative period (Martin, 1996). The aim of this visit is to make a physical and psychological nursing assessment to facilitate ITU care planning, while minimizing the patient and family's fear and anxiety by providing information about the unit and offering the opportunity to ask questions. Some units offer the patient a visit to the ITU. This should be on an individual basis, depending on the wishes of the patient and the suitability of the ITU environment at that particular time.

Patient comments

'My greatest concern is the urine catheter, and how they get it in and out.'

'I found it reassuring that a nurse will be with me all the time, and will explain any procedures that need to happen, and can anticipate my needs.'

The physiotherapist will visit each patient prior to theatre to talk about her role in post-operative recovery. She will assess respiratory function and teach the importance of deep breathing and coughing. Incentive spirometry may be introduced to clear the lungs of any pre-operative atelectasis and to familiarize the patient with its use. To optimize post-operative physiotherapy, it is advisable for the named nurse to confirm that the patient can adequately demonstrate deep breathing and coughing.

Patient comment

'All these visits I am receiving from the staff, does this mean that I am in a high risk group?'

The patient will need an explanation of the purpose of any multidisciplinary team visit he receives. High-risk patients are considered to be diabetics, or those who have had a recent stroke, have lung or renal disease, or have an ejection fraction of less than 20% (Possanza, 1996).

Patient comment

'A friend's neighbour had this operation 10 years ago. He told me that he wasn't allowed anything to drink for 3 days after the operation'.

Misinformation from well-meaning friends can heighten the patient's anxiety; the patient will need to be informed of current practice and the reason for post-operative fluid restriction.

Immediate pre-operative care

Shaving and skin preparation are usually performed the evening prior to surgery using antibacterial, antifungal skin cleanser and shampoo. The patient is kept nil by mouth for 6 hours prior to theatre, and pre-medication is given approximately 1 hour before theatre. Following this, the patient will remain in bed. It may be advisable to inform the family that the whole procedure will take approximately 3–4 hours. If the family choose to stay in the hospital, a suitable environment should be provided and progress reports given at regular intervals.

On arrival in the anaesthetic room, the patient is attached to the monitor by ECG leads in order to observe the heart's rate and rhythm. A peripheral saturation (Sa_{O_2}) probe, placed onto any digit, will record oxygenation and, together with a non-invasive blood pressure (NIBP) measurement, give the anaesthetist information on the patient's cardiovascular status. Oxygen delivered via a facemask will be commenced. A peripheral venous cannula is introduced, allowing access for colloid and drug therapy.

The patient is now ready to be anaesthetized and intubated. Once this is accomplished, the patient is mechanically ventilated.

Preparation continues and arterial access is achieved most commonly via the radial artery (ensuring that Sa_{O_2} monitoring is attached to the opposite hand, as this may affect trace readings). Next, central access is required, using a triple-lumen central line via the internal jugular or subclavian vein. The distal port is then transduced and attached to the monitor, thereby providing the anaesthetist and surgeons with pressure readings of right atrial pressure, blood pressure, heart rate and Sa_{O_2}.

Sterile temperature probes are placed and secured, the first via the nasopharynx, which will reflect the temperature of the brain, and the second in mid-oesophagus, which will reflect the temperature of blood in the posterior heart.

An orogastric/nasogastric tube will be introduced, and finally a silastic urethral catheter is inserted, allowing the total output of urine to be measured.

STUDENT ACTIVITY

From memory, draw a simple diagram of the heart, label the main structures and identify the direction of blood flow through them. Which contain oxygenated and which deoxygenated blood?

Cardiopulmonary bypass

CPB uses the heart–lung machine to provide an extracorporeal circulation. It removes desaturated (venous) blood from the heart, filters it, oxygenates it, cools it or warms it, and then pumps it back into the body via the aorta (Fig. 7.3).

The heart-lung machine consists of:

- *The venous reservoir.* Venous blood returning to the heart from the systemic circulation to be oxygenated is redirected from the right atrium via a venous cannula. Blood from the pericardium is returned to the reservoir, via pump-assisted suction, and filtered prior to entering the reservoir.

- *The oxygenator.* Desaturated blood is passed over a membrane, in place of the lungs, where oxygen is taken up and carbon dioxide displaced. Blood is then 'pumped' forward by a roller pump, in place of the left ventricle, controlled by the perfusionist.

- *The heat exchanger.* This is where systemic temperature control is determined, warming or cooling the blood.

The blood is then directed forward to be returned to the systemic circulation.

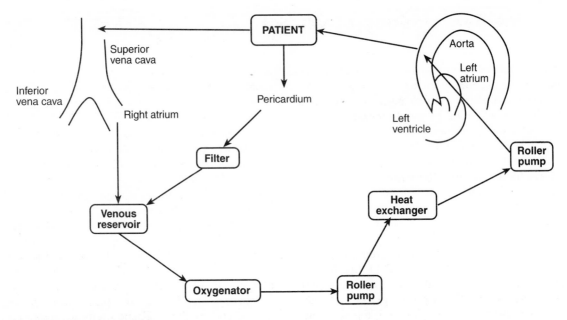

Figure 7.3 Heart–lung machine

Arterial cannulation is directly into the ascending aorta. Venous cannulation into the right atrium and inferior vena cava takes superior and inferior vena caval blood flow to the reservoir. The arterial cannula is always inserted first and connected to the bypass circuit prior to venous cannulation. Ventilation is stopped once full flow is established, the lungs then deflating.

Myocardial preservation during surgery is extremely important. In order to minimize damage due to the ischaemia caused by diverting the heart's own blood supply from the right and left coronary arteries away from the field of operation, steps have to be taken to protect the heart muscle. This is achieved by:

- systemic hypothermia induced via the heat exchanger, reducing the central temperature to approximately 18–32°C according to the particular surgery;
- topical cooling – external cooling to the surface of the heart with, for example, cold Ringer's solution or iced saline into the pericardial cavity;
- internal cooling – cold cardioplegia injected into the aortic root or coronary ostia. This solution has a high potassium concentration and, in combination with the extreme cold,

will initiate cardiac arrest. A completely arrested, non-fibrillating heart, has minimal oxygen requirements.

Hypothermia reduces the metabolic processes within the body, allowing relative hypoxia to be better tolerated. For example, the brain at a temperature of 37°C will tolerate anoxia for only approximately 3–4 minutes prior to irreversible damage. Tolerance improves to 8–12 minutes, however, if the temperature of the brain is reduced to 30°C.

The CPB circulation needs to be fully anticoagulated to prevent blood clotting in the circuit. Large doses of heparin are given to achieve this.

The pump and suction systems of the CPB, and the direct exposure to oxygen, induce red cell damage (haemolysis), which may add stress to the liver and kidneys trying to metabolize and excrete red cell products.

Once surgery is complete, all the air is removed from the heart and replaced with blood. When the procedure ends, the patient is rewarmed to 37°C. Ventilation, temperature and rhythm must be reinstated and acceptable prior to the completion of CPB. The venous line is slowly occluded to allow the heart to fill and recover from ischaemic arrest. Arterial flow is reduced and left ventricular performance monitored closely. Inotropic support may be used in the recovery phase.

The remaining blood from the circuit will be returned to the patient at the end of the procedure, and diuretics may be used to concentrate the circulating volume and increase packed cell volume.

Complications

Complications include:

- tearing of the aorta;
- bleeding;
- air embolus;
- calcium / plaque embolus;
- aortic dissection.

Intensive therapy unit

The patient is received into ITU by the nurse who conducted the pre-operative visit. Attention should be paid to:

- anticoagulation prior to surgery;
- hypertension treated with beta-blockers;
- treatment with digitalis;
- allergies;
- previous embolic episodes;
- special requests made by the patient, for example concerning glasses or dentures, or those identified by relatives; dealing with these may go a long way to reducing post-operative fear and anxiety.

Patient comment

'You promise to put my dentures back in as soon as I wake up . . . don't let anyone see me without them . . . I'd be so embarrassed.'

An ITU bed will have been organized during patient preparation. Particular bedside equipment should include;

1 two wall suction points for chest drainage and the clearance of secretions;
2 an intubation tray;
3 roller clamps and chest drain clamps;
4 a drainage bag for the naso- or orogastric tube;
5 ventilator and infusion pumps/syringe drivers.

Surgical and anaesthetic notes, instructions and prescriptions will state:

- the operation performed;
- the clinical status of the patient during the procedure;
- relevant past medical history;
- pacing requirements where necessary;
- the colloid transfused in theatre and the blood loss from drains;
- intropic support or vasodilator therapy requirements;
- the parameters to be achieved.

The accepting nurse now has enough information to allow forward planning and anticipate complications.

The patient arrives in ITU under the care of the anaesthetist. Great effort will have been made to avoid entanglement of the infusion and monitoring lines. The patient is attached to the ventilator, and transducer lines are connected to the ITU monitor and re-zeroed. Infusion pumps or syringe drivers are placed appropriately and checked as soon as possible against prescription charts for correct dosage and administration. Baseline observations of cardiovascular status and respiratory function are now recorded.

Visual assessment offers the first measurements of what care the patient may need:

- monitor traces;
- chest expansion;
- patient's colour and warmth.

The skin is felt to assess warmth and perfusion. The cooler the peripheries, the higher the resistance offered against the heart, with reduced circulating volume needing to be replaced as the patient warms up.

Chest drains and their number (usually 1–3; commonly pleural and mediastinal) are noted. They should be connected to wall suction under a pressure of 5–7 kPa (50 mmHg). Their arrival level is noted and quarter-hourly measurements commenced, reducing in frequency as drainage subsides. Management of chest drains is dealt with in the section on thoracic surgery (see pp. 161–163).

Wound sites, such as sternal dressings, harvest sites for donor grafting, drain sites and ports of entry for intravenous lines, must be observed for patency or signs of early infection, ensuring that dressings are dry and secure. The urinary catheter chamber is emptied and subsequent urine output measured every hour. Naso- and orogastric tubes should be placed on free drainage once their position has been checked.

Respiration

The patient is attached to the ventilator, routinely preset to deliver 40% oxygen. Initial assessment of chest expansion and air entry is noted, ventilation observations being commenced and repeated at hourly intervals. These recordings include:

- tidal volume (TV);
- minute volume (MV);
- respiratory rate (RR);

where:

$$RR \times TV = MV$$

Manipulation of these values produces and controls the individual's optimum carbon dioxide and oxygen tensions. It is imperative to ensure that alarm limits are set and armed, and that humidification has been provided.

It is sometimes necessary to have a post-operative chest X-ray.

Arterial blood analysis, via the arterial line, will be recorded regularly as determined by the patient's condition and progress (Cornack, 1996; Szaflarsk, 1996).

On return from theatre, analysis will be required approximately 15 minutes after connection to the ventilator to assess its efficacy. Due consideration must be given to those patients with longstanding cardiac and pulmonary dis-

eases, who may show different arterial blood gas values.

Normal arterial blood gas values (Oh, 1987)

pH	7.35–7.45
O_2 (Pao_2)	11.3–13.3 kPa
CO_2 ($Paco_2$)	4.8–5.9 kPa
Bicarbonate (HCO_3)	22–25 mmol/L
Base deficit/excess	+2 to −2

Physiotherapy is not normally needed in the immediate post-operative period. If the patient's air entry becomes noisy, or airway pressures increase above those normally acceptable for that patient, 100% oxygenation via the ventilator for several minutes, followed by the introduction of a suction catheter, will allow further assessment and the removal of loose secretions.

Effective nursing care of the patient receiving ventilatory support will include the following:

1 Ensure adequate ventilation by:

- regular arterial blood gas analysis;
- regularly listening to air entry and observing chest expansion;
- removal of secretions;
- recording ventilatory observations.

2 Position the endotracheal tube comfortably, checking tightness of the ties around the patient's face and neck and ensuring secure placement without tautness or dragging. The endotracheal tube has proved to be a great source of distress for patients who remember some of their short stay within ITU. Inability to speak and a sore throat have also been identified as particular causes of discomfort (Pennock et al., 1994).

Patient comment

'I had been warned that the tube would be unpleasant but that proved to be an understatement.' (Cited by Heath, 1989)

3 Undertake care of the oral mucosa by regular oral hygiene to keep the mouth fresh, and apply Vaseline to the lips.

Extubation

The majority of post-cardiac surgical patients will be ready for extubation within 4–6 hours. Acceptable criteria for this procedure are that the patient:

- is cardiovascularly stable with optimum haemodynamic readings;
- must be warm and well perfused with an axillary temperature above 36°C;
- has minimal blood loss into the chest drains;
- has good respiratory function;
- has a negative crystalloid balance;
- has no obvious neurological deficits.

By this stage, the patient will have been seated upright, thus aiding chest drainage and ventilation. Sedation is then reduced or withdrawn so the patient is awake enough to obey simple commands, such as squeezing a hand and wriggling their toes. This may also give the first indication of any neurological deficit.

Patients must be able to generate their own breaths on a rebreathing circuit. Once this is achieved, they are extubated, with removal of the orogastric tube. Forty per cent oxygen via a facemask is commenced and quarter-hourly respiratory observations charted. Air must be audible to all quarters, with equal chest wall expansion. Arterial blood gas tensions should be measured 20–30 minutes later and thereafter as indicated by results.

Oxygen has a drying affect on the oral mucosa and is frequently a major source of concern to the patient in the immediate post-extubation period.

Patient comment

'My throat and mouth were so dry and uncomfortable I remember wondering if they would ever recover. The mouth wash did help briefly but what I really needed was a huge cold drink of water.'

Mouth care is therefore essential to the comfort of the patient and must be performed with great frequency. Another frequent concern is thirst.

The nurse plays a crucial role in the active prevention of post-operative complications such as chest infection. The lungs may still suffer from areas of atelectasis existing post-bypass, pre-existing pulmonary disease, and further collapse from shallow breathing using only the apices or breathing using the abdominal muscles because of pain caused by the large surgical incision. This reduces air entry to the bases, which may predispose to consolidation. The solution is effective analgesia and physiotherapy.

Pain relief

Sedation after theatre will vary, one drug of choice being propofol because of its short duration of action and low withdrawal effects. It has no pain relief properties but induces unconsciousness. Pain relief, together with an appropriate anti-emetic, may be administered in several ways, for example:

- voltarol 100 mg suppository; together with
- domperidone 30 mg suppository.

However, caution is necessary in the use of voltarol as renal impairment may ensue; thus measurements of pre-operative renal function, i.e. urea and creatinine, must be within normal limits.

Urea	3.0–8.0 mmols/L
Creatinine	50–120 μmols/L

(Oh, 1987)

Voltarol is contra-indicated in patients with a history of asthma.

In addition to voltarol, incremental intravenous boluses of morphine sulphate (e.g. 1–5 mg), as required, are beneficial. Anticipation of pain prior to treatment or movement aids comfort. A morphine infusion may occasionally be necessary. Patient-controlled analgesia (PCA) systems, as discussed in Part One can be beneficial.

Because of the large amounts of morphine that may be required, close observation of respiratory function is essential to avoid respiratory depression. Monitoring of respiratory rate and Pa_{CO_2} will indicate the effectiveness of respiration.

Patient comment

'She looked so busy, I didn't like to disturb her by asking for painkillers, but then I remembered, that was exactly what I was supposed to do!'

When effective pain relief is established, regular deep breathing and coughing will become easier for the patient. Regular repositioning of the patient, allowing increased chest expansion, will be more comfortable.

Cardiovascular system

Cardiac output is calculated and determined (Bojar, 1994) by:

Heart rate (HR) × stroke volume (SV) = 4–8 L/min

HR is dependent on rhythm, and SV is determined by:

- preload;
- afterload;
- myocardial contractility.

Effective management optimizes cardiac output by ensuring correct manipulation of the above variables by close monitoring and assessment. A trend is established on the observation charts by recording cardiovascular measurements at quarter-hourly intervals, decreasing to half-hourly and subsequently hourly as the patient stabilizes.

The patient is rewarmed using artificial heat delivered by a warming blanket. Rewarming leads to a decrease in peripheral resistance, which in turn reduces blood pressure. The aim is to rewarm the patient while maintaining the prescribed filling and arterial pressures. This avoids labile pressures, which may put undue stress upon the suture lines. Rewarming should be gradual.

Blood losses into the drains should be balanced against colloid infusions to reduce hypovolaemia. Drainage of more than 1 ml/kg should be viewed with caution and clotting times checked. Drainage tubes must be viewed for clots and may be 'milked' to remove these. Assessment proceeds in finding a balance between management of blood loss and providing an optimum level of cardiac output.

Renal system

Many post-CPB patients have a large circulating volume of cardioplegia and priming fluid that needs to be excreted. This will often be induced by diuretic therapy administered prior to arrival in ITU. A large diuresis may therefore be evident, resulting in concentration of the circulating volume, raising the packed cell volume (PCV) and reducing the need for blood as colloid replacement. Another effect of diuretic treatment is the reduction in extracellular potassium. Potassium is essential to myocardial cell function and its level must be maintained at around 4.5 mmol/L (normal levels being 3.8–5.0 mmol/L). When the diuresis settles and haemostasis is achieved, a urine output of greater than 0.5 ml/kg/hour is required.

Crystalloid replacement is determined as follows:

- 70 kg woman = 70 ml total fluid infused in 1 hour;
- 70 kg woman = 35 ml minimum urine output in 1 hour.

Gastro intestinal tract

The oro- or nasogastric tube should remain on free drainage until extubation, when it is also generally removed. Blood glucose levels are recorded initially in the post-operative period to identify stress hyperglycaemia and repeated at intervals determined by the results.

Once the patient is extubated, regular anti-emetics are administered as required, as the analgesic employed may induce nausea and vomiting. When a good strong cough, with clear speech, is present, oral fluids may be introduced. Patients are generally too sleepy and not hungry following extubation, so food may not be introduced until the day after surgery. Patients with, for example, a history of gastric ulceration should have their medication continued.

Investigations

Once the patient has settled onto the ventilator, arterial blood gas analysis is undertaken to assess the efficacy of ventilation. The following are measured simultaneously (normal values are given below):

- Haemoglobin · · · · · · · · · 13–18 g/dl (male); 11–16 g/dl (female)
- Packed cell volume/ haematocrit · · · · · · 45
- Activated clotting time · · · · · · · · 92–128 seconds
- International normalized ratio · · · · · · 0.8–1.2
- Activated partial thromboplastin time ratio · · · 0.2–1.2
- Platelets · · · · · · · 150–400 × 10^3
- Sodium · · · · · · · · 136–148 mmol/L
- Potassium · · · · · · 3.8–5.0 mmol/L

The aim is to normalize all values.

A 12-lead ECG is recorded and compared with the pre-operative recording to identify further ischaemia and confirm adequacy of graft patency. It also confirms the patient's heart rhythm. A chest X-ray may also be requested.

Further nursing considerations

Once the patient is deemed to be cardiovascularly stable, sitting upright will aid drainage via the chest drains and improve ventilation. Good eye and oral hygiene continues to be essential, and assessment of the patient's pressure areas is imperative as soon as possible.

Once extubated, the patient should be placed or positioned onto his right side (i.e. left side uppermost) to aid drainage and lung expansion. Deep breathing and coughing, assisted by effective analgesia, must be encouraged throughout to help reduce plug formation and initiate clearance of secretions. Passive and active movements must be encouraged to reduce clot formation and pooling of blood in the veins. However, it is also important to allow the patient to rest as much as possible, so interventions should be kept to a minimum.

Psychological support

Psychological support is paramount to the patient's holistic well-being. The unconscious patient should be informed of what will happen, when and how, what it may feel like and whether

it will hurt. Where the patient is, how he is progressing, what the surgery was and, most importantly, that he is safe must be repeated. Introducing and re-introducing oneself prior to treatment and handling may help to reduce anxiety and promote a sense of familiarity (Tucker, 1993). The extremely noisy environment of ITU can cause confusion, especially at night, which may totally disorientate the patient. Disruption of sleep patterns, combined with unfamiliar noise, serves to heighten anxiety. The nurse must play a major role in promoting a sense of well-being and safety. Gentle touch, hand-holding, etc., in combination with repetition of time and place, and explanations of events and noises, in particular monitor alarms, will help to welcome and calm the patient (Laitinen, 1996).

Day 1 post-surgery

The patient's fluid allowance is increased up to 2 L per 24 hours, and breakfast may be offered.

Chest drainage should now be minimal and haemoserous on inspection. Removal can now be carried out. This is extremely painful and uncomfortable, and it is thus essential to reduce this discomfort. An intravenous bolus of morphine, together with Entonox, is very effective (Lawler, 1995).

Patient comment

'They didn't use that "gas and air" when I had the first valve replaced, that time the pain was really sharp worse than I've known, I was really worried about this lot, but it was much easier this time'.

Entonox should be administered for approximately 2 minutes to allow accumulation of its analgesic properties. The patient is instructed to take deep breaths and to hold a breath as agreed. The drain is removed on breath-holding, and a purse string suture is secured. Drains are removed under this positive intrathoracic pressure to reduce the risk of air entering the thoracic cavity, creating a pneumothorax. This may be checked by X-ray.

Patients are then reviewed and assessed by the physiotherapist, and, with the aid of a rolled-up towel, the patient pressing it against his chest on coughing to support the wound, respiratory function is progressed.

A further 12-lead ECG will be recorded and blood samples taken for:

* arterial blood gases;
* full blood count;
* urea and electrolytes;
* clotting screen – for patients who have had valve surgery.

The patient can now be prepared for transfer to the ward. Removal of central access and the urethral catheter will sometimes precede transfer.

Arterial lines should be removed and pressure applied to the artery for a minimum of 5 minutes

STUDENT ACTIVITY

Draw a diagram of the ECG over one complete cardiac cycle. Label each wave and identify which part of the cardiac cycle it represents.

to reduce haematoma formation before transferring the patient to the ward.

Patient comment

'The nurse told me before my operation that I would be on the ward the next day, but I didn't really believe her, after all, I was having open heart surgery, but I was and I was amazed how good I felt considering what I'd been through'.

Complications

1 *Respiratory*:

* pulmonary oedema;
* pleural effusion;
* mediastinal haematoma;
* pneumothorax.

2 *Cardiovascular*. Of the many potential cardiovascular complications, the following are the most profound:

* arrhythmias;
* low-output syndrome;
* cardiac tamponade;
* bleeding.

3 *Renal system*. A reduction in cardiac output will impair renal perfusion. Reduced perfusion with prolonged hypotension predisposes to further renal impairment. In addition, reduction in renal blood flow is caused by hypothermia and vasopressive agents.

4 *Central nervous system*. Damage here may result from a number of factors:

* ischaemia from hypotension, reducing cerebral perfusion and causing hypoxia;
* emboli, producing cerebrovascular incidents of varying severity, resulting from air, clots or calcium plaques released during valve surgery.

Other effects include:

* paranoid delusions;
* disorientation;
* hallucinations.

Major causative factors include:

* sleep deprivation;
* confusing sensory input;
* constant aggressive nursing care.

Treatment is effective pre-education and re-inforcement of information with constant communication and support. Ensuring that the patient has periods for sleep and relaxation during treatment (Dyer, 1995) also helps.

Transfer from ITU to ward

The timing of transfer to the ward depends on the patient's post-operative course in ITU. Generally,

for the patient whose recovery has been uncomplicated, transfer from ITU may be as little as 4–6 hours post-operatively to a designated high-care area, or the morning after surgery to a post-operative cardiac ward. Adjusting to transfer can be stressful. With adequate pre-operative preparation, the move can be seen as a positive step in terms of physical recovery.

Patient comment

'I don't remember very much about being in ITU, but I do remember the relief I felt when I arrived back on the ward. I felt as if the first hurdle was over.'

The patient is usually received back to the ward in a location that will allow close observation. The patient may arrive with an internal jugular catheter, pacing wires, a peripheral intravenous cannula and urinary catheter in situ, most of the invasive monitoring equipment having already been removed. Patient management is now directed towards rehabilitation, as well as post-operative recovery and the prevention or early detection and treatment of complications (*see* Part One on general post-operative care). The patient will probably be extremely tired after the events of the previous 24 hours. The ITU nurse will inform the ward nurse of the post-operative course to date, particularly emphasizing factors that may affect subsequent planned care. The patient will usually be nursed in bed for the first day.

Observation of vital signs

Observation of heart rate, blood pressure and temperature is usually made 4-hourly unless significant changes occur. Observation of haemodynamic instability remains vital because the patient's physiological state will not yet have returned to normal; for example, it will take several days for blood pressure to return to its pre-operative level (Bojar, 1994). ECG changes are frequently seen as a result of the pericardium being opened. Continuous ECG monitoring may be required, for example if new myocardial ischaemia is diagnosed. The incidence of perioperative myocardial infarction is thought to be in the region of 5–10% (North, 1988). Atrial fibrillation is common, especially in the elderly. If the rate is high, cardiac output may be reduced. Atrial fibrillation may also predispose to thrombus formation in the left atrium, and increases the risk of stroke.

Pacing using temporary epicardial wires may be required to control brady- or tachyarrythmias, more commonly following valve surgery in which surgical damage to the conduction system may precipitate complete heart block (Keenan, 1995). A permanent pacing system may be required if normal conduction does not resolve. The temporary pacing wires are usually removed on the sixth or seventh post-operative day.

Delayed tamponade can occur 1–3 weeks after surgery. It may be a result of haemorrhage but is often associated with a pericardial effusion and the administration of anticoagulants or antiplatelet agents. It is usually treated by pericardiocentesis.

Fluid management

The patient's fluid balance is accurately measured to prevent complications of hypo- or hypervolaemia, for example pulmonary oedema resulting from fluid overload. A urinary catheter usually remains in situ until the second post-operative day to facilitate accurate fluid balance measurements. Adequate intravascular volume and haemoglobin values need to be maintained. The haemoglobin level should rise gradually as post-operative diuresis continues. However, this may not occur, owing to the shortened lifespan of the red blood cells because of CPB and owing to the estimated loss of 30% of transfused red blood cells within 24 hours of the completion of transfusion (Bojar, 1994). Blood transfusion or iron supplements may be required. Thrombocytopenia may occur, as described above, but should resolve within several days.

As soon as the patient is able, he is weighed; any increase in body weight above the pre-operative value is considered to be caused by fluid retention. The patient will be informed of a '2 L in 24 hour' fluid restriction and a diet restricted to 2 g sodium. This will continue until the pre-operative weight is achieved; it is especially important if there was pre-operative evidence of heart failure, poor left ventricular function or regular diuretic therapy. If indicated, blood samples are taken to measure urea and electrolyte levels.

Respiratory management and mobilization

Nursing observation and assessment of respiration are made. The patient may initially require oxygen therapy as a result of impaired oxygenation following the anaesthetic, intermittent positive-pressure ventilation (IPPV), fluid overload and chest wall discomfort, with consequent 'splinting'. The patient may develop a pyrexia in the first 48–72 hours following surgery, often caused by atelectasis resulting from mucous plugging and poor respiratory effort.

Physiotherapy following cardiac surgery is an integral part of patient management. Exercises to prevent atelectasis and pneumonia include deep breathing, coughing and 'huffing', to improve lung expansion and encourage expectoration. Advice is given regarding positioning in bed, posture, early mobilization and active leg exercises to prevent deep vein thrombosis. The patient is advised to repeat these exercises once every waking hour.

Patient comment

'The physiotherapist told me that I might experience a stiff neck and shoulders due to the bad posture I've developed because of the wound. The shoulder exercises are very helpful.'

On the second post-operative day, gentle mobilization begins, the patient usually sitting out of bed for short periods. On the third and fourth days, mobilization increases, and the patient is encouraged to dress in his own clothes to promote rehabilitation. The physiotherapist will supervise stair-climbing prior to discharge.

Analgesia

Effective analgesia is an essential part of care to aid chest physiotherapy and early mobilization.

The type and degree of pain cannot be predicted, pain and perception can be affected by a diversity of psychological factors such as the threat of CHD itself, anxiety, perceived lack of control, inaccurate expectations and the anticipation of pain (Ferguson, 1992). The type of analgesic varies between cardiac centres but might be a combination of codeine phosphate and Co-proxamol. Pain may be experienced from the mediastinal and saphenous vein harvest incisions. The latter may be accompanied by numbness, pins and needles and some local swelling. The wounds are covered with a dry dressing or left exposed. Elastic support stockings should be worn and the limb elevated. The need for analgesia is anticipated throughout.

Patient comment

'I thought that the operation had failed. As I walked to the bathroom, I had chest pain similar to angina.'

Chest pain can be a symptom of significant complications, for example pericarditis, pneumothorax, myocardial ischaemia, and, rarely, pulmonary embolism and should be investigated. However, the cause is often musculoskeletal pain, which is usually sharp and well localized and may be accompanied by a burning sensation (Bojar, 1994). The patient should be reassured that this is a normal part of the healing process.

Prevention of infection

A broad-spectrum intravenous antibiotic is prescribed to reduce the risk of opportunistic infection and may be continued until all the invasive lines have been removed. The most common sites for infection are wound, urinary tract, lung and endocardium. Predisposing factors are listed in Table 7.3. Sternal wound infections occur in approximately 2% of patients (Bojar, 1994), and wound scoring systems can be utilized (Hall and Hall, 1996). A wound infection may be localized tissue breakdown and cellulitis or an extensive infection involving the sternum or mediastinum.

Table 7.3 Factors predisposing to the development of a wound infection in the patient following cardiac surgery

- Diabetes
- Poor nutritional state
- Obesity
- Low cardiac output
- Post-operative re-exploration for bleeding

If the infection is major, wound debridement and irrigation with povidine iodine will be required. Severe infections of the saphenous vein harvest incision occur infrequently, but, in a recent study, impaired healing had occurred in 43.8% of patients studied (Wipke-Tevis *et al.*, 1996). In most instances, the wound will remain clean and the healing process continue. The sutures from the chest drain sites are usually removed on the sixth or seventh day.

Mood fluctuations

Many patients experience mood changes, which may include fatigue and pain (Gillis, 1984), loss of concentration, and anxiety or depression (Artinian and Duggan, 1995). Anticipating these can help to reduce the patient's distress. These symptoms generally come and go, usually disappearing within 2–3 months.

Discharge planning

(*See* the checklist in Part One).

Health education and lifestyle modifications should be introduced while the patient is in hospital and more willing to consider change (Mullinax, 1995).

On the fifth post-operative day, the patient is reassessed by the surgical team. This involves a physical assessment, EGG, chest X-ray and repeat blood tests, on which basis the patient may be considered fit for discharge either to the referring

Patient comments

'I thought I would never feel well again. I wanted to sleep all the time, and when I tried to walk around the ward, the pain seemed to be getting worse rather than better.'

'I went to 'phone my husband, and I couldn't even remember my own 'phone number'.

In some patients, a variety of neurological symptoms, collectively known as post-pump psychosis, can occur. Presentation is as diverse as confusion and insomnia, to hallucinations and delusions. It has multiple causative factors, including CPB and a long bypass time, inadequate perfusion, hypoxia, microemboli and medication (Tucker, 1993). Treatment involves correcting and identifying causative factors and providing reassurance and support. Some patients require psychotropic medication for agitation.

Medication

Medication will be reviewed by the cardiologist. For CABG patients, low-dose aspirin is prescribed to reduce platelet aggregation and prolong graft patency (Underhill *et al.*, 1989). Oral diuretics may be prescribed to discourage fluid retention and reduce myocardial workload, especially if left ventricular function is poor. For those patients who have received a prosthetic valve, heparin may be prescribed initially and warfarin long term.

physician, to convalescence or home. If the patient is not yet fit for discharge, he is reassessed daily.

The patient may need help in understanding what his medication is for, its side-effects and any relevant interactions; for example, excessive alcohol should not be taken with warfarin. A list of drugs and the times they should be taken is often helpful. For those patients who have had valve replacement, the importance of warfarin and attending the anticoagulation clinic is stressed, as is the necessity to take prophylactic antibiotics for dental treatment or minor surgical procedures.

Expected progress during recovery is discussed. The patient may consider himself completely cured and may have unrealistic expectations about the future. Many patients will experience problems during convalescence, including changes in physical condition and emotional reactions (Jaarsma et al., 1995). Recovery may at times seem slow, and some days will be better than others, which can affect the patient's perception of his recovery. Many patients lack confidence about going home and pursuing their normal daily activities, and it is often helpful for them to have a companion for the first week or two at home, providing physical help and reassurance.

Patient comment

'The nurse said that I can bathe and shower as often as I like. I thought that the water may affect the time the wound takes to heal.'

The patient's named nurse will spend time reviewing symptoms that can be regarded as normal and those for which the GP should be contacted, such as excessive chest pain, palpitations, shortness of breath and an infected wound. The patient can be taught self-examination of the wound.

Patient comment

'I felt confident going home knowing what the first signs of infection were likely to be should the problem arise. The nurse also reassured me that the deep wound sutures are secure and that this flaking of skin that I've had won't affect the healing of the wound.'

Written material is usually offered in addition to verbal advice to provide an effective discharge service. Audiotapes have also been effective in achieving this goal (Moore, 1996).

Patient comment

'It was useful to be given literature telling me what I could and could not do. It gave me the answers to questions that I would never dare ask. It suggested that sexual intercourse should not be resumed for approximately 4 weeks.'

Convalescence

The patient is given a telephone advice number, for example to a rehabilitation nurse or local heart support group, which may be used during convalescence, rehabilitation and beyond.

Patient comment

'My GP thinks I'm fine, but I know that I'm not. It was really useful to talk to the rehabilitation sister; she seemed to understand my problem and gave me some useful advice.'

The convalescence period is generally considered to be about 6–8 weeks. CHD is a multifactorial disease with interrelated risk factors, some of which can be altered or controlled, and it is hoped that the patient will maintain the necessary lifestyle changes during convalescence. Family members may also require support. The spouse may be anxious about the discharge home and the responsibility of caring for the patient.

Wife's comment

'He seemed so tired, and I constantly felt responsible for his pain. I wanted to fetch and carry for him, but he wouldn't let me. I thought he was doing too much.'

Activity and exercise

The patient will be aware that exercise and increased physical fitness are advantageous in preventing CHD (Horgan et al., 1992). The patient is advised to stay at home for the first 2 days, and on the third day to have a 5 minute walk. Deep breathing and coughing exercises can also be continued. A steady increase in the amount of exercise and adequate periods of rest should be incorporated into the day. Support stockings should be worn during the day for the first 4 weeks, and the legs should be elevated whenever possible. Some discomfort and shortness of breath may be experienced with increasing exercise, but this will improve. The patient is advised to increase his activity by 5 minutes each day. He will soon be able to assess his own progress and recognize his own limitations, and will begin to incorporate light activity. It is generally considered safe to increase activity gradually as tolerated, avoiding some sports and the lifting of weights greater than 4.5 kg for 3 months following surgery as this may interfere with sternal healing (Bojar, 1994). By 8 weeks, many patients are walking up to 3–4 miles each day.

Patient comment

'I thought that I would never be normal again, so after I had been home a week I started to push myself to do more.'

It has been identified that, after a week or so at home, patients will begin to 'test themselves' in an attempt to regain some independence and to confirm that the surgery has worked (Gillis, 1984).

Driving may be resumed 4–6 weeks after surgery. Patients whose occupation involves driving heavy goods vehicles will need to inform the DVLC of their surgery. Many patients experience a feeling of heaviness or discomfort around the shoulders and arms when first driving.

Dietary advice

The patient is advised to continue a low cholesterol, low sodium, high fibre diet, reducing the consumption of saturated fatty acids or replacing them with monosaturated or polyunsaturated fatty acids. A blood cholesterol level will be recorded by the patient's GP later in the postoperative course. Referral to the dietitian may be appropriate if the patient is overweight as weight loss helps to reduce hypertension and hyperlipidemia, thus lowering the risk of further heart disease. Cholesterol-lowering medication is especially useful in patients who have a combination of risk factors or familial hypercholesterolaemia. Thomas (1990) suggests that a combination of dietary manipulation and cholesterol-lowering medication can produce a slowing of the progression of CHD and lead to the regression of coronary artery lesions.

Cigarette smoking

If the patient continues to smoke pre-operatively, great emphasis should be placed on giving up. Smoking is associated with early graft closure in post-CABG patients. The risk of death from CHD is reduced when smoking is stopped (Underhill et al., 1989).

Eight weeks after surgery, the patient will attend a follow-up clinic. Some patients see this as a milestone, proof that they are recovering. Recovery is assessed, ECG, chest X-ray and blood samples are checked, and medication adjusted. Suitability to participate in a rehabilitation programme is assessed, including an exercise stress test.

Rehabilitation

Cardiac rehabilitation aims to assist the patient to make the necessary lifestyle modifications to pursue and maintain optimal health. Many cardiac centres offer a formal rehabilitation programme, although this is not nationally consistent, and some patients may have to depend on written information alone (Newens et al., 1995). A rehabilitation programme is usually organized by a rehabilitation nurse and physiotherapist, and the 6–8 week course is usually offered free. It involves health education, exercise, medication advice, coping strategies, support groups and stress and relaxation classes. Considerable emphasis is placed on building confidence in pursuit of these lifestyle changes. Should patients be considered unfit to participate in exercise, they can attend the rehabilitation programme for relaxation, education and socialization.

Patient comments

'My husband came with me to the classes. He didn't join in with the exercises, but he did listen to the health issues that were discussed. It meant that he could give me the encouragement that I needed at home.'

'For months after surgery I felt useless. It was terribly disappointing. I wanted to run and play with my grandchildren, but felt that I couldn't.'

The future

Patient outcome

If myocardial tissue is fully perfused and muscle function good, a complete or substantial relief of symptoms should be expected (North, 1988). Late complications can occur, for example post-pericardiotomy syndrome, in which damaged pericardial tissue triggers an autoimmune response, resulting in inflammation of the pericardium and pleura (Underhill *et al.*, 1989). This can occur weeks or months after surgery and can contribute to tamponade, constrictive pericarditis or early vein graft closure (Bojar, 1994).

Long-term results are influenced by the redevelopment of atherosclerosis. This may affect the native arteries or the bypass conduits. The control of high-risk factors can improve results (Bojar, 1994). The highest incidence of graft occlusion occurs within the first year after CABG surgery and is mainly attributed to technical problems or thrombosis at the distal graft anastomosis (Underhill *et al.*, 1989).

With time, significant physical, psychological and social recovery will be made following CABG (Papadontonaki and Paul, 1994; Artinian and Duggan, 1995). Many patients are ready to return to work 8–12 weeks after surgery, depending on their occupation. Women tend to experience more difficulty in physical recovery and have poorer perceptions of their physical health

following discharge (Artinian and Duggan 1995).

Patient comment

'I had difficulty climbing the stairs and doing the housework. I felt as if I would never get back to normal.'

In a prospective study of quality of life in male patients before and after CABG surgery, there was an appreciable improvement in general health, symptoms and activity following surgery, 73% being in employment and a further 8% being fit for work but unable to find employment (Caine *et al.*, 1991). However, other studies do not reflect such positive results (McAllister and Farquhar, 1992, Papadontonaki and Paul, 1994; Artinian and Duggan, 1995; Baric, 1995). Recovery may depend on such factors as:

- pre-operative health status and how the patient and his family have adapted to long-term ill-health;
- pre-operative employment, including redundancy or early retirement on the grounds of ill-health;
- the length of time on the waiting list;
- the availability of a formal rehabilitation programme;
- personal expectations of health;
- adaptation to and preference for staying in the 'sick role'.

Advances in cardiology

Advances in cardiology may be seen in terms of more sophisticated diagnostic procedures. These may include the increased diagnostic use of MRI to differentiate between normal or scarred myocardial tissue and the use of positron emission tomography (PET), which traces radioactive fluoride or carbon to assess blood flow to the heart muscle.

An increase should be seen in the usage and success of minimal invasive techniques, for example radifrequency catheter ablation in the management of potentially life-threatening dysrrythmias (Keenan, 1994), with a subsequent reduction in comparative surgery.

Improved surgical techniques

New developments and improved surgical techniques and post-operative care should improve mortality rates for those patients who require open-heart techniques. For example, a lack of donor organs for heart transplant has led to the development of dynamic cardiomyoplasty (Metcalfe and Cox, 1996), a procedure involving wrapping skeletal muscle around the heart and electrically stimulating it to contract with systole, thus augmenting the ventricular function of a failing heart. Other surgical developments include minimally invasive coronary artery surgery (MICAS) or 'keyhole surgery'. This technique has been employed for single-vessel disease but is currently in its infancy (Glennen and Metcalfe, 1996).

Another surgical technique under development is xenotransplantation – complete organ donations from genetically altered pigs. To avoid the complication of rejection by a transplant recipient, the gene patterns of the transgenic pig will be altered structurally to resemble human genes as closely as possible; this development will have far-reaching ethical implications (Wilkinson, 1996).

NON-CARDIAC THORACIC SURGERY

Introduction

Non-cardiac thoracic surgery encompasses a wide range of symptoms, diagnostic procedures, treatments and complications. Therefore surgery and treatment for cancers of the lung and oesophagus only will be discussed, to demonstrate the principles of care.

To date, there are no formal screening services available in the UK for early detection of either cancer, so diagnosis and subsequent treatment may be offered at a fairly advanced stage of the disease. Surgery then becomes palliative rather than curative for many patients. Further complicating this prognostic picture is the age group most commonly affected, who will inevitably present with other co-morbidities as part of the ageing process (Sims, 1988).

Lung cancer

The male death rate from lung cancer is declining, but that among women appears to be increasing (Held, 1995).

The most common cause of lung cancer is smoking, which accounts for approximately 80% of all diagnoses (Department of Health, 1992).

Primary lung cancer is one of the most common forms of malignancy in The West, being the most frequent cancer in men and the third most frequent in women (Department of Health, 1992)

Other risk factors include exposure to asbestos and radon, air pollution, passive smoking and a diet low in vitamins A, C and E (anti-oxidants) (Held, 1995). Survival from diagnosis at 5 years is approximately 5% (Department of Health 1992). Metastases are usually away from the immediate lung area and may be found in the brain, bones, liver, kidney and remaining lung. Various cell types are implicated, with differing degrees of malignancy and varying responses to treatment.

Diagnosis

Early detection is difficult. Patients may only become symptomatic at a later stage of the cancer unless the tumour is spotted on a chest X-ray taken for the investigation of unresolving chest infections.

Signs and symptoms of lung cancer include:

- recurrent cough;
- sputum (which may be flecked with blood);
- wheezing;
- dyspnoea;
- weight loss;
- chest pain;
- a hoarse voice if the recurrent laryngeal nerve is involved.

Investigations

NON-INVASIVE

- A chest X-ray is taken, noting the position of the trachea and observing the lung field. Tumours will be seen as areas of high density.
- A sputum specimen is sent for microscopy, culture and sensitivity (MC&S) and cytology.
- A computerized tomography (CT) or MRI scan is helpful in detailing localization of the tumour and any infiltration of the liver.

INVASIVE

- Bronchoscopy allows biopsy sampling and brushings of the cells to be aspirated for MC&S and cytology. Rigid bronchoscopy requires a general, and fibreoptic bronchoscopy a local, anaesthetic.
- Percutaneous lung biopsy is indicated when the tumour is peripheral and cannot be biopsied at bronchoscopy. The tumour is accessed using a needle aspiration under X-ray guidance.
- Mediastinoscopy requires a general anaesthetic. It involves a small suprasternal incision, allowing close examination by endoscope of the mediastinal lymph nodes; enlargement may indicate cancer.
- Anterior mediastinotomy allows biopsy of lymph nodes not accessible during mediastinoscopy and involves an incision along the second intercostal space.
- Blood cell count, alkaline phosphate and serum calcium levels, and liver function tests may reflect abnormalities suggesting metastasis.

The results of the investigations allow further assessment of treatment by staging the extent of tissue and structure involvement (Bojar, 1994; Held, 1995).

Treatment

Surgical removal is by excision of the tumour and surrounding lymph nodes or lung tissue:

- pneumonectomy – removal of the lung;
- lobectomy – removal of the lobe;
- segmentectomy – removal of the segment.

Preparation for surgery

Admission is generally 2 days prior to surgery, which is at most 2–3 weeks from diagnosis. In addition to a general pre-operative medical and nursing assessment, patients undergoing pulmonary resection require pulmonary function tests in order to assess suitability for pulmonary resection in terms of adequate pulmonary function post-surgery. For optimum results, pulmonary function must be optimized pre-surgery, treatment including bronchodilators, antibiotics to treat existing infection, physiotherapy and the cessation of smoking. Arterial blood gases, in association with pulmonary function tests, are the best indicaters of respiratory compromise; appropriate therapy must then be commenced.

Thoracotomy incisions are immensely painful owing to surgical division of the respiratory muscles. Incentive spirometry will be helpful in education for good recovery. The physiotherapist will teach the correct arm and shoulder exercises for the affected side to reduce the risk of developing a 'frozen shoulder'. The patient should, however, be aware that his shoulder will be painful to move. Active exercises must be encouraged also to reduce the incidence of deep vein thrombosis. Anti-embolitic stockings may be applied.

Aims of physiotherapy

Correct breathing exercises + coughing to:

- open all lung fields
- reduce atelectasis
- reduce the risk of infection
- remove secretion build-up

Reassurance must be given when discussing pain control and the variety of methods available. Information on the chest drain, present on return from theatre, includes, that it is there to drain fluid from the surgical field and will usually be removed the day after surgery. Breathing may feel restricted as a result, but the patient must persist with deep breathing in order to expand his lung. The chest drain will not impede mobilization, which is a crucial part of recovery.

Relaxation techniques may provide the patient with control over his own progress and, together with pre-operative education, may help to reduce his anxiety, fear, pain and dyspnoea. Very high levels of psychological support are required by the patient and family, demanding additional knowledge and expertise from the nurse (Bernhand et al., 1991, McCarron, 1995).

Patient comment

'I know that I need this operation, but will I be all right after this surgery? My wife already has enough on her plate without me adding to them'.

The operation

In the anaesthetic room, the patient is intubated using a double-lumen endotracheal tube, allowing the unaffected lung to be sufficiently ventilated, while isolating the lung requiring surgery, leading to its collapse. This allows exploratory and surgical handling. Antibiotic therapy will be introduced on induction.

The patient is placed onto his side with the affected lung uppermost, and an incision – a posterolateral thoracotomy – is established at the 5th intercostal space.

How much of the lung is removed depends upon several factors. If the tumour is classed as small to moderate and is contained within one lobe, a lobectomy or even a segmentectomy is indicated. If the tumour has invaded another lobe or structure, more extensive surgery, leading to a pneumonectomy, will be required. However, in a patient with poor lung function, only the tumour may be removed.

Post-operative care

The patient is usually recovered in theatre and may be in the recovery room for 2–3 hours, where he will be extubated unless his condition dictates otherwise.

On admission to the ward, the patient is nursed in an upright position. Information on blood loss, volume replacement and analgesia is necessary for assessment.

RESPIRATORY SYSTEM

Close respiratory observation from arrival is essential. Air entry, chest expansion and respiratory rate must be recorded frequently. Special concern is indicated because of the thoracotomy incision, which along with the effects of a general anaesthetic, decreases lung function.

Flexible bronchoscopy may be performed prior to extubation to remove secretions that have collected. This may be repeated on the ward if clearance of secretions becomes a problem. However, as deep suctioning may cause trauma to the suture line, it should be avoided. Removal of blood and secretions helps to promote lung expansion and reduce atelectasis.

Coughing and deep breathing exercises will also help to expand the lung and reduce atelectasis, which is also an important factor in helping to seal alveolar and bronchial air leaks. Therefore, deep breathing and coughing must be commenced as soon as possible and repeated frequently to promote good recovery.

Oxygen should be well humidified; nebulized bronchodilators or mucolytic agents may prove beneficial, as will nebulized saline. Oxygenation will be assessed using pulse oximetry.

The use of a face mask and system that promotes CPAP will also encourage the airways to remain open because the pressure generated does not allow a negative pressure to be created.

CARDIOVASCULAR SYSTEM

Recordings of temperature, heart rate and rhythm on an ECG, blood pressure, assessment of circulation and measurement of blood loss, frequently repeated, will identify a trend that will chart progress, allowing an early indication of inadequate perfusion by detecting hypovolaemia and haemorrhage.

These patients are frequently already compromised from the effects of coronary artery disease, and may be further compromised, especially if left pneumonectomy was required. This is due to the surgical handling with possible pericardial resection. The result may be atrial fibrillation.

Posturing of these patients may also be delayed because of the risk of the heart herniating through the pericardial window.

Further compromise is associated with fluid overload resulting in pulmonary oedema, which is more of a problem if there is only one lung remaining. Cautious fluid balance with fluid restriction is essential.

POSTURING

On arrival in the ward, the patient will be placed in an erect position to aid chest expansion, allow the diaphragm to 'drop' and promote deeper breathing and coughing.

The patient recovering from *lobectomy* can be moved from side to side from approximately 6 hours after surgery if his condition allows. However, recovery should begin with the affected side uppermost, promoting lung expansion on the operated side by offering the least resistance to air flow on inspiration. Unrestricted respiration in this position will increase air loss into the chest drains from the pleural space, thereby helping to recreate a negative pressure within the pleura. When the patient is placed with the unaffected side uppermost, least resistance is offered by that lung, with reduced ventilation to the affected lung. Therefore, the patient should not be positioned with the affected side down for too long.

After *pneumonectomy*, the patient is nursed erect until the drain is removed, generally the following day. Pressure relief is then reduced, varying the pressure as best able with the help of a pressure-reducing mattress. The patient is never positioned on the side with the drain. Once the drain is removed, the pneumonectomy patient should not be placed with the affected side down at first, especially if he required a pericardial window during surgery (left pneumonectomy) as he is at risk of his heart herniating through this. Mediastinal shift may occur if fibrosis within the pulmonary space is insufficient.

The bronchial stump is at risk of breakdown (bronchopleural fistula) if 'bathed' in the fluid collection (exudate) that fills the pulmonary space. This exudate, which begins with bleeding into this space, occurs within the first 36–48 hours and fills approximately half of the pulmonary space. Following this, the volume is increased by

Mediastinal shift

- One lung is collapsed, creating an increased positive pressure
- This in turn pushes the mediastinum towards the opposing chest wall (mediastinal shift)

As a result:

- the remaining lung is compressed
- the heart is compressed
- there is 'kinking' of the great vessels

This emergency situation needs:

- advanced cardiopulmonary resuscitation
- needle aspiration to secure a patent chest drain

inflammatory exudate, and, by the twelfth day, the level has reached the 4th rib. Gas collection within this cavity will be reduced by the absorption of oxygen, and the pulmonary space subsequently becomes full, a negative pressure being established. Serial X-rays will chart this process.

Complications

A *bronchopleural fistula* is a communication between the airways and the pleura that develops on breakdown of the bronchial stump. It occurs in lobectomy patients and can prove fatal in post-pneumonectomy patients. The exudate may spill over into the 'good' lung, effectively drowning the patient.
Presentation is:

- increasing expectoration of copious secretions that may be 'rusty' in appearance;
- pyrexia;
- tachypnoea (the sudden onset of shortness of breath);
- a corresponding reduction in Sao_2 on pulse oximetry;

- surgical emphysema;
- tachycardia;
- a large-volume air leak into the drains;
- shock.

A chest X-ray will show tracheal deviation, indicating mediastinal shift (*see* above box). A diminished fluid level will also be evident.
Treatment is with:

- an upright position;
- oxygen;
- a chest X-ray;
- the insertion of chest drains (should they have been removed);
- possibly rib resection and the insertion of an empyema drainage tube and bag;
- surgical repair.

Sputum retention occurs rapidly and constitutes an emergency.
Presentation is:

- a reduction in Sao_2, consistently below 86%;
- increasing $Paco_2$ resulting in restlessness and confusion;
- a reduction in Pao_2;
- exhaustion;
- ineffective weak cough;
- increasing use of the accessory muscles;
- cyanosis.

Treatment:

- Flexible or rigid bronchoscopy may be performed on the ward for the removal of secretions.

- A mini-tracheostomy (insertion of a small tube through the cricoid cartilage under local anaesthetic) allows passage of a suction catheter into the trachea to remove sputum build-up. It also allows the patient to continue self-ventilation through the nose and mouth without relying on the patency of the mini-tracheostomy.

Oesophageal cancer

This form of cancer accounts for fewer deaths. However, combined with all other cancers, it contributed to approximately 25% of deaths in 1991 (Department of Health, 1992).

In 1987 (OPCS figures), a ratio of 3:2 deaths occurred (2633 male : 1906 female), the majority of patients being of middle or older age.

The survival rate from diagnosis is generally poor, with 60% post-surgical survival at 5 years without metastatic spread, reducing to 5% at 5 years from diagnosis if metastic spread has occurred. Suitability for surgery and treatment is determined by assessment and staging of the cancer (Bojar, 1994; Daniel, 1994).

Risk factors include smoking and alcohol consumption, ingestion of repeated hot liquids and reflux oesophagitis. Many patients will have been unwell for some time so their general health may be poor with severely reduced nutritional status predisposing them to a high risk of infection and reduced tissue healing.

Signs and symptoms include:

- dysphagia (difficulty in swallowing);
- odynophagia (painful swallowing);
- weight loss;
- haematemesis;
- heartburn.

Investigations

1 Non-invasive:

- chest and contrast X-rays;
- barium meal;
- CT or MRI scan.

2 Invasive:

- oesophagoscopy and biopsy;
- oesophageal ultrasound;
- laparoscopy and/or thoracoscopy, allowing staging of the cancer;
- bronchoscopy, if the tumour is level with the carina (where the trachea branches into two bronchi).

Treatment

Treatment is by:

- surgical resection or bypass;
- laser therapy, which is effective with early diagnosis;

- intubation of the oesophagus with an endoluminal stent, for example a Celestin tube. This is most often used as a palliative treatment for inoperable tumours, or for patients who present with a weakened cardiopulmonary state, rendering them poor candidates for surgery.

Preparation for surgery

Preparation for oesophageal surgery involves improving nutritional status. If the patient has been unable to swallow, a nasogastric tube may have been passed at oesophagoscopy and enteral feeding commenced. If the patient is managing to swallow without too much discomfort, a low-residue diet, supplemented with high-calorie, high-protein drinks, is encouraged.

> **Patient comments**
>
> 'I don't feel hungry, just sick, but I do try to eat the meals they provide and drink those drinks. The nurse explained how important it was to my recovery.'
>
> 'I do want this operation, so that I will have some relief in swallowing and so I will try and drink as much as I can'.

Discussion about altered eating habits after surgery is important for the patient in understanding the operation itself. Explaining that there is an increased incidence of diarrhoea after surgery, owing to altered gastric function, will allow time for him to prepare himself. Reassurance that this is normal must be given, as must information on diet and helpful drugs (e.g. Lomotil or codeine phosphate).

The physiotherapist will discuss deep breathing exercises, for thoracotomy patients, and chest drainage.

The day before surgery, the patient is given free fluids only (including nutritional drinks). A bowel preparation, for example, Picolax, may be prescribed, together with an antibiotic such as neomycin if reconstruction of the alimentary tract, using a resected portion of colon is necessary. This avoids contamination at surgery and subsequent infection (*see* Chapter 8).

Patient comment

'If I don't have the operation then I'll die soon, but if I do have the operation, then I'll still die, but in a couple of years. Not a lot of choice is there, really?'

The operation

The procedures performed depend on the size, position and infiltration of the tumour. Three common ones are described below.

LEFT OESOPHAGOGASTRECTOMY

This is usually performed for tumours of the lower oesophagus and stomach. A thoraco-laparotomy approach (chest and abdomen) allows access to the oesophagus, enabling mobilization above the site of the tumour and access to the upper abdomen, freeing the stomach for transplantation once the oesophageal tumour has been resected (oesophagectomy). A partial or total removal of the stomach is required if the tumour has invaded the stomach, with anastomosis to the remaining portion of oesophagus (oesophagogastrectomy). This is achieved by 'pulling up' the stomach through the diaphragmatic hiatus and attaching it to the remaining oesophagus once the tumour has been resected. Alternatively, a section of bowel may be used to connect the remaining oesophagus and stomach, with the advantage of preserving a degree of peristalsis and thus reducing reflux.

IVOR LEWIS OESOPHAGECTOMY

This operation is preferred when the tumour presents in the mid-oesophagus; it requires two procedures.

The first stage of the operation uses a laparotomy approach to the upper abdomen, allowing mobilization of the stomach and enlarging the hiatus. The abdomen is then closed and the patient placed onto his left side for a right thoracotomy incision, allowing the oesophagus to be mobilized. The stomach is brought through the diaphragmatic hiatus into the chest. The tumour in the oesophagus is then resected and an end-to-end anastamosis of oesophagus and stomach completed. This, however, has the disadvantages of no longer leaving a reservoir for food, and loss of peristalsis with the reduction of oesophagus, so there is an increased incidence of reflux.

THREE-STAGE PROCEDURE

For tumours presenting in the upper thorax and lower cervical oesophagus, a three-stage procedure may be required. The first stage is via a laparotomy, as above, followed by a right thoracotomy incision. The third stage involves an end-to-end anastomosis in the neck through a cervical incision. The advantage of this procedure is that, should the anastamosis break down and leak, the fluid will be contained within the neck rather than the mediastinum.

Post-operative care

Following this type of surgery, patients are recovered in ITU. They generally arrive already extubated but may require ventilation for a short time to reduce the risk of aspiration. After oesophageal surgery, the patient must not be nursed flat but at an angle greater than 45° in order to reduce the incidence of aspiration pneumonia. This may occur from 'overspill' of gastric contents into the lungs, now a problem because the stomach has been lifted into the chest.

RESPIRATORY SYSTEM

It is essential to encourage deep breathing and coughing in order to displace air and blood from the pleural cavity into the chest drains. The thoracotomy incision (and laparotomy if used), in combination with anaesthetic and analgesic agents, induces shallow respiration, which leads to atelectasis and increases the risk of infection and sputum retention.

CARDIOVASCULAR SYSTEM

The patient must be observed for signs of haemorrhage and shock.

GASTROINTESTINAL TRACT

A nasogastric tube will be in place and must be kept on free drainage, and hydration with intravenous fluids will occur for some days while the patient is nil by mouth. Recovery regimens will vary from surgeon to surgeon.

Example of a recovery regimen for the gastrointestinal tract

- 3 days nil by mouth:
  - nasogastric tube (NGT) on free drainage
  - intravenous infusion
- Day 3: sips of water
  - frequently aspirate the nasogastric tube to monitor absorption, progressing to:
- Day 4: free fluids, including high-protein, high-calorie soups and drinks
  - nasogastric tube/intravenous infusion removed if oral intake adequate
- Days 5–6: pureed diet introduced
- Days 7–9: minced diet introduced, progressing to soft diet

The dietitian, invaluable to the recovery of these patients, will be involved from an early stage, helping to re-educate the patient about suitable food. It is important to eat small but frequent meals, especially after partial or total gastrectomy, which result in the inability to cope with large meals.

Patients who have undergone total gastrectomy may also benefit from the additional support of total parenteral nutrition in the immediate post-operative phase.

Leaflets and guidance about feeding should always be available on the ward and patients' questions answered.

Complications

OESOPHAGEAL LEAK

Cervical anastamosis breakdown and subsequent leakage are contained within the neck. However leakage of the intrathoracic anastomosis via a tear or through breakdown secondary to infection is a much more urgent complication. An oesophageal leak carries a 50% mortality (Bojar, 1994), so treatment must be swift. Presentation is with:

- pyrexia;
- tachycardia;
- chest pain;
- surgical emphysema;
- increasing chest drainage;
- shock.

Confirmation is by:

1 contrast chest X-ray;
2 a widening mediastinum;
3 barium meal.

Treatment consists of:

- nil by mouth status;
- intravenous antibiotics;
- intercostal drainage;
- surgical exploration and repair;
- total parenteral nutrition.

Post-operative care in thoracic surgery

Pain Management

A thoracotomy incision via layers of respiratory muscle, at times including rib resection, results in extreme pain. Good recovery depends upon the patient's ability to avoid chest infection by deep breathing and effective coughing. This encourages full expansion of the lung, effective drainage and early mobilization. Pain results in ineffective respiration, a poor ineffectual cough and a reduced ability or willingness to perform arm and shoulder exercises, breathe deeply or mobilize early. As a result, secretions build up, leading to hypoxia and infection. Subsequent respiratory distress may require ventilatory support in ITU. Additionally, deep vein thrombosis may result. Not least, ineffective pain relief causes distress and needless suffering to the patient and family.

Pain relief is available in many forms, which may be used in combination. Intravenous, intramuscular and patient-controlled opiates are effective but need to be given in large, frequent doses and are associated with:

- drowsiness;
- nausea and vomiting;
- hypotension;
- depressed respiratory function.

The epidural route is frequently used and is effective (Faber, 1990), thus aiding respiratory function and recovery. However, Richardson *et al.* (1993) have recorded side-effects of 'nausea and vomiting, urinary retention, pruritis and delayed respiratory depression'.

Extrapleural analgesia has proved to be the most effective, producing the fewest side-effects (Sabanathan *et al.*, 1990; Richardson *et al.*, 1993). It provides safe, continuous pain relief after surgery and may be used with additional methods (e.g. intramuscular and patient-controlled analgesia), opiates being required in much reduced doses with fewer cumulative side-effects. The effectiveness of extrapleural analgesia results from placement of the catheter into the paravertebral space, allowing local anaesthetic to act directly on the exposed intercostal nerves. It is thought that this unilateral blockade of the sympathetic chain may also reduce the hormonal and neural metabolic response to surgery (Giesecke *et al.*, 1988, cited by Sabanathan *et al.*, 1990). Removal of the catheter occurs approximately 2–5 days post-surgery (Sabanathan *et al.*, 1990), a codeine-based analgesic being substituted.

Patient comments

'I was told before the operation that I would be in a lot of pain, and I was worried about being sick: I usually am after anaesthetic. It was difficult to take big breaths and cough and uncomfortable but the pain was not as bad as I'd expected.'

'The pain was unbearable, I couldn't move and all I could hear was someone telling me to take deep breaths, I wanted to scream at them, but I couldn't, it was too painful.'

Underwater seal drainage system

An underwater seal drain is used to remove air or fluids from the mediastinum (after cardiac surgery) and from the pleura. A chest drain is placed intercostally to deal with collections of air (pneumothorax) or fluids (pleural effusion). The chest drain and tubing connect to the drainage system and exit underwater (Fig. 7.4), allowing the flow of air and fluid into the water on expiration. On inspiration, the sterile water in the drain rises (swinging) slightly but not enough to allow air back into the pleura. The drain must always be kept below the level of the patient's chest to ensure that the water swinging in the tube does not enter the chest. It also allows gravity to aid

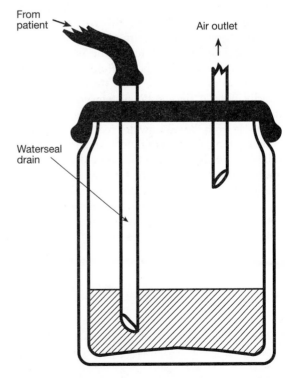

Figure 7.4 Underwater seal drain: one-bottle system

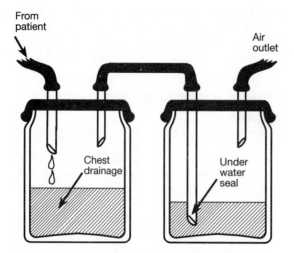

Figure 7.5 Underwater seal drain: two-bottle system

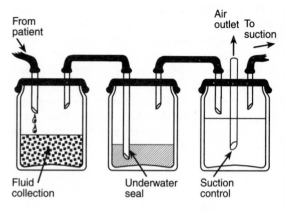

Figure 7.6 Underwater seal drain: three-bottle system

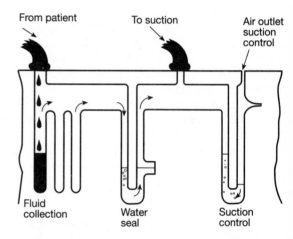

Figure 7.7 Enclosed unit encompassing the three-bottle system

drainage. Air expelled or displaced by fluid exits through an outlet tube at the top of the drain, which serves to equalize the pressure between the bottle air space and the atmosphere. Alternatively, the outlet port may be attached to suction (20–50 mm H_2O) to increase drainage and improve lung expansion (or to clear blood from the mediastinum, reducing the risk of cardiac tamponade after cardiac surgery).

The disadvantage of using this single-bottle system is that the volume of fluid may impede the flow of air down the tube, thus reducing its effectiveness. A two-bottle system will limit this impedance. It involves a drain that enters a separate bottle from the underwater seal (Fig. 7.5), thus allowing the collection of fluid to enter via a short tube. The air displaced in the bottle then exits via another short tube attached to the underwater seal bottle. By adding a third bottle (Figs 7.6 and 7.7), better control of suction is achieved. Various combinations of drainage system are now available, but the basic principles are the same.

Air expelled into the system on expiration produces intermittent bubbling, which will diminish once all the air is removed. If intermittent bubbling continues, an air leak is likely within the pleura. However, should bubbling be continuous, the leak is probably within the chest drain system. This may be at the insertion site, so sutures and dressings should be checked, as should the connection ports between the chest drain, drainage hose and bottles.

When suction is not used, swinging in the drain should be visible. If it is not, either the lung has re-expanded or the tubing is not patent. The tubing should always be 'free' and not attached to the bedclothes, or coiled where fluid may

---

STUDENT ACTIVITY

Take a glass full of clear or pale liquid and a straw. Gently blow bubbles into the liquid. Suck slightly on the straw until you can see a fluid level half way up it. Vary the power of your suction and see what happens to the fluid level.

collect and negate use of the system. If suction is used, swinging is not visible; once suction is disconnected, it should resume on inspiration. A chest X-ray will confirm re-expansion.

It is necessary to ensure that the entry site dressings are dry and intact.

Encouraging the patient to breathe deeply, cough and mobilize will force air from the pleura and promote lung expansion. Drains should not limit mobilization. Any suction tubing should be long enough to allow movement around the bed. Should the patient need to move further away suction may be discontinued and the drain carried by the patient or nurse as long as it remains below the patient's waist.

Patient comment

'I joked that I was carrying my handbag, but I was scared moving around that I might catch it on something and pull it out.'

Fear of mobilizing should be discussed with the patient.

Clamping of chest drains (UWS) should occur in only three circumstance (Erickson, 1989):

1 to locate an air leak – bubbling will stop when the clamp is between the airleak and the UWS
2 when changing a drainage bottle
3 as a trial before drain removal – monitor the patient's respiratory status and take a chest X-ray

Post-operatively, thoracic patients will have two chest drains: an apical drain to remove air and a basal drain to remove fluids.

Basal drains are generally removed on the first post-operative day, once drainage has minimized and a chest X-ray has ruled out evidence of fluid around the lung. The apical drain will be removed approximately 24 hours after the air leak diminishes when a chest X-ray shows a fully expanded lung.

Pneumonectomy patients usually have a single drain or, increasingly, none at all. The drain is clamped at all times, unlike other intercostal drains, and released for approximately 1 minute every hour to prevent mediastinal shift and maintain the centrality of the trachea. Thus these drains must never be placed on suction. The patient is X-rayed on the first day post-surgery to check fluid level in the pulmonary space and placement of the mediastinum. The drain is then removed. By assessing the centrality of the trachea on general observation and monitoring the patient's recovery progress, early indications of mediastinal shift can be noted.

Removal of intercostal drains is a sterile procedure carried out after inspiration, either with the patient holding his breath, thereby creating a raised intrathoracic pressure and reducing the risk of air entry into the drain site, or as he exhales deeply (Valsalva manoeuvre), with the same effect. A pursestring suture placed on insertion of the chest drain is quickly tied, and the patient may breathe freely again. A dry dressing is then applied.

Pain relief should be administered approximately 20–30 minutes in advance if existing analgesia is insufficient.

Patient comment

'The nurse told me that the drain coming out might be painful, so I prepared myself, but it wasn't so bad. The lady who took my blood hurt me more!'

Complications

TENSION PNEUMOTHORAX

Tension pneumothorax is created when there is an air leak into the pleura but the drain is not patent or has been clamped, thus removing an exit point. This increase of air into the pleura collapses the lung, creating an increasing positive pressure. This, in turn, pushes the mediastinum towards the opposing chest wall (mediastinal shift), compressing the remaining lung and the heart, and 'kinking' the great vessels. This is an emergency situation.

Indications of it are:

- dyspnoea;
- chest pain;
- hypoxia;

- respiratory distress;
- collapse of the patient;
- electromechanical dissociation;
- death.

Treatment comprises:

- advanced cardiopulmonary resuscitation;
- needle aspiration/patent chest drain.

SURGICAL EMPHYSEMA

This occurs around the site of insertion and is a sign of air infiltration. It presents with 'rice krispies under the skin' (Megaeret, 1994) – crackling that can be both heard and felt. A small area of this is harmless and will be absorbed. However, should the affected area spread to the face and neck, airway integrity may be compromised, and intubation and ventilation may be necessary.

Discharge

Patients are discharged from the ward approximately 10 days after surgery if recovery is uncomplicated. At this stage, patients are fairly mobile, and the usual pre-discharge assessments are made. Outpatient appointments will be for 6 weeks post-discharge. Written information regarding potential problems should be given, along with advice to contact the GP should any difficulties arise, for example should post-oesophagectomy patients experience further difficulties in swallowing, weight loss or abdominal discomfort, or should post-lobectomy patients experience further dyspnoea, heamoptysis or chest pain.

Summary

1 The incidence, investigations, indications and diagnosis of the most common surgically treated cardiac and thoracic problems are outlined.

2 Specific preparation includes assessment of the patient's physical, psychological, orientation and information needs prior to major surgery.

3 Peri-operative care, including CPB, is summarized.

4 Monitoring and support in ITU and the ward are outlined.

5 Aims of post-operative care and possible complications are listed. The principles of chest drainage management are reviewed.

6 Probable progress, including transfer, discharge, convalescence and rehabilitation, is anticipated.

CASE HISTORY

Mr O'Keefe, a self-employed electrician aged 48, is a heavy smoker and takes very little exercise, preferring to drive his van even short distances. He enjoys a fried breakfast most days.

Now he has been placed on the waiting list for CABG. To make the best use of this time, what are the most important changes that Mr O'Keefe could make to improve the operation's chances of success?

Review Questions

1 What is the pulse pressure and why is it significant?

2 What does CPB replace?

3 Why is cooling the patient necessary during cardiac surgery?

4 Why is the measurement of urinary output a significant part of post-operative monitoring?

5 What is the effect of the patient's emotions on his respiratory rate?

6 What would happen if an unclamped underwater seal drainage bottle were raised above the level of the patient's chest?

References

Artinian, N.T. and Duggan, C.H. 1995 Sex differences in patient recovery patterns after coronary artery bypass surgery. *Heart and Lung* **24**(6), 483–93.

Baric, L. 1995 *Health promotion and health education*, Module 1, *Problems and solutions*. Altrincham: Barns.

Bernhand, J., Phil, L. and Ganz, P.A. 1991 Psychological issues in lung cancer patients, Part 1. *Chest* **99**, 216–23.

Bojar, R.M. 1994 *Manual of perioperative care in cardiac and thoracic surgery*, 2nd edn Massachusetts: Blackwell Science.

Caine, N., Harrison, S.C.W., Sharples, L.D. and Wallwork, J. 1991 Prospective study of quality of life before and after coronary artery bypass grafting. *British Medical Journal* **302**, 511–17.

Cheetham, D. 1993 Pre-operative visits by ITU nurses: recommendations for practice. *Intensive and Critical Care Nursing* **9**, 253–62.

Coombs, M. 1995 *The cardiac patient: nursing interventions*, Chapter 2, Assessment of cardiac patient. London: CV Mosby.

Cornack, M.A. 1996. Making sense of arterial blood gases and their interpretation. *Nursing Times* **92**(6), 30–1.

Daniel, B.T. 1994 *Gastrointestinal cancers*. In: *Oncology nursing*, 2nd edn. Philadelphia: Mosby Year Book.

Department of Health 1989 *Working for patients*. London: HMSO.

Department of Health 1992 *The health of the nation. Strategy for Health in England*. London: HMSO.

Department of Health 1994 *The health of the nation. Coronary heart disease: an epidemiological overview*. London: HMSO.

Donaldson, R. and Donaldson, L. 1993 *Essential public health medicine*. Lancaster: Kluwer Academic.

Endacott, R. 1993 Cardiovascular assessment. *Nursing Standard* **8**(7), 23–6.

Erickson, R.S. 1989 Mastering the ins and outs of chest drainage, Parts 1 and 2. *Nursing* **19**(5): 36–44; **19**(6): 46–50.

Faber, L.P. 1990 Epidural analgesia: different strokes for different folks. *Annals of Thoracic Surgery* **50**, 862–3.

Ferguson, J.A. 1992 Pain following coronary artery bypass grafting: an exploration of contributing factors. *Intensive and Critical Care Nursing* **8**(3), 153–62.

Ferraris, V.A. and Ferraris, S.P. 1996 Risk factors for postoperative morbidity. *Journal of Thoracic and Cardiovascular Surgery* **111**(4), 731–41.

Fox, K. 1996 Hypertension and heart disease. *Nursing Standard* **10**(23), 52.

Gilliss, C.L. 1984 Reducing family stress during and after coronary artery bypass surgery. *Nursing Clinics of North America* **19**(1), 103–12.

Glennen, S. and Metcalfe, H. 1996 Minimally invasive cardiac surgery (MICS). *Nursing Standard* **11**(5), 54.

Hall, J.C. and Hall, J.L. 1996 Wound scoring system put to the test. *Nursing Times* **92**(37), 13.

Held, J.L. 1995 Caring for the patient with lung cancer. *Nursing* 25 Oct, 34–43.

Hoffman, R.M. and Garewal, H.S. 1995 Antioxidants and the prevention of coronary heart disease. *Archives of International Medicine* **155**, 241–6.

Horgan, J., Bethell, H., Carson, P. et al. 1992 Working party on cardiac rehabilitation. *British Heart Journal* **67**, 412–18.

Jaarsma, T., Kastermans, M., Dassen, T. and Philipsen, H. 1995 Problems of cardiac patients in early recovery. *Journal of Advanced Nursing* **21**, 21–7.

Jones, J. 1996 Exercise: a review. *Nursing Standard* **23**(10), 53.

Keenan, J. 1994 Radio frequency catheter ablation. *Nursing Standard* **9**(10), 50–1.

Keenan, J. 1995 Temporary cardiac pacing. *Nursing Standard* **9**(20), 50–1.

Lawler, K. 1995 Entonox: too useful to be limited to childbirth? *Professional Care of Mother and Child* **5**(1), 17–8.

McAllister, G. and Farquhar, M. 1992 Health beliefs: a cultural division. *Journal of Advanced Nursing* **17**, 1447–54.

McCarron, E.G. 1995 Supporting the families of cancer patients. *Nursing* 25 Jun, 48–51.

Martin, D. 1996 Pre-operative visits to reduce patient anxiety: a study. *Nursing Standard* **10**(23), 33–8.

Megaeret, S. 1994 S.T.O.P. and access chest tubes the easy way. *Nursing* Feb, 52–3.

Metcalf, H. and Cox, W. 1996 Cardiomyoplasty. *Nursing Standard* **11**(5), 49–51.

Moore, S.M. 1996 The effects of a discharge information intervention on recovery outcomes following coronary artery bypass surgery. *International Journal of Nursing Studies* **33**(2), 181–9.

Mullinax, C.H. 1995 Cardiac rehabilitation programs and the problem of patient dropout. *Rehabilitation Nursing* **20**(2), 90–2.

Nelson, S. 1996 Pre-admission education for patients undergoing cardiac surgery. *British Journal of Nursing* **5**(6), 335–40.

Newens, A.J., Bond, S., Priest, J. and McColl, E. 1995 Nurse involvement in cardiac rehabilitation prior to hospital discharge. *Journal of Clinical Nursing* **4**(6), 390–6.

North, N. 1988 Psychosocial aspects of coronary artery bypass surgery. *Nursing Times* **84**(1), 26–9.

Oh, T.E. 1987 *Intensive care manual*, 2nd edn. Sydney: Butterworth.

Owen, H. 1994 Mobile cardiac catheterisation. *Nursing Standard* **8**(22), 55.

Papadontonaki, A. and Paul, S.M. 1994 Comparison of life before and after coronary artery bypass surgery and percutaneous angioplasty. *Heart and Lung* **23**(1), 45–52.

Parkinson, D. 1995 Oxygen free radicals: in search of a unifying theory of disease. *Intensive and Critical Care Nursing* **11**(6), 336–40.

Penkofer, S. 1993 Women and heart disease. *Nursing* **23**(6), 42–6.

Pennock, B.E., Crawshaw, L., Maher, T., Price, T. and Kaplan, P.D. 1994 Distressful events in the ICU as perceived by patients recovering from coronary artery bypass surgery. *Heart and Lung* **23**(4), 323–7.

Possanza, C.P. 1996 Coronary artery bypass surgery. *Nursing* **26**(2), 48–50.

Quinn, T. and Jones, C. 1996 Electrocardiography. *Nursing Times* **92**(19), 5–8.

Richardson, J., Sabanathan, S., Eng, J. et al. 1993 Continuous intercostal nerve block versus epidural morphine for post thoracotomy analgesia. *Annals of Thoracic Surgery* **55**, 377–80.

Sabanathan, S., Mearns, A.J., Bickford Smith, P.J. et al. 1990 Efficacy of continuous extra-pleural intercostal nerve block on post thoracotomy pain and pulmonary mechanics. *British Journal of Surgery* **77**(2), 221–5.

Sanderson, R. and Kurth, C. 1983 *The Cardiac patient: a comprehensive guide.* Philadelphia: WB Saunders

Shuttleworth, A.L. 1996 Coronary heart disease. *Professional nurse* **11**(6), 386–90.

Sims, S. 1988 Cancer and aging. *Nursing Times* **84**(27), 26–8.

Szaflarsk, N.L. 1996. Emerging technology in critical care: continuous intra-arterial blood gas monitoring. *American Journal of Critical Care* **5**(1), 55–65.

Thomas, M. 1990 Coronary regression. *Nursing Standard* **4**(52), 50–1.

Thomas, S. 1994 Cardiac catheterisation. *Nursing Standard* **8**(22), 50–2.

Tortora, G.J. and Grabowski, S.R. 1993 *Principles of anatomy and physiology,* 7th edn. New York: HarperCollins.

Tucker, L.A. 1993 Post-pump delirium. *Intensive and Critical Care Nursing* **9**(4), 269–73.

Underhill, S.L., Woods, S.L., Sivarajan Froelicher, E.S. and Halpenny, C.J. 1989 *Cardiac nursing,* 2nd edn. Philadelphia: JB Lippincott.

Vaca, K.J. and Moskoff, M.E. 1994 Cardiac surgery in the octogenarian: nursing implications. *Heart and Lung* **23**(4), 13–22.

Wilkinson, M. 1996 At the edge of knowledge. *Nursing Times* **92**(43), 27–8.

Wipke-Tevis, D.D., Stotts, N.A., Skov, P. and

Carrieri-Kohlman, V. 1996 Frequency, manifestations, and correlates of impaired healing of saphenous vein harvest incisions. *Heart and Lung* **25**(2), 108–16.

Witztum, J.L. 1994 The oxidation hypothesis of atherosclerosis. *Lancet* **344**, 793–5.

Further reading

Abern, J., Fildes, S. and Peters, R. 1995 A guide to blood gases. *Nursing Standard* **9**(49), 50–2.

Alton, R. 1994 Arrythmias associated with cardiopulmonary arrest. *Nursing Times* **90**(19), 42–4.

Belshaw, M. 1989 Temporary transvenous pacing. *Nursing Times* **85**(1), 39–41.

Bhagat, K. 1994 Beta blockers in cardiology. *Nursing Standard* **9**(10), 54.

Blinkhorne, K. 1995. Prepared for a smooth recovery? *Nursing Times* **91**(28), 42–4.

Bradshaw, P. and Bradshaw, G. 1995 Time for reappraisal. *Journal of Community Nursing* **9**(12), 19–22.

Carter, L. and Lamerton, M. 1996 Understanding balloon mitral valvuloplasty: the Inoue technique. *Intensive and Critical Care Nursing* **12**(3), 147–54.

Chambers, J. 1995 Thoracic aortic dissection. *Nursing Standard* **9**(35), 50–1.

Colizza, D.F. 1995 Action stat series: Dislodged chest tube. *Nursing* **95**(25), 33.

Cornock, M. 1996 Making sense of central venous pressure. *Nursing Times* **92**(40), 38–9.

Elliot, P. 1994 Nutritional factors in blood pressure. *Journal of Human Hypertension* **8**(8), 595–601.

Feneck, R.O. 1996 Cardiac surgery and intensive care. *British Journal of Intensive Care* **5**, 155–61.

Fosse, M.A. 1989 *Thoracic surgery.* London: Austen Cornish.

Gift, A.G., Spearing, Bolgiano, C. and Cunningham, J. 1991 Sensations during chest tube removal. *Heart and Lung* **20**(2), 131–6.

Girling, D.K. 1990 Cardiopulmonary bypass, Parts 1 and 2. *Hospital Update* **10**, 799–804; **11**, 875–80.

Gupya, S. and de Belder, A. 1994 ACE inhibitors. *Nursing Standard* **9**(10), 53.

Imai, K. and Nakachi, K. 1995 Cross sectional study of effects of drinking green tea on cardiovascular and liver diseases. *British Medical Journal* **310**, 693–6.

Keenan, J. 1995 Temporary cardiac pacing. *Nursing Standard* **9**(20), 50–1.

Lascelles, K. 1995 Permanent pacemakers. *Nursing Standard* **9**(20), 52–3.

Lloyd, C. 1990 Prevention in practice. *Nursing Standard* **4**(52), 47–8.

Massey, D. and Meggit, G. 1994 Recovery units: the future of post-operative cardiac care. *Intensive and Critical Care Nursing* **10**(1), 71–4.

Nolan, M.F. and Wilson, M.C.B. 1995 Patient controlled analgesia: a method for the self administration of opioid pain medications. *Physical Therapy* **75**(5), 374–9.

O'Hanlon-Nichols, T. 1996 Commonly asked questions about chest tubing. *American Journal of Nursing* **96**, 60–4.

Place, B. 1996 Inotrope therapy. *Nursing Times* **92**(35), 55–7.

Riley, J. 1995 Fast track cardiac care. *Nursing Standard* **9**(49), 55–6.

Rogers, H. 1994 Making sense of cardiac catheterisation. *Nursing Times* **90**(36), 45–7.

Smyth, D. 1990 Thrombolytic therapy. *Nursing Standard* **4**(52), 54–5.

Walsh, M. 1989 Making sense of chest drains *Nursing Times* **85**(24), 40–1.

Weiland, A.P. and Walker, W.E. 1986 Physiologic principles and clinical sequelae of cardiopulmonary bypass. *Heart and Lung* **15**(1), 34–8.

Useful address

British Heart Foundation 14 Fitzhardinge Street, London W1H 4DH.

Gastrointestinal surgery

Somduth Parboteeah

Introduction

The focus of this chapter is on the nurse's role in helping patients undergoing common gastrointestinal surgery to achieve optimal recovery and rehabilitation. It deals with the care and treatment of a range of surgical operations in a hospital setting. The features common to all the pre-operative and post-operative procedures will be discussed initially in order to avoid repetition, and only specific care will be described for each of the surgical procedures.

Anatomy of the gastrointestinal tract

For detailed information on structure (Fig. 8.1) and function, the reader is advised to consult a textbook such as Wilson and Waugh (1996).

Features common to gastrointestinal surgery

Pre-operative fasting

The practice of pre-operative fasting for patients undergoing surgery under general anaesthetic, or under local anaesthetic with a possibility of proceeding to a general anaesthetic, such as laparoscopic cholecystectomy, is essential in order to prevent aspiration. During induction of anaesthesia, the stomach contents can be regurgitated and, if inhaled into the lungs, the semi-digested food particles will cause inflammation, resulting, in adult respiratory distress syndrome (ARDS), which has a high mortality rate.

To prevent aspiration, the patient is starved for 6 hours of solids and for 4 hours of liquids (Rodgers, 1994). Those patients having surgery in the morning are usually starved of solid foods from midnight and are allowed clear fluids until 6 am. Patients undergoing surgery on the afternoon list are allowed a light breakfast and clear fluids until 11.00 am. Some hospitals may have their own 'in-house' policies to maintain safe practice. Patients undergoing gastrointestinal surgery such as ileostomy may be starved for longer periods and allowed only fluids for some days to ensure that the gut is empty prior to operation.

Elderly patients who are starved may become dehydrated by the time they reach the operating room and may develop complications of electrolyte imbalance. They may also experience hunger and tiredness, and complain of a dry mouth. The nurse must ensure that unnecessary fasting is avoided. Prolonged starvation can also contribute to pre-operative stress.

Post-operative hypovolaemic shock and renal failure patients are more prone to developing deep vein thrombosis, pulmonary embolus and pressure sores.

Pre-operative nutrition

Adequate nutrition is particularly important in the pre-operative period. Patients who are malnourished are unable to tolerate surgery, resulting in poor wound healing, oedema owing to low protein intake and a generally greater risk of pressure sores, weakness and tiredness, leading to poor mobility and an increased length of hospital stay. Effective nutrition also optimizes the patient's recovery. There is overwhelming evidence of undernutrition in hospital patients (Allison, 1995), and nutritional management should be an integral part of patient care.

Patients admitted for gastrointestinal surgery may have already experienced a long period of ill-health or disability. Therefore all patients should have a detailed nutritional assessment using an appropriate tool in order to identify those at risk. Nutritional assessment should be undertaken in the outpatient clinic prior to admission, enabling any supplements to be given for several weeks before surgery.

If patients are malnourished on admission, the nurse should co-ordinate the multidisciplinary team to encourage food intake in the pre-operative period, which may be for 24 hours. High-protein, high-calorie nutritional supplements may be prescribed. If a long period of starvation is necessary, it is advisable to seek

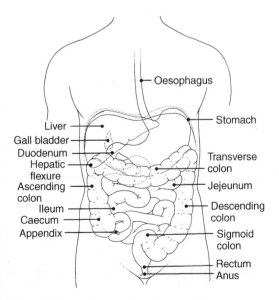

Figure 8.1 Digestive tract in body outline

Oesophagus

Liver
Gall bladder
Duodenum
Hepatic
flexure
Ascending
colon
Ileum
Caecum
Appendix

Stomach

Transverse
colon

Jejeunum

Descending
colon

Sigmoid
colon

Rectum
Anus

alternative methods of ensuring that nutritional needs are met.

Pre-operative bowel preparation

Good preparation of the bowel prior to gastro-intestinal surgery is essential for the following reasons:

- It decreases the incidence of post-operative complications by reducing spillage of infected faecal contents in the peritoneal cavity.
- An empty bowel is much easier to handle during surgery.
- It is more comfortable for the patient in the immediate post-operative period and later prevents constipation.

Patients undergoing gastric surgery do not require bowel preparation, but a stimulant laxative such as glycerine suppositories or an enema is administered to empty the bowel if the patient is constipated. This will prevent defaecation during induction and surgery. Specific bowel preparation for surgery of the lower gastrointestinal tract is detailed in Table 8.3, page 176.

Pre-operative skin preparation

Skin preparation is carried out before surgery:

- to reduce the number of resident micro-organisms;
- to inhibit their rapid rebound growth;
- to prevent post-operative complications such as wound infection, a particular risk in gastro-intestinal surgery.

On the day of surgery, the patient should be encouraged to have a shower using an antiseptic skin cream or lotion such as Hibiscrub. The treatment of skin with antiseptic detergents significantly reduces skin flora (Garibaldi, 1988). Patients should also be encouraged to wash their hair. Bathing should be avoided as it increases the risk of cross-infection from the hospital bath. Patients should then wear a clean hospital gown and their bed linen should be replaced.

Management of a nasogastric tube for gastrointestinal surgery

A Ryle's or Levin tube is passed via the nose into the stomach, to decompress the stomach and keep it empty. It may be used to reduce post-operative vomiting and when paralytic ileus is present. This is achieved by free drainage (siphoning) into a collection bag, combined with intermittent aspiration or suction. The nature and volume of output is carefully noted and recorded.

An intravenous infusion will be in progress while the patient is nil by mouth, and it is important that frequent mouth care is performed, particularly in the debilitated patient, to prevent oral infection and keep the mouth more comfortable.

Once the patient has returned from theatre, the tube will be kept on free drainage and aspirated at frequent intervals. When he is no longer nauseated, normal bowel sounds have returned and drainage from the tube is minimal, it can be clamped or spigoted and aspirated at 4–6 hourly intervals. Oral fluids are now gradually reintroduced. In the first 24 hours, the patient is given 15–30 ml water hourly for mouth comfort and hydration, and nasogastric drainage is monitored. If it is minimal and the patient has passed flatus, fluid is gradually increased from 30 to 60 to 90 ml per hour, progressing to free fluids. If there is no nausea or vomiting, the tube can be removed. Once the patient is tolerating adequate amounts of fluid to prevent dehydration (30 ml/kg body weight per day), intravenous infusion is discontinued. The patient may begin a light diet once he has opened his bowels.

Management of wounds and drains

(*See* Part One for general principles.)

Wound drains are removed when drainage is minimal. Dressings are checked daily and renewed as necessary. Clips or sutures are removed after 7–10 days, depending on the rate of healing.

Gastrectomy and partial gastrectomy

This involves the removal of part or all of the stomach. It can be carried out as an emergency procedure, for example for uncontrollable haemorrhage or perforation. Alternatively, it may be elective, as for gastric malignancy and chronic ulceration failing to respond to medical treatment.

Peri-operative management

The patient is admitted the day before surgery as full patient assessment and investigations are carried out in the OPD. The patient may require one or more of the following:

- endoscopy with or without biopsy;
- barium meal;
- abdominal ultrasound or CAT scan;
- full blood count and assessment of clotting times;
- further blood tests to detect electrolyte imbalance;
- chest X-ray and ECG depending on the age of the patient.

The emergency patient is taken to theatre as quickly as possible. An analgesic such as morphine is given as soon as a diagnosis has been made and the consent form signed. An intravenous infusion is commenced, and antibiotics may be administered. The patient is nil by mouth, and any vomitus or stool is monitored for blood. If the patient becomes hypovolaemic, plasma expanders will be administered to raise the blood pressure. Close monitoring of blood pressure and pulse is essential to detect complications. During this time, the patient and family may be very anxious and require much reassurance.

For an elective procedure, the patient requires a careful explanation of surgery and aftercare. The incision for gastric surgery is high in the abdomen, and the physiotherapist should visit the patient and teach deep breathing exercises to prevent post-operative pulmonary complications. The patient will also be taught leg exercises to prevent the complications of bedrest.

If malnutrition, dehydration or electrolyte imbalance has been identified with a history of chronic or anorexic symptoms, medical treatment and a supplemented diet or total parenteral nutrition may be required prior to and after surgery. Patients frequently indicate that they 'have been unable to eat properly for some time'; some patients may have had only a very soft or a liquid diet because of nausea, vomiting, pain and fullness. This is particularly important as numerous studies have shown that malnutrition is common in patients undergoing surgery and that it often goes unrecognized and untreated (Hill *et al.*, 1977). Malnutrition can contribute to a reduced rate of recovery and the development of surgical sepsis. If anaemia, either iron deficiency or pernicious, is diagnosed, the patient may require a blood transfusion (*see* below).

To optimize post-operative recovery and minimize septic complications, the patient may require bowel preparation if he is constipated, depending on his condition and the surgeon's preference. This may include 'fluids only' and the administration of a phosphate enema the day before surgery.

Partial (polya-type) gastrectomy

In partial gastrectomy, usually about 50% of the stomach is removed. This includes a small cuff of the duodenum, the pylorus and the antrum (Fig 8.2). The stump of the duodenum is sutured and the side of the jejunum anastomosed to the distal end of the stomach.

In subtotal gastrectomy, about 60–75% of the stomach is removed, including the small cuff of the duodenum and the pylorus. The duodenum or side of the jejunum is anastomosed to the remaining part of the stomach, thus restoring intestinal continuity.

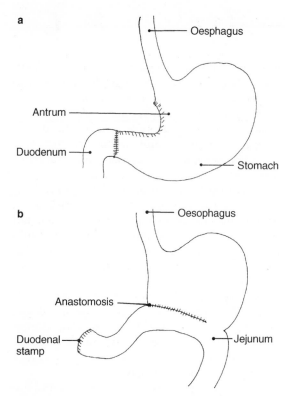

Figure 8.2 About two-thirds of the distal part of the stomach is to be resected and the rest anastomosed to the duodenum (a) or jejunum (b). Also known as polya gastrectomy.

Specific post-operative management

When recovery from anaesthesia is complete, the patient is nursed in a sitting position for comfort, easy drainage of the stomach and to aid expansion of the lungs.

The patient will remain nil by mouth for 5 or more days to allow healing of the anastomosis. During this time, he will have a nasogastric or gastrostomy tube on free continuous drainage into a collection bag. After 24 hours, the tube may be aspirated at 4–6 hourly intervals and the contents inspected. Some blood, usually altered (brown in colour), may be present in the first 12 hours, but excessive haemorrhage (500+ ml) and frank fresh blood should be reported to the surgeon immediately. Patients often complain of the discomfort of the nasogastric tube: 'I hate having the tube in my nose'. Nursing staff must be careful to ensure that the tube is secured and avoid accidentally pulling it. The nasogastric or gastrostomy tube will be removed when the patient is no longer nauseated and there is minimal drainage.

Once normal bowel sounds have returned, indicating that peristalsis has recommenced, the patient can start drinking small measured quantities (30 ml) of water. He will then progress to free fluids (water only). A light diet, initially consisting of ice cream, soup, small light meals (excluding salads), milk puddings, porridge and scrambled egg, should be planned to meet individual needs. The patient may be concerned about eating a solid diet: 'I am afraid to eat', 'I might be sick and I don't feel like eating anyway'.

The intravenous infusion will continue until the patient is able to tolerate an adequate amount of fluid to maintain hydration and electrolyte balance. The patient is given an average of 3000 ml of intravenous fluids per 24 hours. Antibiotics may also be given intravenously for 5–7 days. The wound drain is removed at approximately 3–5 days as it may show breakdown of the anastomosis.

The patient should be advised that he may experience some initial dietary problems (Table 8.1). Regurgitation after a meal is a common problem after gastric surgery, and the patient should be advised to eat food slowly and chew thoroughly, taking frequent light meals with protein and calorie supplements, particularly if he was malnourished or nil by mouth for an exten-

Table 8.1 Symptoms of Dumping Syndrome

The patient may complain of:

- weakness
- faintness
- palpitations
- a feeling of fullness
- nausea
- diarrhoea

Symptoms may start while eating a meal or 5–10 minutes after a meal. The attack may last for 20–60 minutes

ded time. The patient should continue regulating his diet, as outlined above.

The patient may also suffer from 'dumping syndrome', which tends to lessen or disappear completely with the passage of time. Its symptoms are caused by (Brunner and Suddarth, 1992):

- the entrance of food directly into the jejunum without undergoing natural digestive changes;
- hyperosmolar fluid causing fluid to be drawn into the gut;
- the sudden rise of glucose in the bloodstream;
- the rapid emptying of the stomach contents into the small intestine, initiating an intense gastrocolic reflex.

The doctor will request blood tests to assess whether the patient is anaemic, possibly due to vitamin B12 deficiency. Gastric surgery interferes with the secretion of intrinsic factor, which binds vitamin B12 and makes it more readily absorbed in the ileum, thus aggravating the health and recovery of an anaemic patient. Anaemia due to vitamin B12 deficiency does not develop for 2 years or more after a total or partial gastrectomy and can be corrected by regular vitamin B12 replacement. Iron deficiency anaemia may result from duodenal interference; iron supplements are given, and the patient is advised that the stools will appear black.

The patient is normally discharged 7–10 days post-surgery, providing he is tolerating an adequate diet. Elderly patients may require a longer hospital stay or transfer to a residential home to convalesce.

An outpatient appointment will be made for 4–6 weeks later. The patient should be advised to avoid heavy lifting, shopping, gardening and strenuous activity in order to allow the muscles to heal and prevent herniation. At the outpatient appointment, the doctor will advise on return to work, normally within 3 months, at which point complete recovery should have taken place.

Regular follow-up may be required if further treatment is needed. Blood will be taken regularly to check haemoglobin levels. Vitamin B12 will be given by intramuscular injection, as arranged by the GP.

Vagotomy and pyloroplasty

Truncal vagotomy and pyloroplasty is the surgical treatment performed for peptic ulceration when there is an indication of failure to heal or stenosis caused by scar tissue.

Peri-operative management

The patient may be admitted at least 1 day prior to surgery, but patients with chronic disease or anorexia, who may be debilitated, may need extra time to correct malnutrition and/or electrolyte imbalance, thus ensuring optimum recovery after surgery.

The following special investigations may be carried out in the outpatient clinic:

- barium meal;
- gastroscopy;
- occult blood in the stools, indicating gastric bleeding;
- full blood count and blood cross-match;
- chest X-ray;
- ECG.

The patient will require a clear explanation of the operation and aftercare, including the careful control of pain using analgesics. An intravenous infusion will be in progress to maintain post-operative hydration, a nasogastric or gastrostomy tube will remove gastric acid and prevent vomiting during the paralytic ileus phase, and a tube drain may also be in situ.

The physiotherapist will visit the patient to advise about breathing and leg exercises to prevent pulmonary infection and circulatory complications such as deep vein thrombosis.

The stomach must be empty following a period of starvation for 4–6 hours prior to surgery. It is more comfortable for the patient post-operatively if the bowels have been cleared by the use of an appropriate laxative.

A vagotomy entails a mildline incision, isolating and dividing the vagus nerve, which abolishes the neurogenic production of acid in the stomach and slows gastric motility. As this interferes with gastric emptying, it is often accompanied by a pyloroplasty – enlargement of the exit of the stomach to encourage gastric drainage (Fig. 8.3a).

In a selective vagotomy (Fig. 8.3b), the vagal fibres to the stomach are divided and the possible effects of visceral denervation outside the stomach avoided. Pyloric denervation still takes place, resulting in gastric stasis, so pyloroplasty must be performed.

Highly selective vagotomy (Fig. 8.3c) involves isolating the branches of the vagus nerve and retaining intact those supplying the pyloric sphincter, dividing the remaining nerves; this reduces the vagal phase of acid secretion but does not affect motility.

Post-operative management

The patient will be starved for the first 24–72 hours post-operatively because of paralytic ileus and also to allow healing. During this time, the patient will have a nasogastric tube in situ (*see* features common to gastrointestinal surgery above for management).

The intravenous infusion will be continued until the patient is able to tolerate a fluid intake adequate to maintain hydration. Antibiotics may be given via this route.

The patient should be advised that he may initially have some dietary problems and should continue regulating his diet. The dietitian will visit the patient to discuss a dietary regimen as outlined in Table 8.2.

The wound drain is removed after 48–72 hours, with minimal discomfort to the patient. He is discharged home 7–10 days post-operatively or earlier.

Early and/or late complications may develop:

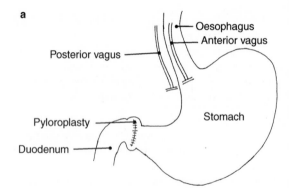

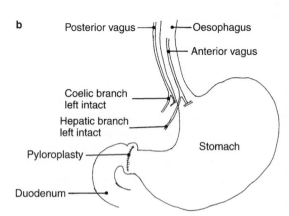

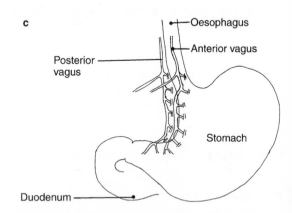

Figure 8.3 (a) Truncal vagotomy and pyloroplasty. (b) Selective vagotomy and pyloroplasty. (c) Highly selective vagotomy.

1 *Early complications*:

- paralytic ileus;
- mechanical intestinal obstruction/twisted bowel;

Table 8.2 Principles of dietary advice

- Eat small light meals
- Meals are taken at frequent intervals
- Supplements if patient is malnourished
- Avoid large volume of fluids
- Eat more carbohydrates
- Avoid high glucose meals

- transient dysphagia (because of the delay in stomach emptying).

2 *Late complications*:

- fistulae;
- dumping syndrome;
- anaemia;
- weight loss;
- bilious vomiting;
- diarrhoea.

An outpatient appointment will be made for 4–6 weeks, and the doctor may request a full blood count to check for iron deficiency anaemia (see p. 173). The patient is advised to avoid heavy lifting or straining for between 6 weeks and 3 months in order to prevent herniation. Return to work and full activity can be planned for approximately 3 months.

Partial gastrectomy and polya reconstruction interfere with the duodenal absorption of iron, and a microcytic anaemia may develop. If patients are unwilling to eat a normal diet, weight loss is common, and they may suffer from the effects of malnutrition – muscle loss, low albumin level, oedema, impaired immunity, poor wound healing and apathy.

The loss of the function of the pylorus allows bile to reach the stomach and may cause atrophic gastritis associated with bilious vomiting (Dudley, 1989).

Colectomy

Colectomy is the resection of part of the colon for a complete or partial obstruction of the bowel, as for carcinoma. A restorative colectomy (without the formation of a stoma) can be performed providing attention is directed towards constructing an anastomosis that has a good blood supply. This can be carried out as an elective or an emergency procedure. *See* Table 8.4 (page 179) for pre-operative investigations.

Peri-operative management

The patient will be admitted 1 or 2 days before elective surgery. If he has a history of chronic disease or anorexic symptoms, dehydration, malnutrition or electrolyte imbalance, medical treatment may be required as well as a supplemented diet to ensure optimum recovery.

Strict bowel preparation (Table 8.3) is the key to safe gastrointestinal surgery and is essential for the following reasons:

- It minimizes any post-operative septic complications by reducing the spillage of faecal matter in the peritoneal cavity.

- It ensures that the bowel is free of faeces, thus facilitating handling of the bowel during surgery.

- It enables safe anastomosis. Emergency surgery without bowel preparation may require stoma formation owing to faecal contamination and the inability to perform a safe anastomosis.

In an emergency situation, the patient will be admitted and taken to theatre as soon as possible. A limited number of essential investigations will be performed depending on the patient's general status. An intravenous infusion is commenced, and an antibiotic may be administered. The patient will be nil by mouth, and a nasogastric tube may be inserted if he feels nauseated, has been vomiting or fluid levels are seen on the X-ray. Analgesia is given and a stoma site marked as a precaution.

Table 8.3   Regimen for bowel preparation for bowel surgery

Method A

1 Early admission, the day before surgery at approximately 7.30/8.00 am
2 A strong aperient – Picolax at 8 am and 2 pm
3 The patient is encouraged to drink at least 3 L of fluid. He can have nourishing fluids, e.g. Fortisips (at least three cans)
4 The patient is only allowed clear soup and jelly for food
5 The patient may require intravenous fluids from midday for hydration and electrolyte balance
6 The patient is to remain nil by mouth from midnight but could have water until 6.00 am for morning lists or 11.00 am for afternoon lists

Method B

1 Admission 2 days pre-operatively
2 A strong aperient – Picolax at 2.00 pm on the first day, followed by a low-residue diet from midday. Nourishing fluids may be given for the evening meal
3 Then as per Method A for the second day

Method C

1 Early admision – 2 days before surgery
2 Give 'Clean Prep', one sachet per litre of water at 10.00 am and 2.00 pm on the first day
3 On day 2, give four sachets of 'Clean Prep' in 4 L of water until the stools are clear. This procedure will clear the bowel and does not cause colonic spasm and pain. The patient can have nourishing fluids on both days and remain nil by mouth from 6 hours prior to surgery.

Surgery will depend on the position of the growth or abnormality and whether or not obstruction is present. The available operations are illustrated in Fig. 8.4 a–c. A long right or left paramedian incision is usually the best approach as wide access is essential.

Management of a stoma will be discussed below.

Post-operative management

An intravenous infusion will be in progress to maintain hydration as the patient will be nil by mouth for at least 4–7 days or until bowel sounds are heard, usually around 5–7 days depending on the extent of bowel manipulation. Until then, the patient may have a nasogastric tube in position to prevent vomiting during the paralytic ileus phase (*see* features common to gastrointestinal surgery, above, for the management of a nasogastric tube).

The first bowel action may be altered blood or watery bile, and the patient should be informed

of this so that he is not alarmed and reassured that it will settle in a couple of days. If diarrhoea becomes a problem, an antimotility drug such as Imodium may be prescribed.

The patient will be able to progress gradually to a light and then a normal diet. High-calorie, high-protein nutritional supplements may be required to accelerate recovery and healing, especially if the patient is debilitated or malnourished. Patients comment that they have, 'lost appetite and do not feel hungry like they used to'. In such cases, appropriate measures should be taken to meet the patient's nutritional needs.

After surgery, an abdominal washout is often performed and one or two drains inserted. A suction drain is used during the first 24 hours to remove the excessive drainage, which can be up to 500 ml. A second gravity drain is kept in situ for 3–5 days. The wound drain should cause little discomfort on removal. The wound will be dressed as necessary, and the clips or sutures will be removed between the seventh and tenth day when the wound is healed.

The physiotherapist will visit the patient at

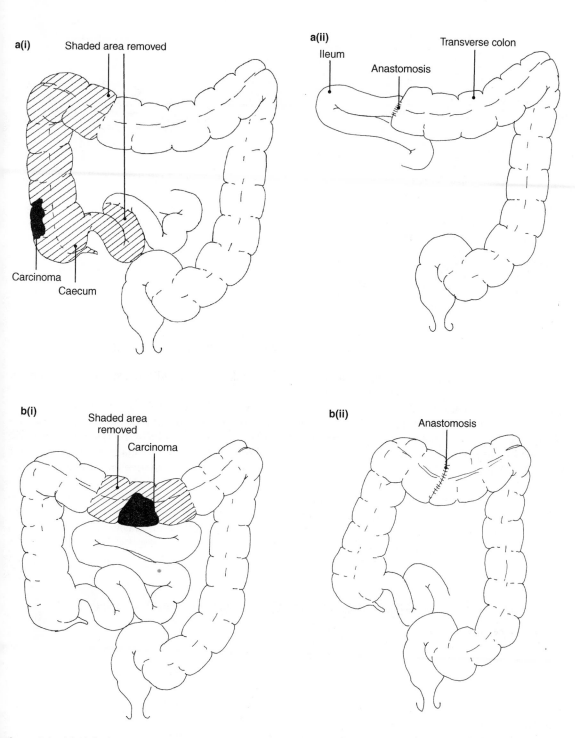

Figure 8.4 (a) Right hemicolectomy for carcinoma of the caecum before (i) and after (ii) ileotransverse colonic anastomosis. (b) Transverse colectomy for carcinoma before (i) and after (ii) end-to-end anastomosis

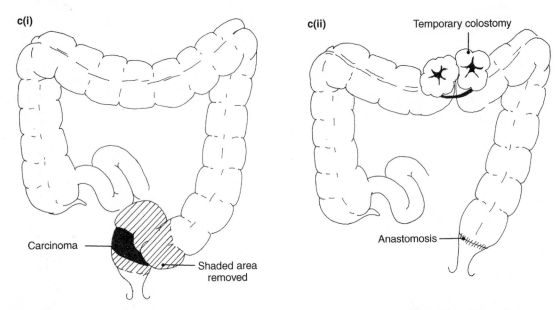

c(i)

Carcinoma

Shaded area removed

c(ii)

Temporary colostomy

Anastomosis

Figure 8.4 *continued*   (c) Excision of sigmoid colon and upper rectum for carcinoma (i) and end-to-end anastomosis (restorative resection) following excision of sigmoid colon and upper rectum for carcinoma (ii).

least daily to encourage mobilization and deep breathing exercises to prevent the complications of bedrest. These activities should be reinforced by the nursing staff. Unless contraindicated, the patient should wear anti-embolic stockings and be given subcutaneous heparin while in hospital. Antibiotic therapy may be continued for up to 5 days.

The patient is normally discharged from hospital approximately 10 days after the surgery or as soon as he is able to tolerate an adequate diet and is independent. The patient is advised not to undertake any heavy lifting, straining, gardening, etc. for 8–12 weeks.

An outpatient appointment will be arranged for 4–6 weeks so that doctors can assess the patient's progress and discuss his return to work. If the patient has a manual occupation, longer convalescence or alternative employment may be advised.

Some patients who have had a malignant condition or one predisposing to malignancy will need regular follow-up checks and possibly also require further treatment.

Surgery involving the formation of a colostomy or ileostomy

Surgery involves the formation of a temporary or permanent stoma by bringing the open end of a healthy colon or ileum to the surface of the abdomen to form an exit for waste matter. This may be an elective or an emergency procedure to treat various conditions that require the bowel to be rested, to relieve obstruction or to allow healing.

A temporary colostomy may be required:

- to relieve acute intestinal obstruction or perforation;
- for bowel trauma;
- in rectal or anal surgery;
- to allow healing of anastomosed bowel;
- to allow healing of a fistula;

• to allow healing of deep sacral pressure sores where faecal contamination is a problem.

A permanent colostomy may be performed when the large intestine, rectum or anus is diseased or damaged, thus necessitating excision or bypass. It encompasses:

• pan-proctocolectomy and anterior resection of rectum with the formation of a permanent colostomy for chronic extensive Crohn's disease or carcinoma of the rectum or anus;
• trauma to the spinal cord, resulting in perineal nerve damage.

A temporary ileostomy may be carried out as an elective or emergency procedure for the treatment of various conditions, such as extensive carcinoma of the large bowel, providing a temporary bypass away from the operated area. The sphincter muscles and anus may be left intact for the formation of an ileal pouch at a later date (see below).

A permanent ileostomy may be performed, when the whole of the colon has been removed as well as the rectum and the anus, for conditions such as chronic inflammatory bowel disease failing to respond to medical treatment.

Peri-operative management

In acute conditions such as bowel perforation or acute intestinal obstruction, emergency surgery will be carried out as quickly as possible with minimal pre-operative preparation. With elective surgery, the patient may be admitted 2–3 days prior to surgery for investigations (Table 8.4) and a full assessment.

Table 8.4 Pre-operative investigations for patients undergoing bowel surgery

• Barium enema
• Sigmoidoscopy/colonoscopy
• Ultrasound
• Full blood count and clotting times
• Electrolyte balance
• Blood grouping and cross-matching
• Stoma siting and counselling
• Chest and abdominal X-rays
• ECGs

In an emergency situation, the patient will be taken to theatre as quickly as possible. An analgesic should be given immediately after initial assessment and signature of the consent form. Clear explanation must be given. An intravenous infusion is commenced and antibiotics may be administered, during which time much reassurance is necessary Vital signs are monitored to detect hypovolaemia and septicaemia.

Post-operative care will include:

• pain management;
• 15–30 ml of water orally to maintain mouth comfort;
• a nasogastric tube to prevent vomiting;
• an intravenous infusion to maintain hydration;
• wound drains;
• care of the stoma;
• care of the perineal wound and perineal drain;
• management of a urinary catheter;
• chest physiotherapy.

Careful siting of the stoma by the stoma therapist will ensure that the appliance does not interfere with activities of daily living when the patient returns home. A more in depth discussion of stoma care is included below.

Rigorous pre-operative assessment will take place, especially for those with a history of chronic disease, weight loss and anorexia. Any nutritional deficits or electrolyte imbalances need to be corrected as a catabolic state can be detrimental to a patient undergoing major surgery, significantly affecting morbidity and mortality (Allison, 1995). Bowel preparation (Table 8.3) will be required to reduce post-operative complications and lessen the spillage of faecal matter into the abdominal cavity; surgery on an unprepared bowel carries a high risk of sepsis. Prophylactic antibiotics may be given with the premedication and on induction.

For patients who may have a form of irritable bowel disease, rigorous aperients may be inappropriate, in which case a gentle aperient may be prescribed and the patient restricted to oral fluids for 24 hours prior to surgery.

The physiotherapist will visit the patient to teach deep breathing and leg exercises.

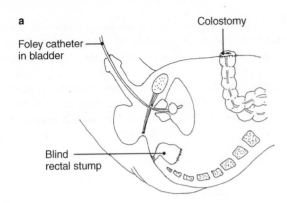

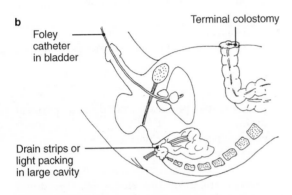

Figure 8.5 (a) Hartmann's operation resection of the rectum, with the blind rectal stump preserved for reconstructive surgery. (b) Abdominoperineal excision of the rectum. Formation of a permanent colostomy, with rectum and anus removed.

TEMPORARY COLOSTOMY (HARTMANN'S OPERATION)

This involves excising the problem area, for example the growth or obstruction, and bringing the proximal end of the colon to the surface of the abdominal wall to form a stoma (Fig 8.5a). The rectal stump is closed for later reconstructive surgery. The distal end can also be brought to the surface to form a loop colostomy (transverse colostomy or defunctioning colostomy) or can be closed and left in position.

PERMANENT COLOSTOMY (ABDOMINOPERINEAL RESECTION)

The diseased part of the bowel, as well as the rectum with its mesentery and anus, is removed

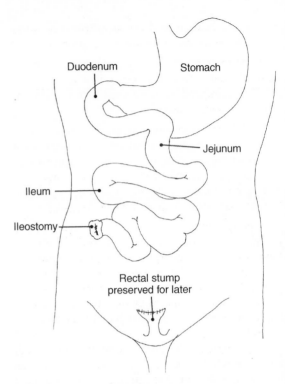

Figure 8.6 After ileostomy

(Fig. 8.5b). The distal end of the remaining bowel is then brought out of the abdominal wall to form a colostomy.

TEMPORARY LOOP ILEOSTOMY

The affected portion of the bowel is excised and the rectum is retained and closed off. The distal end of the ileum is then brought out onto the surface of the abdominal wall as a terminal ileostomy (Fig 8.6).

Post-operative management

Now that the 'eversion' technique of ileostomy construction is almost universally employed, post-operative faecal output from the ileostomy is low in the first few days after surgery. When the ileostomy first functions, the daily output is small, increasing on each subsequent post-operative day. Over the days, a satisfactory equilibrium is reached (otherwise the body will

Table 8.5 Features of the return of peristalsis

1 The patient does not complain of nausea
2 The abdomen is less distended
3 The patient starts to pass flatus freely
4 Bowel sounds are present

become dehydrated) so the nurse must closely monitor for fluid and electrolyte imbalance of patients who develop a high ileostomy output (1000 ml per 24 hours).

Indications for the cessation of paralytic ileus are listed in Table 8.5.

STUDENT ACTIVITY

Listen with a stethoscope to your own bowel as an indication of normal sounds.

Paralytic ileus may last between 4 and 7 days, until which time the patient may have an intravenous infusion and a nasogastric tube; this will be on free drainage and aspirated 4 hourly. For management of a nasogastric tube, see features common to gastrointestinal surgery, above.

Patients return from theatre with a urethral catheter in situ as urinary retention is common. Epidural surgery can also affect bladder control. While immobile, drainage will be monitored and recorded. The catheter will be removed as soon as the patient is able to pass urine independently. (For management of a urinary catheter, *see* Chapter 10.)

The patient will be able very gradually to progress to a normal diet, and the dietitian may need to visit the patient and family to give advice. Protein and calorie supplements may be necessary to hasten the recovery of the debilitated patient. If the patient is unable to tolerate a diet adequate to satisfy the basal metabolic rate, enteral or parenteral feeding may be considered.

The wound drain is removed after 3–5 days or when bowel sounds are present. This should cause little discomfort to the patient as long as he has been told what will happen.

A perineal drain is often in situ as fluid gravitates down to the suture line, causing maceration and wound breakdown. If there is a perineal wound, it may be open or closed and will require

Table 8.6 Clinical features of peritonitis

1 Symptoms:

- abdominal pain
- nausea
- vomiting

2 Signs:

- pyrexia
- abdominal tenderness
- absent bowel sounds

3 Later:

- abdominal distension
- hypotension
- shock
- respiratory, renal and cardiac failure

Table 8.7 Antiperitonitis regimen (also known as 'drip and suck' regime)

- Nil by mouth
- Nasogastric tube
- Antibiotics
- Intravenous infusion

regular attention. The perineal area should be kept clean and dry, and the dressing changed as often as necessary. Dressings are held in place with a pad or disposable pants, which may cause some discomfort, particularly in the sitting position. Some patients complain of phantom rectal sensations and feeling a need to defaecate.

Antibiotic therapy may be continued for up to 5 days to reduce the risk of peritonitis. The nurse should monitor closely for signs and symptoms of peritonitis (Table 8.6) as there is an increased risk of mortality if it develops. Antiperitonitis measures are illustrated in Table 8.7.

Patients who are malnourished prior to surgery will require particular attention to their skin, especially to areas prone to pressure sores. Patients should be encouraged to mobilize as soon as their condition allows. The physiotherapist will give advice and support the patient to mobilize. Pressure-relieving aids such as air mattresses may be used and total parental nutrition may be required until the patient is able to eat.

Specific stoma care

The patient facing stoma surgery is confronted with the prospect of a change in appearance and the loss of control of elimination, which can be a severe blow to self-esteem and give rise to fears of rejection by family, friends and the patient's sexual partner. Thus understanding of the psychosocial implications of stoma surgery is essential to the delivery of good nursing care.

Patients awaiting stoma surgery require careful preparation. In the pre-operative phase, the initial encounter between the patient and the stoma care or ward nurse provides an opportunity to discover the patient's feelings towards the proposed surgery. Education of the patient and family should start as soon as possible, and the stoma care/ward nurse should work with them to resolve any difficulties at once rather than later on. At this stage, any time spent with the patient and relatives is time well spent in achieving a successful outcome.

The stoma care nurse may bring a 'stoma care box' to show the patient the different appliances available and enable the patient to choose the most comfortable fit. This box is kept by the patient and used in his colostomy care.

Siting of the stoma is one of the most important pre-operative tasks undertaken by the stoma nurse and is considered to be the first step in ensuring that patients enjoy optimum quality of life after operation (Black, 1985). Following an emergency admission, a suitable stoma site may be established just before surgery, but with elective surgery, this may be performed at a convenient time a few days prior to surgery.

The most suitable site is marked after sitting, standing and bending. The following should be considered:

1 The stoma site needs to be visible for managing appliances.
2 It should not interfere with the patient's occupation or leisure activities.
3 Waistbands of trousers or skirts should not impinge on the site.

4 Abdominal bulges, creases and bony sites should be avoided as these contribute to 'bag disasters'.
5 Stoma bags should not cover the suture line.

> ## STUDENT ACTIVITY
>
> Partially fill a stoma bag with 200 ml fluid and stick it onto your own abdomen for at least 2 hours, with your clothes on top. Try to perform a range of activities at home and at work.

Leakage of faecal matter and skin excoriation, as well as difficulty in managing the bag, have been associated with badly sited stomas. The fear of spilling faecal matter and of odour can be a major problem, and it may not be easy to reassure that disasters with the bag will not happen. Patients dread unexpected disaster and should be reassured that help is available and that, with time, most will learn to cope quite well with the situation.

A pre-operative visit from a stoma patient who has successfully adapted to living in the community may be beneficial. Seeing a patient who is not wearing baggy, smelly clothes can give an immense boost before surgery and alleviate much fear and anxiety. Frank discussion about living with a stoma should be encouraged.

For patients who undergo emergency stoma surgery, the transition is more stressful as there is not enough time to prepare patients adequately, both physically and psychologically, prior to surgery. Their horror has been succinctly summed up in the following comment from one patient who underwent such an experience: 'When you wake up, you realize that your body is not the same any more and it affects you'.

Immediately after operation, the stoma may be swollen and protruding. After a while, it will reduce in size, protruding just enough to enable faeces to pass directly into the bag. As the stoma has no sensation, it is important for the nurse and patient to prevent accidental injury. An ileostomy should protrude as it has a spout deliberately formed to prevent excoriation.

Immediately following surgery, the patient will have a transparent drainable bag to allow the stoma to be observed, checking for size, colour (pink and healthy), shape and swelling. The drainage collecting in the bag should also be

Table 8.8 Nursing actions to help the patient gain confidence

- Explain that the stoma will initially be swollen but will eventually become smaller
- Show the stoma through the transparent bag first
- Empty the bag regularly to avoid possible disasters
- Accept the patient's concerns as being genuine

monitored. The daily output from the stoma varies with the surgery. When ileostomies first function, the daily output is small, rising on each subsequent post-operative day until a plateau volume of about 200–600 ml is reached (Hill, 1983). It is only with an extensive resection of the terminal ileum that the ileostomy output in the early post-operative period is higher. As diet is introduced, faecal matter will be discharged, which may be very liquid at first.

As soon as patients have recovered sufficiently and have no intravenous cannula in place, they should be encouraged to participate in their own care (where appropriate) so that they can become independent in managing their stoma before discharge and regain their feelings of self-worth. The primary care/stoma care nurse should gradually reduce her involvement in practical management of the stoma, allowing the patient to gain more control. The patient should be encouraged to make even the simplest of choices in order to maintain his dignity.

Many patients are horrified at first sight of their stoma: 'I didn't think it was going to look so dreadful'. Careful preparation is essential to reduce the impact (Table 8.8). It is important for involved nurses to show no signs of distaste and be aware that patients may be watching their reaction. Deodorizing drops or sprays may be used when emptying bags.

The patient will be advised that some foods, for example onions, cabbage, baked beans and sweetcorn, may cause problems such as excessive flatus and pain and should thus be avoided. Experimentation on which foods and alcoholic drinks can be tolerated should be encouraged.

Discharge planning is important; one way in which nurses can help is to suggest in advance the time or day of discharge. Patients then turn the possibility over in their minds and begin to make arrangements in order to be ready for discharge. During this period, they should model how they will manage outside hospital, for example dressing in day clothes and venturing to other hospital areas to re-learn interaction in normal social situations, thus gaining confidence.

Discharge from hospital is usually approximately 2 weeks after surgery or as soon as the medical and nursing staff are satisfied that the patient can manage his stoma. If the patient is very debilitated, the partner or another family member may need to learn how to change the stoma appliance.

Before discharge, the patient should receive advice from the stoma therapist regarding skin care, especially as the stoma will start to shrink after about 3–4 weeks following surgery. Patients should know how to dispose of used appliances and how and from where to order supplies. They should be given written details of how to contact the stoma care nurse, along with prescription details. It is essential that equipment is ordered at least 2 weeks in advance from the chemist or supplier. The patient may be exempt from prescription charges; this should be organized through the GP.

An outpatient appointment will be arranged for 6 weeks so that progress of both patient and stoma can be assessed. Arrangements may be made at this time for later readmission to hospital to close a temporary colostomy and restore bowel continuity. Normally after a period of convalescence, the patient can return to work – at a minimum of 8 weeks for those with a sedentary job. Those with manual occupations may be advised to have a longer convalescent period and/or seek alternative employment. Some patients with malignant conditions may require regular follow-up checks even when asymptomatic.

It may be 2–3 months before the patient is able to return to normal activity, including sexual activity. Existing sexuality may be impaired owing to loss of libido or impotence. Sexual activity may also cease if the partner feels revulsion towards the stoma or is afraid of causing harm. Those patients who have a temporary stoma may decide to wait until the stoma has been reversed before resuming sexual relations. Patients with stomas may be advised to empty their bag to avoid any disasters, and some patients may prefer to secure the bag.

For male patients, libido may be a problem, while women may worry about their attractiveness. Male patients who have become impotent should be counselled. A penile implant could be carried out to improve self-esteem. Women may find intercourse difficult as a result of displacement of the vagina or pain from scar tissue. Women experiencing difficulty with intercourse may be advised to change sexual position; alternatively, a gynaecological opinion may be sought. Sexual difficulties may also occur in male patients following abdominoperineal resection. Difficulty with ejaculation is more common than impotence, and sexual counselling should be offered, beginning in the peri-operative phase.

Only a few contact sports, for example karate, rugby and boxing, are inadvisable for patients with stomas. Depending on the reason for the surgery, women are able to bear children, but are advised to have a caesarean section as the normal process of childbirth may damage the stoma.

The stoma nurse may visit the patient at home to ensure that he is coping and to give support and reassurance. Details of helplines and ostomy associations may enhance security.

Closure of colostomy/ ileostomy

Those patients eligible for closure of their stoma will be readmitted after 3–6 months, or later if their general health has been poor. Pre-operative management will be the same as for patients undergoing stoma surgery, except that no strong aperients are given and nourishing fluids are encouraged.

Formation of an ileo-anal pouch

After resection of the diseased colon, a pouch is constructed from the patient's terminal ileum and attached to the anus (Fig. 8.7a,b), allowing defaecation in the normal manner. When the pouch is formed depends on the condition of the

patient and on the surgeon's preference. Some patients may have either a two- or a three-stage operation, but the inability to set a timescale should be stressed.

1 Three-stage operation:

- colectomy/ileostomy and formation of stoma;
- formation of ileo-anal pouch;
- closure of stoma.

2 Two-stage operation:

- colectomy/ileostomy, formation of stoma and ileo-anal pouch;
- closure of stoma.

PERI-OPERATIVE MANAGEMENT

The patient will come into hospital fully aware of the next stage of the operation. Pre-operative preparation and post-operative management for this procedure are the same as for patients undergoing stoma formation.

Post-operatively, the patient should be able to perform anal defaecation and be faecally continent. Bowel movements may initially be frequent, as the faeces will be loose, and may be difficult to control. This is temporary, and as the ileum adapts (which may be up to 1 year), the faeces will become thicker as a result of eating normally again. Discharge from hospital occurs as soon as the patient is able to open his bowels normally and is continent at night. It is important to maintain a high standard of anal hygiene.

Most patients do not need to restrict their diet, but some are unable to tolerate rich spicy meals or alcohol as these may put a strain on the pouch.

The ileo-anal pouch may undergo asymptomatic morphological changes such as shortening of villi, crypt hyperplasia and chronic inflammatory cell infiltration, in the neorectum. There is also an increase in anaerobic bacterial flora in the pouch as a consequence of faecal stasis. As a result of exaggerated immunological responses, a proportion of patients will develop pouchitis. It has been suggested that, in patients suffering from ulcerative colitis, this may represent the recurrence of ulcerative colitis in the neorectum

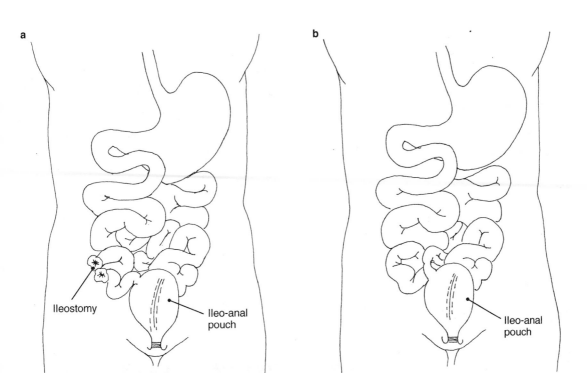

Figure 8.7 Two-stage operation for formation of ileo-anal pouch. (a) Stage 1: ileostomy. (b) Stage 2: closure of ileostomy.

(Nicholls, 1994). Patients may complain of pain, pyrexia and a change in bowel routine. They should contact their GP or hospital for treatment.

Most patients will be able to return in time to their normal sporting activities, and it may take 2–3 months before normal sexual activity can be resumed. Women becoming pregnant will be advised to have a caesarean section to avoid damaging the sphincter muscles.

Cholecystectomy

Abdominal cholecystectomy

Cholecystectomy is removal of the gallbladder, usually for gallstones, chronic infection or congenital abnormalities. Laparoscopic cholecystectomy, or 'keyhole surgery', will be described below.

PERI-OPERATIVE MANAGEMENT

An obese patient will require advice about weight reduction and be given a low-fat diet to prevent pain, inflammation of the gallbladder and stones from being passed from the gallbladder into the common bile duct. She should be advised to stop the oral contraceptive pill at least 6 weeks before surgery (Keane *et al.*, 1991) or receive full prophylactic measures to prevent complications.

The patient is assessed for surgery in the OPD, and the following special investigations may be performed to find the exact location of the stones:

- cholecystogram;
- ultrasound;

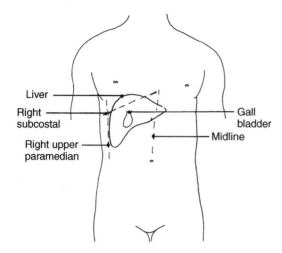

Figure 8.8 Common incisions for abdominal cholecystectomy

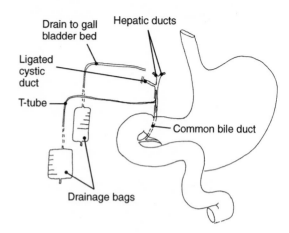

Figure 8.9 T-tube in situ following exploration of common bile duct and cholecystectomy

- an endoscopic retrograde cholangiopancreatogram (ERCP).

Further urine tests may be required if routine urinalysis indicates the presence of urobilinogen, signifying obstruction of the biliary tract.

A full blood count and clotting times are essential as there may be a reduction in prothrombin production, which may affect the clotting mechanism. If this occurs, intramuscular vitamin K may be prescribed. Blood should also be grouped in case transfusion is necessary.

The incisions most commonly advocated for abdominal cholecystectomy, illustrated in Fig. 8.8. are:

- right upper paramedian;
- right subcostal;
- midline.

The incision may be transverse or horizontal, depending on the surgeon and the shape of the abdomen. The gallbladder is identified, and the cystic duct and cystic artery divided and ligated. The gallbladder is dissected away from the liver bed and removed.

The common bile duct may be explored to ensure its patency and confirm that stones are not trapped. This involves performing a T-tube cholangiogram – the introduction of a fine cannula into the common bile duct and the injection of radio-opaque fluid. Following exploration of the common bile duct, a T-tube (Fig. 8.9) will be inserted and left in situ attached to a drainage bag.

POST-OPERATIVE MANAGEMENT

When the patient is awake and stable, she will be helped into the sitting position to encourage full expansion of the lungs, which is of paramount importance considering the position of the wound. The patient is encouraged to walk within the first 24 hours.

In the immediate post-operative period, a (patient-controlled) analgesic pump or continuous intravenous infusion of opiates such as morphine should be used to manage the patient's pain as good pain control will enable the patient to continue with deep breathing and mobilization, as taught by the physiotherapist. Morphine preparations tend to produce spasms of the sphincter of Oddi. If repeated doses are used, addition of an antispasmodic drug such as atropine 0.6 mg should be considered (Keane *et al.*, 1991). TED stockings and subcutaneous heparin may be used.

An intravenous infusion will be in progress to maintain fluid and electrolyte balance while the patient remains nil by mouth. Providing the patient is not feeling nauseated, she may commence oral fluids. Once adequate amounts of fluid can be tolerated, the infusion will be discontinued. After this, the patient can progress to a light diet. Urinary output should be monitored to ensure adequate diuresis.

The tube draining the gallbladder bed is usually removed 48–72 hours post-operatively. If bile spillage has occurred, the drain is left in situ for longer. The wound should be checked daily and dressed as necessary.

The T-tube, if present, remains in situ for about 8–10 days to allow oedema of the common bile duct to resolve, by which time the patient's general condition should be satisfactory. Approximately 300–500 ml of bile should drain in the first 24 hours, the amount decreasing as patency of the common bile duct returns. Management of the T-tube should include:

- an accurate record of output;
- supporting the drainage bag to prevent traction;
- an aseptic procedure for changing or emptying the bag;
- daily cleaning of the skin site;
- checking for bile leakage around tube entry site.

After 8–10 days, the T-tube is clamped for 24–48 hours and, providing there is no nausea or pain, a post-operative T-tube cholangiogram is performed to ensure that there are no residual stones in the common bile duct or hepatic radicles. If the common bile duct is patent and the patient has no signs of steatorrhoea, removal of the tube can be covered by an analgesic such as pethidine 50–100 mg given half an hour in advance or nitrous oxide (Entonox) administered during the procedure. A dressing is then applied and checked regularly as there may be some leakage of bile; if this occurs, the dressing should be changed. The wound sutures are removed between the 7th and 10th day depending on the rate of healing.

Post-operative atelectasis occurs in more than half the patients (Gunn, 1986) and pre-operative physiotherapy, cessation of smoking and, in some patients, antibiotic cover are required.

After a simple cholecystectomy, the patient will be discharged about 7–10 days after surgery. If the common bile duct has been explored, discharge is delayed to about the twelfth post-operative day.

The patient is advised not to undertake any

Table 8.9 Complications of cholecystectomy

- Bile leakage as a result of a slipped ligature
- Biliary peritonitis, depending on the amount of bile leaking into the peritoneum
- T-tube blocked, kinked or accidently pulled out
- Vascular damage of the portal triad
- Post-cholecystectomy syndromes

heavy lifting or strenuous exercise for at least 6 weeks to prevent wound herniation. There is no need for a specific diet, although it is healthy to remain on a low-fat one (*see* Part One).

COMPLICATIONS

Cholecystectomy is one of the most common biliary operations and usually results in improved quality of life for the patient. However, when complications (Table 8.9) occur, they are usually the result of technical errors (Dudley, 1989).

As the gallbladder has been removed, there will be no concentrated squirt of bile into the duodenum after a meal. Instead, there will a steady trickle of bile as it is formed, which may cause the patient to have loose stools for up to a year afterwards. Fortunately, the gut usually adapts within this time.

An outpatient appointment is arranged for 6 weeks, and the doctor will advise the patient on returning to work.

Laparoscopic cholecystectomy

This is removal of gallbladder through small incisions in the abdominal wall using laparoscopes.

PERI-OPERATIVE MANAGEMENT

The patient is admitted on the day of operation, the assessment and investigations having been performed in the OPD. The investigations and pre-operative preparations are the same as for cholecystectomy, so that if stones are present in the common bile duct or there is any difficulty, an abdominal approach is used. The operation is carried out under general anaesthesia, and the

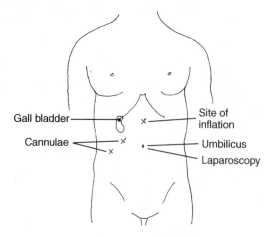

Figure 8.10 Laparoscopic cholecystectomy

nurse should give a full explanation of the procedure and its aftercare.

Four small incisions (Fig. 8.10) are made in the patient's abdomen to take the laparoscope and laser probe, and to provide access for suction and a drainage tube if required. During the procedure, carbon dioxide is used to insufflate the patient's peritoneal cavity. The cystic duct and artery are freed before being clipped and divided. The gallbladder is freed from the liver and removed via the ports. It is then emptied of its contents by suctioning before it is pulled out in one piece.

Laparoscopic cholecystectomy takes longer than traditional 'open' cholecystectomy – an average of just over 1 hour compared with 40 minutes (Hope, 1992). The patient remains anaesthetized for longer and is more at risk of anaesthetic complications. The incisions may have dissolving sutures or skin closure strips, so no suture removal is required. If there are no complications, the benefits include:

- early mobilization and full mobility by the next day;
- no manipulation of the gastrointestinal tract, so the patient starts eating by the next day;

- rapid wound healing and early discharge.

If stones are present in the common bile duct or inflammation has caused the gallbladder to stick to surrounding structures, making it too difficult to remove, an abdominal operation is performed (*see* above).

POST-OPERATIVE MANAGEMENT

Regular analgesics will be given as the patient may have some abdominal discomfort and complain of shoulder pain, which is referred pain along the phrenic nerve caused by gas trapped under the diaphragm. It is important that the patient is helped into the sitting position as soon as possible.

An intravenous infusion will be in progress until the patient is able to tolerate enough fluid to maintain hydration without suffering nausea. Nasogastric tubes can often be omitted or removed soon after surgery. The patient can commence a light diet as soon as she is able, usually on the first post-operative day. Early mobilization is important to prevent complications of bedrest.

The patient is usually discharged 1–2 days after the procedure and can often return to work within 2–4 weeks (Dubois *et al.*, 1990). The hospital stay may be prolonged if there is a drainage tube in situ.

Patients should be advised to contact the GP or hospital if they feel unwell or develop pyrexia or abdominal pain. There are always dangers associated with puncture of the gastrointestinal tract, for example hypotension, peritonitis and haemorrhage. Patients are given an outpatient appointment for 4–6 weeks for assessment of their symptoms. They will still feel tired and weak after surgery, although they have few signs of the procedure. The patient should not do any heavy lifting, hoovering, etc. for 3–4 weeks.

Pancreatoduodenectomy

This involves removal of part of the pancreas. It is carried out as an elective procedure for malig-

nancy of the head of pancreas and is the treatment of choice for operable malignant tumours.

Table 8.10 Investigations for pancreatic disorders

- Gastroduodenoscopy
- Ultrasound
- CAT scan
- Percutaneous pancreatic biopsy
- Endoscopic retrograde cholangiopancreatogram

Peri-operative management

The patient is admitted at least 2 days prior to surgery for assessment and investigation. If pre-operative assessment and investigation (Table 8.10) have been carried out in the OPD department prior to admission, the patient is admitted the day before surgery.

A careful explanation of the operation and aftercare will be given. Drains, multiple intravenous infusions, epidurals for pain management and a nasogastric tube to decompress the stomach, preventing nausea and vomiting, should be expected. The incision for pancreatoduodenectomy is high in the abdomen, and the physiotherapist should teach the patient breathing and leg exercises to prevent post-operative complications.

If the patient's nutritional status is poor, an attempt should be made to improve it. Constipation may require a laxative or an enema to ensure clear bowels.

Any pre-operative pain should be assessed, and analgesics given to control it. It may be appropriate at this time to work out a strategy for managing post-operative pain. The patient may be shown how to operate the patient-controlled analgesia (PCA) pump and taught how to use it effectively. Any fears and anxieties about this should be handled sensitively, and the patient should be reassured that if PCA fails, other methods of pain control will be instituted.

Diabetes should be stabilized with soluble insulin and dextrose solutions. Blood glucose should be recorded 4 hourly or more frequently to ensure that the patient does not develop hypo- or hyperglycaemia.

When the carcinoma is localized with no evidence of metastases, Whipple's procedure may be performed, as shown in Fig. 8.11. This involves

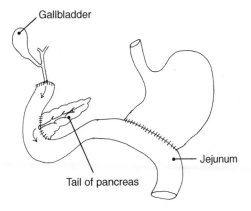

Figure 8.11 Whipple's procedure: resection of the head of pancreas, duodenum and antrum of the stomach. Reconstruction is carried out to maintain homeostasis: pancreatojejunostomy, gastrojejunostomy and choledojejunostomy

resection of the antrum of the stomach, duodenum, varying amounts of pancreas and often the gallbladder. Anastomoses are constructed between the stomach, common bile duct, pancreatic duct and jejunum.

Post-operative management

A patient with pre-operative diabetes will have an infusion of insulin and intravenous dextrose to maintain blood glucose levels within normal limits (4–6 mmol/L). Initially blood glucose levels will be measured every hour and the insulin infusion regulated to maintain them within normal limits. When levels are stable, measurements may be decreased to 2–4 hourly. Close monitoring of the patient is essential to ensure that she does not suffer from hypo- or hyperglycaemia (Table 8.11) on weaning from an intravenous infusion of insulin to subcutaneous insulin injections and dietary measures.

Regular analgesia will be given via continuous intravenous infusion as this method has been shown to be most effective. As soon as the patient is awake and observations are stable, the patient will be helped into the sitting position, well supported by pillows, and encouraged to take deep breaths.

Table 8.11 Clinical features of hypo/hyperglycaemia

1 *Hypoglycaemia*
- Rapidly falling blood glucose – sweating, tremor, tachycardia and palpitations
- Slowly falling blood glucose – headache, confusion, lightheadedness, numbness of the lips/tongue, slurred speech, inco-ordination, staggering gait, double vision, drowsiness and convulsions/coma

2 *Hyperglycaemia*

Clinical features are polyuria, polyphagia, polydipsia, dehydration, malaise, visual changes, headache, abdominal pain, nausea and vomiting, deep laboured breathing, drowsiness and coma

Table 8.12 Principles of a diabetic diet (British Diabetic Association, 1992)

1 Maintain blood glucose within the normal range of 4–7 mmol/L*

2 Optimize quality of life and decrease symptoms:
- thirst
- polyuria
- tiredness
- lethargy

3 Prevent long-term complications at micro- and macrovascular levels:
- retinopathy
- neuropathy
- nephropathy
- cardiovascular events

4 Diet should aim to be:
- low in sugar
- high in carbohydrates
- high in fibre
- low in fat
- low in salt

5 Patients should have regular meals with a variety of foods from the four main food groups. Cereal, bread, pasta, potato and rice/chappatis should form the main part of the meal

* This may sometimes be set at a different level depending on what is appropriate for improving that particular patient's quality of life.

The intravenous infusion will continue until the patient is able to tolerate an adequate amount of oral fluid to maintain hydration; she should be given an average of 3000 ml in each 24 hours. Antibiotics will be given for 5–7 days.

The wound drain will remain in position until output is minimal and is then removed, at approximately 3–5 days. The dressing should be checked daily and dressed as necessary, the sutures being removed after 10–12 days.

The patient will continue to remain nil by mouth for the first few days as manipulation of the gut will result in paralytic ileus. During this time, the patient will have a nasogastric or jejunostomy tube on free drainage. The tube may be aspirated at 4–6 hourly intervals and the contents accurately measured and recorded on the fluid balance chart. When bowel sounds return and the patient starts drinking small amounts of water without nausea, the nasogastric tube is removed. The patient will start on a light diet of soup and ice cream and will require advice about her diabetic diet (Table 8.12), being helped to select appropriate food from the hospital menu. The dietitian and diabetic nurse will visit the patient before discharge.

The physiotherapist will visit the patient to assist with breathing exercises and mobilization.

An outpatient appointment will be made for 4–6 weeks. The patient should be advised to convalesce slowly and exercise gently until after the outpatient appointment, at which return to work and activities of living can be discussed. Patients may require regular follow-up or further therapy.

Prognosis

The 5-year survival after radical surgery for those patients with peripapillary carcinoma is 40% (Dudley, 1989).

Abdominal hernia repair

A hernia is the protrusion of an organ or part of an organ through an opening in the cavity in which it is normally contained. Abdominal herniae may be congenital or acquired; there are several different types:

- inguinal;
- femoral;
- umbilical;
- incisional.

It is rare for a hernia to strangulate, i.e. for the blood supply to the contents of the hernia sac to be obstructed. Acute intestinal obstruction and gangrene (Table 8.13) may ensue, or the bowel may rupture, causing peritonitis. In such a situation, emergency surgery is required and nursing care is much more complex. Surgery may involve formation of a stoma (see above). Constipation should be excluded as a possible cause.

Peri-operative management

For elective surgery, the patient is admitted 1 day previous to or on the day of surgery as no special investigations are required. A careful examination by the doctor will ascertain whether the hernia is reducible or irreducible. The hernia is examined with the patient in the standing and supine positions. A hernia that disappears in the supine position is defined as a reducible hernia; the patient will also be asked to cough to see whether the hernia appears with a rise in intra-abdominal pressure. The medical staff then mark the site of the hernia with an indelible pen.

In the emergency situation, the patient is taken to theatre as quickly as possible. An analgesic is given as soon as an initial assessment has been made and the consent form signed. An intravenous infusion is commenced to correct dehydration, and antibiotics may be administered. During this time, much reassurance (see Chapter 1) from the nurse is necessary.

A clear explanation of per-operative preparation, surgery and aftercare must be given by the nurse, for example that any pain will be controlled with analgesics, that there may be an intravenous infusion in progress for a few hours, depending on the complexity of surgery, and that there will be a dressing over the wound. The operation site must be shaved on the day of the surgery. The patient may be seen by the physiotherapist, who will advise on breathing exercises and how to support the wound when coughing or mobilizing post-operatively. It is important to ensure that the patient is not suffering from a severe persistent cough as this may damage the integrity of the repair. For the same reason, active and passive smoking are discouraged.

The surgical repair performed depends on the position and type of hernia; treatment may include:

- herniorrhaphy – repair by suture of 'darning' weakened muscle layers;
- herniotomy – excision of the sac and suturing of the muscle layers;
- hernioplasty – refashioning and strengthening the muscle layers. Often a man-made mesh (e.g. marlex mesh) is used.

Post-operative care

As the patient wakes up, he can be moved into a sitting position, helped by nurses preventing exertion of the newly sutured abdominal muscles. Patients often report that 'The wound felt very tight, hot and painful when I woke up' and that

Table 8.13   Sequence of events leading to strangulation and gangrene

Venous and lymphatic obstruction ⇒ swelling ⇒ arterial supply reduced ⇒ further swelling ⇒ lumen obstructed ⇒ gangrene

'Moving around was no fun at all.' Careful positioning of the pillows is required to provide adequate support.

In the immediate post-operative period, regular intramuscular analgesics (e.g. morphine) are required as there may be muscular pain from the surgery. The dose needed will gradually decrease over a few days. The surgeon will often put local anaesthetic (marcaine) at the wound site or perform a nerve block to reduce post-operative pain.

After an elective hernia repair, small quantities of oral fluids may be commenced and steadily increased to a light diet providing the patient has no nausea. If extensive handling and dissecting of the gut and omentum have occurred, post-operative stomach decompression by means of a nasogastric tube will be required until normal bowel sounds are heard.

The physiotherapist will assist the patient with deep breathing exercises and mobilization.

The wound dressing may be changed within the first few day, further dressings only being applied as necessary. After repair of a lower abdominal hernia in a male patient, it is advisable to wear a scrotal support to prevent any unnecessary strain on the would and newly sutured muscles. This should be worn until the outpatient appointment.

Discharge

Discharge time varies according to the patient the surgeon and the surgery. The patient is often allowed home 2 days after operation, but if it has been a complicated and difficult procedure or healing problems arise, discharge may be delayed. An uncomplicated inguinal hernia may be treated as a day case.

The patient must be advised not to lift at all for 2 weeks and to lift no more than 1 kg for 6 weeks. The physiotherapist should be consulted about the correct way of lifting.

It is important that the patient avoids constipation, coughs or strenuous exercise as these may result in raised intra-abdominal pressure and a recurrence of the hernia. If the patient is prone to weight gain or is obese, the dietitian may suggest a reducing diet to commence 3 months postoperatively. Sexual activity may be resumed following discussion at the outpatient appointment.

An outpatient appointment is arranged for 6 weeks, the wound being assessed and further advice being given about lifting. A change of occupation or hobby may be suggested if heavy manual work is involved. The patient should also be advised not to drive for 3 months as an emergency stop will be extremely painful.

Appendicectomy

This is the removal of the appendix for acute inflammation (appendicitis) with or without generalized or localized pertitonitis (see Table 8.6 above).

Peri-operative preparation

Appendicectomy is usually carried out as an emergency procedure. On admission, the doctor carries out a careful examination, which may include rectal examination to assess the extent of inflammation or infection.

In an emergency, the amount of preparation required depends on the state of the patient. Once the diagnosis has been confirmed, the patient will be given analgesics and his condition monitored until he goes to theatre. Prophylactic antibiotics are usually prescribed pre-operatively and may be given on premedication or induction. An intravenous infusion may be commenced to rehydrate the patient and a nasogastric tube inserted to control vomiting.

If there are signs of peritonitis or if vomiting has been a marked feature, the stomach should be decompressed by nasogastric intubation. The patient should also have an anti-anaerobic antibiotic such as metronidazole (Flagyl), often given as a suppository.

An incision is made in the right iliac fossa, and the appendix is identified and immobilized. A ligature is passed round the base and the appendix removed.

Post-operative management

As soon as the patient's condition allows, he is helped into the sitting position and encouraged to take deep breaths. Analgesia, perhaps in the form of an intramuscular injection or continuous infusion, will be given.

An intravenous infusion will be in progress after emergency surgery until the patient is able to tolerate adequate fluid to prevent dehydration; it also provides a route for the administration of antibiotics. Once bowel sounds are heard and fluids tolerated, the patient may commence oral fluids, and the infusion may be discontinued.

Intravenous access may not be required in an elective procedure and antibiotics will be discontinued in the first 24 hours. In more complex cases of suspected peritonitis, antibiotics will be given for 5–7 days and the temperature monitored at least 4 hourly. There may be a wound drain if the appendix was infected or ruptured.

The wound drain should be treated as infected and be removed 24–48 hours post-operatively; if not, the wound will be dressed as necessary.

The physiotherapist may visit the patient to assist him with deep breathing and early mobilization.

Complications

- Manipulation of the gut may cause dissemination of infected material, precipitating peritonitis.
- Emergency appendicectomy carries an increased risk of wound infection compared with elective appendicectomy.

If complications develop, the patient's stay in hospital is prolonged until they are resolved.

Discharge

If surgery has been elective and the patient remains stable, he may be allowed home 2 days after surgery and the community or practice nurse asked to remove the sutures. In an emergency appendicectomy, the patient will be discharged after antibiotics have been discontinued. The sutures are removed 1 week after surgery, if healing is sufficiently advanced.

Haemorrhoidectomy

Surgery for haemorrhoids (piles), or locally dilated or engorged rectal veins, may be performed if conservative treatment has not been successful and the injection of a sclerosing agent is inappropriate.

Peri-operative management

- The patient is admitted the day prior to or the day of surgery.
- A rectal examination may be performed to

ascertain the extent and position of the haemorrhoids.

- Proctoscopy or sigmoidoscopy may be performed to visualize internal haemorrhoids and to eliminate a higher lesion.
- A full blood count may be necessary, especially if there has been a history of persistent rectal bleeding.
- Patients should be encouraged to have their bowels open before surgery, suppositories or enemas being used to ensure this.

- The peri-anal area should be carefully cleaned, and shaved if necessary.

A full explanation of the surgery and aftercare will be given, including explanation that there will be a rectal pack in position on return to the ward and that this may cause some pain, which will be controlled with regular analgesia.

The patient is placed in a lithotomy position and each of the haemorrhoids isolated, ligated and excised.

Post-operative management

The rectal pack remains in position for 24–36 hours after surgery, depending on the doctor's instructions. It is kept in place by a T-bandage or suitable dressing. Before removal of the pack, the patient should be given an injection of pethidine and helped into a warm bath, the nurse remaining with the patient. After soaking in the warm water for a while, the pack should come out with ease, causing minimal discomfort, although the patient may be extremely frightened. Afterwards, there may be some bleeding for a short time, about which the patient should be reassured. The

area should be rinsed and dried, and a pad, supported with disposable pants, applied.

It is advisable, if possible, not to have a bowel action for 3–4 days post-operatively, as evacuation may be rather uncomfortable and cause some bleeding. It is better if it can be delayed as soft stools can be promoted by administration of an aperient. It is important for the patient to maintain a high standard of anal hygiene to reduce the risk of infection. A low-residue diet should be provided for the first few days.

Discharge

The patient will be allowed home once he has opened his bowels, which should be within 3–5 days of surgery. The following advice must be given to the patient prior to discharge:

1 In case of excessive bleeding, contact your doctor or the hospital.

2 It is essential to avoid constipation.

3 Eat a high-fibre diet and avoid the use of long-term aperients.

An outpatient appointment with the surgeon will be arranged 4–6 weeks post-operatively. In the meantime, the patient can, after convalescing for approximately a week, return to work.

Summary

1 All surgery to the gastrointestinal system carries risks, which may be related to initial malnutrition, handling and opening of the gut or to subsequent starvation.

2 All patients need to be assessed nutritionally to anticipate possible complications such as poor wound healing, pressure sores and chest infection, all leading to a prolonged hospital stay.

3 If malnutrition is identified, nutritional support must be initiated and maintained throughout the hospital stay. Precise post-operative nutritional advice will be needed by these patients.

4 Bowel preparation is directed at reducing the faecal and bacterial content of the bowel, making it easier to handle during surgery and minimizing the risk of infected faecal spillage.

5 Peritonitis may be a risk in many of these operations. The antiperitonitis regimen involves fasting the patient, passing a nasogastric tube, setting up an intravenous infusion and giving antibiotics.

6 Paralytic ileus may follow peritonitis and delay the patient's progress to normal hydration and nutrition.

CASE HISTORY

Fred, a skinny, 18-year-old motorcycle messenger who lives in a bedsit and exists on fast food, is admitted to your ward with a perforated appendix. Identify the essential features of care that he will need in order to be prepared for surgery. What progress is he likely to make post-operatively, and what complications may he be at risk of? Is there any long-term advice that he might need for convalescence?

Review Questions

1 How would you determine a patient's nutritional status? Collect assessment tools from a range of sources and identify features they have in common. Design and test your own.

2 Draw and label, from memory, a simple diagram of the gastrointestinal tract. Check with a textbook and correct any errors.

3 What is the purpose of an nasogastric tube? How is it managed?

4 Why do patients with abdominal incisions tend to be at risk of chest infections?

5 Why is an abdominal wound drain placed away from the suture line?

6 Describe the features of a healthy stoma. Explain these as you would to a patient in your care.

7 Calculate the volume of fluid intake needed using the formula found in this chapter.

References

Allison, S.P. 1995 Malnutrition in hospital patients. *Hospital Update* Feb, 55–61.

British Diabetic Association 1992 *Dietary recommendation for people with diabetes: an update for the 1990's.* London: BDA.

Black, P. 1985 Selecting a site. *Nursing Mirror* **61**(9), 22.

Brunner, L.S. and Suddarth, D.S. 1992 *The Textbook of Adult Nursing* 6th edn. London: Chapman & Hall.

Dubois, F. Icard, P., Berthelot, G.and Levard, H. 1990 Celioscopic cholecystectomy. *Annals of Surgery* **211**(1), 60–2.

Dudley, H.A.F. 1989 *An aid to clinical surgery,* 4th edn. Edinburgh: Churchill Livingstone.

Garibaldi, R.A. 1988 Prevention of intra-operative wound contamination with chlorhexidine shower and scrub. *Journal of Hospital Infection*, Suppl. B(11), 5–9.

Gunn, A.A. 1986 Cholecystectomy, cholecystostomy and exploration of the common bile duct. In: Dudley, H., Carter, D.C. and Russell R.C.G. (eds) *Atlas of general surgery.* London: Butterworths.

Hill, G.L., Pickford, J.A., Young, C.A. *et al.* 1977 Malnutrition in surgical patients – an unrecognised problem. *Lancet* **i,** 689–92.

Hope, P. 1992 Laparoscopic cholecystectomy. *British Journal of Nursing* **1,** 36–8.

Keane, F.B.V., Tanner, W.A. and Darzi, A. 1991 Alternatives to cholecystectomy for gall bladder stones. *Recent Advances in Surgery* **14,** 1–16.

Nicholls, R.J. 1994 Pouchitis – what's new in aetiology and management? In: Sutherlands, L.R., Collins, S.M., Martins, S., McLeod, R., Targan, S.R. (eds) *Inflammatory bowel disease.* Dordrecht: Kluwer Academic.

Rodgers, S.E. 1994 The patient facing surgery. In: Alexander, M.F., Fawcett, J.N., Runciman, P.J. (eds)

The Adult patient, hospital and home. Edinburgh: Churchill Livingstone.
  Wilson, J.W. and Waugh, A. 1996 *Ross and Wil-son's Anatomy and Physiology in Health and Illness.* Edinburgh: Churchill Livingstone.

Further reading

Alexander J.W., Fisher, J.E., Boyajia, M., Palaiquist, J. and Morris, M.J. 1983 The influence of hair removal methods on wound infection. *Archives of Surgery* **118**(347), 51.

Alexander, M.F., Fawcett, J.N. and Runciman, P.J. 1994 *Hospital and home; the adult.* Edinburgh: Churchill Livingstone.

Beck, D.E. and Fazio, V.W. 1990 Current pre-operative bowel cleansing methods: results of a survey. *Diseases of the Colon and Rectum* **33**(1), 12–15.

Downing, R., Dornicott, J.N., Keighley, M.R.B. et al. 1979 Whole gut irrigation: a survey of patient opinion. *British Journal of Surgery* **66**, 201–2.

Gilmore, I.T., Ellis, W.R., Barrett, G.S., Pendower, J.E.H. and Parkins, R.A. 1981 A comparison of two methods of whole gut lavage for colonoscopy. *British Journal of Surgery* **68**, 388–9.

Hewit, J., Reeve, J., Rugby, J. et al. 1973 Whole gut irrigation in preparation for bowel surgery. *Lancet* **2**, 337–40.

Hill, G.L. 1983 Ileostomy function. In: Allan, R.N., Keighley, M.R.B., Alexander Williams, J. et al. *Inflammatory bowel disease*, 2nd edn. Edinburgh: Churchill Livingstone.

Lancet 1983 Preoperative depilation. June 11, 311 (editorial).

Mead, J. 1994 Discharge planning in stoma care. *Professional Nurse*, Mar, 405–10.

Mosby's Dictionary of medical, nursing and allied health, 3rd edn. 1990 St Louis: CV Mosby.

Poulton, L.J. 1991 Preoperative bowel preparation. *Surgical Nurse* **4**(2), 12–14.

Thomas, E.A. 1989 Preoperative fasting – a question of routine. *Nursing Times* **83**, 46–7.

Winkler, R. 1986 *Stoma therapy: an atlas and guide for intestinal stomas.* New York: Thieme.

Gynaecological surgery

Lysette Butler

Introduction

Gynaecological surgery represents an application of the principles of general surgery to disorders of the female reproductive tract, excluding those relating to hormonal dysfunction.

The physical care of gynaecological patients is not demanding, as self-care is usually possible very soon after surgery. This feature of gynaecology creates a very rapid throughput in inpatient areas. The average length of stay in gynaecological wards is 4–48 hours, rising to a maximum of 7 days for more major surgery.

The sense of speed engendered in this way, and the very intimate nature of the surgical procedures, many of them carrying a threat to body image and femininity, make great demands on the patient's psychological health and emotional stability. The nurse must therefore demonstrate considerable sensitivity and communication skill in order to offer the necessary emotional support, based on accurate knowledge and careful consideration of how it should be conveyed.

Vaginal examination

Indications

Vaginal examination yields a considerable amount of information relevant to the management of gynaecological conditions and aids detection of many cancers of the female genital tract. Its use is therefore indicated in the identification of hitherto symptomless 'well-women' disease, in obstetric care to determine the progression of a pregnancy and as an aid to diagnosis when a patient has presented with symptoms that may be attributable to the reproductive tract.

Implications for the patient

A patient undergoing vaginal examination (VE) requires sensitive support from the nurse. This examination can represent the most gross invasion of a woman's privacy to which she is ever medically subjected. It is also one which is most likely to produce valuable diagnostic evidence. The patient is expected to surrender privacy, dignity and comfort without a qualm for what may seem the uncertain benefits of the examination itself. Furthermore, she may be repeatedly required to make this sacrifice of dignity in pursuit of a diagnosis. Medical and nursing staff should be mindful of the humiliation faced by the patient at this time. Some women have gone as far as to say, when a doctor has been particularly insensitive, that they feel as if they have been 'sexually abused'.

Certain client groups hold very different attitudes toward medical examination. For many, the difficulties associated with vaginal examination prevent them seeking advice until the disease process is far advanced. The reader is referred to special texts for details but is reminded that women from non-Caucasian cultures will not readily be compliant in undergoing vaginal examination and will appreciate appropriate steps being taken to meet their special needs. The recognition of the existence of such special needs will help to build the essential relationship of trust which is required. Menzies (1990) discusses the supportive role of the nurse at this time.

Vaginal examination and nursing care

There are two positions in which vaginal examination may be carried out: first, the vulval area is exposed by parting the knees after they have been drawn up from the supine position, and second, it may be approached from behind with the patient in the lateral position with the knees drawn up. The uppermost leg may need some support in this position, and excessive exposure of the patient must always be avoided.

A good light is essential for the examination, during which a Cusco's speculum is inserted into the vagina (Figure 9.1), a warmed speculum always being preferable to a cold one: 'The fact that the speculum was warmed helped me to relax.' The speculum is slowly opened so that the vagina and cervix are clearly visible. Findings at this point and results of previous investigations will determine how the doctor proceeds; further tests may be carried out or additional samples of tissue or fluid taken.

Following removal of the speculum, digital examination combined with abdominal palpation is performed. The examining fingers within the vagina, pressing on the cervix, and the examining hand over the abdomen (bimanual examination)

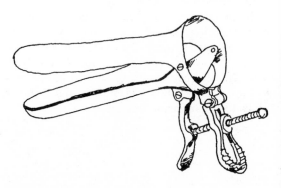

Figure 9.1 Cusco vaginal speculum

allow the doctor to identify the internal organs, revealing abnormalities within the pelvic cavity.

Gynaecological disorders of three particular types may be demonstrated through the use of the vaginal examination:

- Potential malignancies of the cervix can be detected early.

- Anatomical abnormalities of the cervix, vagina and vulva may be visualized.

- Bimanual examination will reveal ovarian and uterine abnormalities. Growths of the uterus

(fibroids) are usually benign. The ovaries may enlarge in the presence of cystic disease.

On completion of the examination, the nurse must ensure that the patient is offered help to get down from the couch, facilities to wash away the lubricant used and anything else needed.

The nurse's major function is to contribute to the patient's feeling of security. The patient will be more likely to relax if she can feel certain that the examination will not be interrupted. She will also be more at ease if exposure is kept to the absolute minimum. Attention to such detail will help to build the confidence needed for effective examination and for subsequent treatment, should it prove necessary.

Minor gynaecological surgery

Minor surgery is defined in terms of the brevity of theatre time and hospital stay. In minor gynaecological procedures, the theatre time may be as little as 10 minutes and the length of hospital stay between 2 and 24 hours. For the patient, however, no surgery is minor, and for the gynaecological patient it may cause emotional distress.

Surgery may be either diagnostic or therapeutic. The advent of the laparoscope and laser treatment has increased the range of conditions that may be managed without prolonged hospital admission.

Admission and pre-operative care

The patient is usually admitted on the day of the operation, having already starved for 6 hours (if general anaesthesia is anticipated). Earlier admission usually results from other health problems.

During the admission procedure, special reference is made to the reproductive physiological function and the effects of any disorder on the patient's view of her own sexuality. Details of the menstrual cycle, vaginal discharge and their influence on everyday life are significant. The

nature of the information the patient is asked to divulge makes further demands on the nurse's discretion, skill and empathy.

It is also beneficial to assess the mobility of the patient's hips and check for any spinal problems so she can safely be placed into the lithotomy position for surgery such as:

- examination under anaesthetic (EUA);
- dilatation and curettage (D&C);
- hysteroscopy;
- evacuation of retained products of conception (ERPC);
- surgical termination of pregnancy (STOP);
- insertion of a Shirodkar suture;
- laparoscopy;
- endometrial ablation;
- vaginal hysterectomy.

STUDENT ACTIVITY

Lie on your bed with one pillow under your head. With the help of a friend, lift both legs at once into the lithotomy position. How do you feel?

It is unnecessary to shave the pubic area before minor gynaecological surgery as the practice produces an increased risk of infection (Winfield, 1986).

Post-operative care

Minor gynaecological surgery requires the same observation of vital signs as does general surgery, with the addition of recording vaginal loss. The nurse must determine the degree of blood loss by frequent examination of the patient's sanitary protection. While, in general surgery, blood loss is often concealed, in gynaecology it may be fairly accurately assessed, although measurement is subjective. It is customarily noted as being 'slight', 'moderate' or 'heavy'.

The pad should be changed on at least every other occasion when slight or moderate loss is observed. Heavy blood loss requires frequent changing of the pad and must be reported to the doctor; it usually indicates continued bleeding. A drop in blood pressure requires a different approach from usual. The legs should be raised with pillows, thus improving venous return without altering the position of the pelvis or masking bleeding.

Pelvic surgery always carries a risk of bladder damage, so it is important for the patient to pass urine before being discharged.

Discharge advice

The use of tampons is contraindicated for at least 2 weeks, until after the next menstrual period, as their use compounds the already present risk of infection if the cervix has been dilated or the operation was linked with a pregnancy. Pregnancy itself renders the cervix soft and susceptible to infection.

Bleeding usually continues for about 10–14 days post-operatively. If it persists or becomes heavy, the patient should consult her doctor. Malodorous loss, a sign that infection might have arisen, should also be reported.

The patient may normally resume work 4–7 days after surgery.

Advice on contraception may be needed by the patient before she leaves the ward; she may resume sexual intercourse after 14 days or when bleeding has ceased, whichever is the later.

Patients needing a further consultation will be seen in the outpatient clinic 6 weeks after discharge, giving the opportunity to assess the effectiveness of surgery and to discuss any further treatment.

Minor surgical procedures

Examination under anaesthetic

EUA can be used to assess the progress of suspected malignant disease; it can be performed when the patient is too nervous to allow effective vaginal examination, and it may offer evidence to help to determine the best surgical approach for subsequent hysterectomy.

The procedure is the same as for vaginal examination without anaesthesia, and the post-procedural care is as described above for all minor surgery. EUA allows the doctor to make a better assessment as the patient's abdominal, vaginal and pelvic floor muscles are relaxed and offer no resistance.

Dilatation and curettage

This requires a short anaesthetic and may be either diagnostic or therapeutic. The cervix is first dilated, and then a curette is passed through it. A sample of the endometrium can be scraped out and sent for histological examination. In cases of heavy menstruation, a D&C will be performed before any other surgery. A polyp can be removed during surgery if it has been found to be the cause of the problem.

POST-OPERATIVE CARE

On her return to the ward, the patient will probably be conscious, although slightly drowsy. Vital signs should be recorded at least once – more frequently if indicated. When fully conscious, the patient should be escorted to the toilet to pass urine. When she is fully conscious, has passed urine and has vital signs within her normal range, she may go home. Discharge advice and outpatient arrangements are as outlined above.

Hysteroscopy

This procedure is commonly carried out at the same time as a D&C, using a rigid or flexible endoscope – a hysteroscope – developed to view the internal cavity of the uterus.

This is generally a diagnostic procedure, although some practitioners remove polyps, small fibroids and even the endometrium itself (*see* section on endometrial ablation and transcervical resection of the endometrium). It can be carried out under either general or local anaesthetic.

The view seen by the camera in the hysteroscope is relayed to a video monitor. The practitioner therefore watches the monitor rather than looking directly through the hysteroscope. The picture is of a very high quality and yields much significant information.

It is a matter of judgement for the gynaecologist and his team to consider the value of inviting the patient to view the screen if local anaesthesia is used. This may provide an opportunity for reassurance and a sense of participation for some patients.

Post-operative care is the same as for a D&C.

Evacuation of retained products of conception

The retention of the products of conception within the uterus following a spontaneous abortion may lead to infection (by activating the normal body responses to foreign protein), with a subsequent reduction in fertility. Therefore, all this material must be removed. The uterus is scraped in the same way as during a D&C.

PRE-OPERATIVE CARE

The patient usually arrives in hospital as an emergency case, having suffered a spontaneous abortion. If she has not starved, the operation is deferred unless there is profuse bleeding, which may happen because of the great vascularity of the endometrium during pregnancy.

A patient who has had a spontaneous abortion is treated as an emergency, and time will dictate what preparation can be made prior to transfer to theatre: it will be the best that can be achieved within the available time.

PSYCHOLOGICAL ASPECTS

The patient who has to face the loss of a pregnancy is facing bereavement and thus needs all the care and attention, both before and after surgery, that should be accorded to anybody in this position. Her partner, too, will be feeling a loss, but he is expected to support the patient regardless of his own feelings, which are not always recognized.

Emotional support for the patient and her partner may be required for a protracted period; various organizations and self-help groups exist, providing long-term support. A follow-up appointment may be offered. (A history of repeated spontaneous abortion suggests that subfertility may be secondary to another condition.)

Surgical termination of pregnancy

The word 'abortion', according to the Stillbirth (Definition) Act 1991, meant termination of a pregnancy before the 24th week of gestation, regardless of how this had occurred. An amendment to the Abortion Act 1967, effective from April 1991, specifies that an *induced* abortion may only take place in the first 24 weeks of gestation.

Most (88%) terminations of pregnancies are performed before the 10th week of gestation. Fetal abnormalities account for most late terminations; their number can therefore be expected to decrease as tests for fetal abnormality become more sophisticated.

Prior to 12 weeks gestation, the termination of pregnancy is a relatively simple procedure similar to a D&C, although great care must be taken not to pierce the uterine wall. Later on, it becomes more complex, as the cervix cannot be sufficiently dilated without causing damage.

Surgery always carries the risk of infection, which may be aggravated by the premature resumption of sexual intercourse, the use of tampons or poor personal hygiene. Prophylactic antibiotics may be prescribed.

POST-OPERATIVE CARE

Hospital admission is likely to be short: the patient is usually discharged a few hours after anaesthetic. Care is similar to that following ERCP.

PSYCHOLOGICAL CARE

The patient will need highly sensitive care at this time. Regardless of the reasons for the operation, she will be trying to deal with a variety of quite unexpected emotions that she may not understand. Her reactions to the situation may be totally unpredictable – for her, her partner and her carers.

While there are no firmly prescribed responses for the nurse to use, she needs to be aware of her patient's emotional turmoil. Her demeanour should be one of gentle, unhurried understanding, without a trace of judgement.

IMPLICATIONS FOR THE NURSE

The 1967 Abortion Act allows doctors, nurses and other health professionals the expression of a conscientious objection to abortion, a right overridden by a duty to care in life-threatening situations. The Act does not remove professionals' responsibility to act in accordance with their respective Codes of Conduct. The onus of responsibility lies with the individual to reveal any conscientious objection at the time of appointment to a situation in which that right may be exercised.

STUDENT ACTIVITY

What, for you, are the implications of exercising the right of conscientious objection to abortion if you were assigned to work on a gynaecological ward? How would you feel if you or your closest female friend was advised to have a termination?

Insertion of a Shirodkar suture

During this procedure, a 'pursestring' suture is inserted around the cervix to prevent it dilating prematurely. It may be used to help patients who have had a history of repeated spontaneous abortions or a cone biopsy of the cervix. The operation is performed between the 14th and 16th weeks of pregnancy. Nursing care is directed at both fetus and mother.

PRE-OPERATIVE CARE

Ultrasound scanning prior to admission will confirm the satisfactory progress of the pregnancy; the fetal heart beat will also be checked and recorded.

Preparation will be as for other minor surgery; the obstetric notes, or a summary of them, should be available for reference.

POST-OPERATIVE CARE

In addition to the regular observations that must be made following minor surgery, the fetal heart must be monitored to detect the effect of anaesthetic gases.

The patient may go home the following day, on condition that she rests. She should be advised against lifting for at least 2 weeks and should watch for any bleeding. At the earliest signs of labour, the patient should go to the maternity unit as the suture must be removed prior to cervical dilatation and the establishment of labour. Failure to remove it at this point can lead to cervical damage.

PSYCHOLOGICAL CARE

A patient undergoing this procedure is inevitably concerned about its outcome and the effect on her unborn child. She also has a medical history that threatens the life of the new pregnancy. The situation calls for good listening skills and great sensitivity. The patient's partner is also likely to be in need of support. Both parties may be reassured by hearing the fetal heart for themselves.

Laparoscopy

A laparoscope – a rigid, metal endoscope – is inserted into the abdominal cavity through a small incision made in the umbilicus in order to view the abdominal organs. Laparoscopy may be performed for diagnostic or therapeutic reasons. Substantial manipulation of the abdominal wall is required to prevent the trocar puncturing the underlying bowel, and, because of this, carbon dioxide is used to insufflate the abdomen to further prevent damage.

Laparoscopy may be useful in determining the causes of pelvic pain or failure to conceive. It is frequently used as access for sterilization, being simple and quick. This procedure is usually carried out under general anaesthetic but can occasionally be done under local anaesthetic for those women who are in good general health, are not overweight and choose to avoid general anaesthesia.

Endometriosis, and adhesions following previous surgery or infection, are amenable to treatment with laser therapy or cautery via the laparoscope.

Ventrosuspension

The uterus is normally anteverted (tilted forward) and anteflexed (folded over on itself), but 1 in 5 women has a retroverted (tilted backwards) uterus, causing severe dysmenorrhoea. Ventrosuspension is performed to correct this abnormal position. It is highly painful because the ligaments maintaining the position of the uterus need to be cut and repositioned. They are then sutured back into their new, anteverted, position. There is therefore a great deal of movement within the pelvis without having removed any pelvic organs. This procedure is now carried out using laparoscopy.

In America, hysterectomies are performed via the laparoscope. The approach for freeing the uterus and cauterizing related structures is through the endoscope; the cervix is dissected from the top of the vagina using a laser, the uterus is removed vaginally, and the vault is sutured.

Although this type of hysterectomy is currently rarely performed in the UK, it may become common by the end of the twentieth century. The advantages are evident: the patient has a much shorter hospital stay, the operation is physically less traumatic and carries reduced risks, and it is cost-effective.

PRE-OPERATIVE CARE

This follows the same procedures as minor surgery, detailed above.

POST-OPERATIVE CARE

After laparoscopy, vital signs are recorded as usual, but pain must be assessed and treated as it occurs. Considerable pain will result from manipulation of the abdomen and from the gas with which it was insufflated. The patient often describes a feeling of having been 'kicked in the stomach by a horse'.

Another commonly experienced pain following laparoscopy is that of pain referred to the tip of the shoulder, usually because gas trapped under the diaphragm causes pressure on the phrenic nerve. The gas introduced at operation does not escape before suturing, so is left to disperse; as this is accelerated by mobilization, the patient should be encouraged to walk about as soon as possible.

To test the patency of the fallopian tubes, blue dye will have been passed through them during operation. If the tubes are patent, the dye will escape into the pelvic cavity and some will eventually reach the urine, colouring it green. The patient must be warned of this in advance.

The patient may return to work 4–10 days after surgery but should refrain from heavy lifting for a period of about 1 week to allow the abdominal muscles to regain normal tone. Intercourse should not be resumed for approximately 2 weeks if the cervix has been dilated as, until it has returned to normal, there is an increased risk of infection. Contraceptive advice should be available.

Each puncture site is likely to be closed with a suture that will dissolve in 8–10 days. If the sutures become uncomfortable or do not dissolve, the patient should consult her GP.

PSYCHOLOGICAL CARE

Each patient's reaction to this surgery will be coloured by the reasons for it. The operation may bring relief as the result of successful therapeutic measures, or greater anxiety and stress because a poor prognosis has been confirmed. In either case, an empathetic approach on the part of the health-care team is essential.

Endometrial ablation

This procedure is revolutionizing gynaecological surgery, using laser techniques to obviate the need for hysterectomy. It is an operation in which the basal layer of the endometrium is removed using laser therapy. This may be sufficient to improve the patient's lifestyle when in the past a hysterectomy would have been necessary (Sadler, 1990). Transcervical resection of the endometrium (TCRE) achieves a similar result but uses a resectoscope to remove the endometrium. In both cases, the patient will have either a substantially reduced menstrual flow or no flow at all, and most consultants will recommend sterilization to prevent any possibility of an ectopic pregnancy.

Both procedures are carried out using a video system, enabling visualization of the operative site, the image being transmitted to the video screen from a camera in the end of the resectoscope.

The physical care required is the same as for a D&C; psychologically, however, the patient needs the same approach as for a hysterectomy since the overall result is the same. Patients also state that 'they do not fully realize what has been done' as there is no scar to see.

Major abdominal gynaecological surgery

The factors distinguishing major from minor surgery are the time spent in the operating theatre, the complexity of the surgery itself and whether or not other organs have been involved. Theatre time may vary between a half and 3 hours, the hospital stay lasting from 2 to 8 days.

These operations have far-reaching implications for the patient and her partner; many, but not all, anticipate a cure.

The Pfanensteil incision is the most commonly used approach for major abdominal gynaecological surgery. A horizontal incision is made above the symphysis pubis across the pubic crown, while the underlying muscle layer is cut vertically along its fibres. This incision heals well because the two layers are cut in different directions, thus reducing the pressure on each. It is also more cosmetically pleasing, as the final scar is hidden by the pubic hair. This gives the incision its colloquial name – the 'bikini line' scar.

Pre-operative care

Particular note should be made of the effects of the disorder and its management on the patient's sexuality and on relationships with her partner.

SKIN PREPARATION

The entire pubic crown is usually shaved prior to the operation; the patient may prefer to do this herself if she can. Minimal shaving is technically feasible, but the wound will be covered with adhesive plaster after surgery, which will be painful to remove if pubic hair remains (Winfield, 1986).

BOWEL CARE

The bowel must be empty at the time of operation because it is adjacent to the operative area. If the bowels have not been opened on the day of admission, glycerine suppositories should be offered. If the patient has a history of constipation, an enema may be necessary.

Special pre-operative investigations

Any prophylactic measures will be carried out as indicated; for example, patients with a history of menorrhagia are likely to need a blood transfusion.

PELVIC ULTRASOUND

With skill, intra-uterine problems may be diagnosed early using pelvic ultrasound and decisions taken regarding the extent and type of surgery that will be most helpful for the patient.

HYSTEROSALPINGOGRAM

This is a radiological examination determining the patency of the fallopian tubes. It has largely been replaced by laparoscopy and is now used only to provide a photographic record when tubal surgery is undertaken.

Post-operative care

Observations of vital signs are carried out for longer than for minor procedures. Pulse, respirat-ory rate and blood pressure must be recorded half-hourly, reducing as the patient's condition stabilizes. If a blood transfusion is in progress, observations will continue until it has been completed.

Vaginal blood loss must be estimated while vital signs are recorded. The interpretation to be placed on blood loss varies with the type of operation performed.

URINARY OUTPUT

Major gynaecological surgery carries a risk of damage to the ureters and bladder and their innervation. Dysfunction must be identified as soon after surgery as possible. The patient is assisted onto a commode within 6 hours of returning from theatre.

If urine has not been passed after 12 hours, and abdominal palpation reveals a full bladder, a catheter may be necessary. It is left on free drainage for 24–72 hours and then removed, allowing the patient to pass urine normally. During this time, all precautions should be maintained in order to ensure a minimal risk of infection. Using a catheter allows the bladder a period of rest and provides time for bruise damage to heal.

BOWEL CARE

Because of their proximity to the operative site, the bowels are also at risk. The patient should not strain at stool because this will increase pressure on the suture line, which may tear. If the patient remains constipated after resuming a normal diet, two glycerine suppositories may be offered to help her regain her normal pattern of elimination. Although one treatment is usually sufficient, care must be taken to ensure that regular bowel activity has returned.

EATING AND DRINKING

Following most major gynaecological surgery, intravenous fluids will be given. Physiological saline or dextrose saline is commonly used to maintain normal hydration until oral intake is established.

The optimum time for the patient to resume oral fluids is on return of bowel sounds, sips of water then being allowed. Eructation, sounds of peristaltic activity and the passage of flatus all provide good evidence that peristalsis is normal. When water can be tolerated without producing nausea, the patient may progress to other fluids. Nausea or vomiting may occur as a side-effect of the anaesthetic gases, but this does not indicate a need for controlled fluid intake. Providing the gynaecological patient takes a minimum of 1.5 L in 24 hours, she may safely be left to drink as she pleases.

PERSONAL HYGIENE

A shower should be taken daily in place of a bath until removal of all the sutures.

WOUND CARE

A wound drain may be in position if there has been substantial bleeding during operation. If so, it is usually removed on the first post-operative day unless heavy drainage persists.

MANAGEMENT OF INFECTION

There is generally little risk of infection following gynaecological surgery; it most commonly occurs at the wound site and vaginal vault. Wound infections are easily identified, but those in the vaginal vault are less apparent. A rise in temperature is often the first indication of the problem, followed by a brown, malodorous vaginal discharge from about the third post-operative day. This causes considerable embarrassment to the patient as it is noticeable to those around her. Infections are treated using appropriate antibiotics.

PAIN

Following gynaecological surgery, many women complain of extreme flatulence, which causes considerable pain, much worse than that caused directly by the surgery. Early mobilization is essential to relieve this pain, and peppermint-based mixtures help to disperse the gas.

> **Patient comment**
>
> **'The wind was the worst bit of the whole experience'.**

PHYSIOTHERAPY

Physiotherapy begins pre-operatively, teaching the patient how best to help herself after operation. Deep breathing and leg exercises are demonstrated, as is moving and getting out of bed without causing pain or tension in the wound.

On the first morning after surgery, the patient will be helped out of bed to sit in a chair. Later in the day, she will take a short walk and will thereafter be encouraged to walk about as much as possible. The physiotherapist will ensure that the patient is able to use stairs before discharge. Unless there is a reason for continued visits, such as respiratory difficulty or problems with mobilization, the physiotherapist's input ceases.

PSYCHOLOGICAL CARE

Although reactions differ widely according to the type of surgery and the patient's personality, there is one feature frequently seen regardless of the nature of the operation. Having made a good immediate post-operative recovery, the patient may feel well and look forward to life without her original problem. On the third or fourth day, however, many women suffer from a form of depression, whose origin may be hormonal; it is commonly known as the 'third or fourth day blues'.

The patient complains of 'feeling low' and is tearful and unable to understand this sudden change in herself.

> **Patient comment**
>
> **'I felt that I couldn't cope with anything and kept dissolving into tears.'**

The inability to understand the process creates even more distress, setting up a vicious cycle of events. Her partner, family, and friends find this disturbing as they interpret it as a set-back in the patient's recovery. If the nurse has previously warned both the patient and her partner that this may occur, it is less frightening when it does. An introduction to someone who has passed through this stage successfully will give some reassurance (Broome and Wallace, 1984).

Discharge advice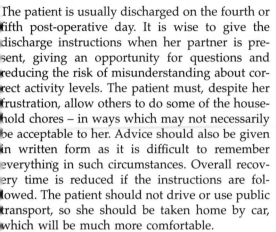

The patient is usually discharged on the fourth or fifth post-operative day. It is wise to give the discharge instructions when her partner is present, giving an opportunity for questions and reducing the risk of misunderstanding about correct activity levels. The patient must, despite her frustration, allow others to do some of the household chores – in ways which may not necessarily be acceptable to her. Advice should also be given in written form as it is difficult to remember everything in such circumstances. Overall recovery time is reduced if the instructions are followed. The patient should not drive or use public transport, so she should be taken home by car, which will be much more comfortable.

The patient will be seen at about 6 weeks following surgery, unless any problems arise. In this case, her GP will determine the proper course of action. Information about relevant self-help organizations should be offered before the patient leaves hospital.

Heavy lifting is contraindicated for at least 8 weeks following major surgery. After this time, the patient may be allowed to carry gradually increasing weights, but she should not lift small children, nor should they be allowed to climb over her.

Mobilization continues to be very important after discharge, so the patient should take a short walk at least twice a day. Some exercise, anything which does not involve lifting or standing for long periods, can be taken indoors, but heavier housework should be reintroduced very gradually. Work at home is allowed if it is carried out sitting down.

It is important for the patient to be given enough detail about levels of activity. If instructions are couched in vague terms ('You must not do too much'), the patient, partner and family will each make their own interpretation, which is unlikely to be correct.

The patient should also realize that she must not push her activity beyond the point at which she begins to feel tired, this signal being an indication to rest. When first home, the patient generally feels too tired to do anything even if she wants to.

Patient comment

'I ran out of energy so quickly at first, it surprised me. I expected to feel better.'

The patient should not return to work before she is advised to do so at the outpatient consultation. The type of work she does, as well as her mode of travel, will dictate the timing of her return, which varies between 6 and 12 weeks after surgery. Return on a part-time basis may initially be beneficial.

Driving is inadvisable for about 4–5 weeks; it is likely to be painful and delay healing.

Sexual activity may be resumed between 4 and 5 weeks post-surgery. Resumption of penetrative sexual activity should not take place before 4 weeks, as this represents an infection risk.

It is unwise to begin strenuous exercise before 4 weeks after surgery, at which point it is gradually introduced. The patient is the best judge of how quickly she may build up to her usual level of exercise, but she should stop if it becomes uncomfortable. Swimming provides good exercise; it can be commenced at about 4 weeks but not before because of the potential for infection in public swimming baths.

A well-balanced diet and fluids may be taken as required, but the patient must not put on weight. Gynaecological surgery does not, of itself, produce weight gain.

While some weakness is to be expected following major surgery, any feeling of ill-health not attributable to this should be reported to the GP.

Few drugs need to be prescribed for the patient on discharge, although she may need continued mild analgesics and must complete any post-operative antibiotic therapy that has been instituted.

All post-operative care and discharge advice is similar in major gynaecological surgery; differences will be described below.

Aims of convalescence

- Steadily increasing activity levels, exercise and weight lifting
- Avoiding constipation, overtiredness, overweight and turning into a 'couch potato'
- Balancing rest and activity
- Eating a balanced diet for healing and body maintenance

Major gynaecological surgical procedures

Laparotomy

This term applies to any procedure in which the abdomen is opened surgically and the internal organs operated on. More specifically, it is used when the surgeon needs to see the condition of the organs in order to reach a decision. He will then proceed to the form of surgery that he considers to be in the patient's best interest. Laparotomy is performed when it has not been possible to reach an accurate diagnosis using other techniques and also to assess the spread of neoplastic disease.

Ovarian cystectomy

A solid or fluid-filled cyst on the ovarian surface may become very large. When it causes problems it is removed by aspirating the fluid through a laparoscope or, in the case of a solid mass, an abdominal incision. The ovarian tissue is usually left intact, and the damaged area is sutured. An oophorectomy is performed only if too much ovarian tissue is disrupted by the mass or if malignancy is suspected. The use of microscopes in surgery now enables the surgeon to save ovaries that once would have been removed.

Ideally, an ovarian cyst is removed without rupturing it. Should this occur, the protein-rich fluid from the cyst may cause adhesions between the pelvic organs. The cyst and its contents are always sent for histological examination.

PRE-OPERATIVE CARE

A pre-operative ultrasound scan will provide evidence of the nature of the cyst and therefore determine the surgical procedure.

POST-OPERATIVE CARE

Discharge is on about the fifth post-operative day. Antibiotics are rarely needed, but histology results should be known prior to discharge so that early treatment can be instituted if malignancy is present.

PSYCHOLOGICAL CARE

When a cyst proves to be non-malignant, the patient is likely to experience a great feeling of relief, and she may be reassured that her fertility remains unaffected.

If malignancy has been demonstrated, the patient, her partner and immediate family members and friends in whom the patient chooses to confide will need proper support to enable them to meet this crisis and regain emotional stability.

It must not be assumed that a poor diagnosis and prognosis must first be divulged to the patient's partner. This runs counter to all notions of confidentiality and also puts the onus upon the partner to be the bearer of bad news (Simons, 1985).

Tubal surgery

The aim of this is to achieve patency of the fallopian tube when an obstruction has been identified. A full assessment will have been carried out.

The nature of the surgery varies in form, being determined by the type of abnormality. Excision of a part of the tube and anastomosis of the remaining tissues may be carried out, or it may be possible to ream out the lumen of the tube to allow the passage of ovum and sperm. Alternatively, the fimbriated ends of the tube may be freed to open the tube up to ova. As the fallopian tubes are only 5 mm in diameter at their widest point, a microscope must be used. This lengthens the operating time and produces further long-term problems, with an increased risk of adhesion formation. Such adhesions can alter the position of the tubes relative to the ovaries so that they will be unable to receive an ovum.

POST-OPERATIVE CARE

Discharge will take place between the third and fifth post-operative days. The significant distinction in advice is that the patient is advised to recommence sexual intercourse *early*, increasing the possibility of conception before adhesions have become established.

PSYCHOLOGICAL CARE

Tubal surgery has a relatively low success rate, only about 20–30% of women achieving and maintaining a pregnancy (Lewis and Chamberlain, 1990). This is the cause of much distress both pre- and post-operatively. Both partners may swing from moods of high expectation pre-operatively to very low ones post-operatively. It is important to maintain a degree of realism about the likely outcome. Self-help organizations exist to help those who are unable to conceive.

Ectopic pregnancy

An ectopic pregnancy is one which has implanted in a site other than the uterus, 99% of them being in the fallopian tubes. The tubes cannot sustain a pregnancy for very long; pain will occur, and the tubes may rupture as the embryo increases in size. Major haemorrhage is a real risk because of the vascularity of the site, and a ruptured tube diminishes fertility. Emergency surgery is therefore essential.

PRE-OPERATIVE CARE

The patient is usually admitted as an emergency and will complain of abdominal pain, possibly some nausea, amenorrhoea and slight vaginal loss. She may not realize that she is pregnant. On examination, the abdomen will be tense, and guarding will be noted.

An ultrasound scan provides evidence of a mass in one of the tubes, which, together with the clinical features, confirms the diagnosis. If, however, vaginal loss and amenorrhoea are absent, the condition mimics acute appendicitis.

The patient is prepared for emergency surgery.

Quarter-hourly monitoring of vital signs and abdominal girth measurement should be carried out to assess internal bleeding.

The aim of surgery is to remove the pregnancy while preserving as much of the tube as possible. A laparoscopy will establish the differential diagnosis, and the surgeon will then proceed to a laparotomy. No attempt is made to repair damage to either tube, as the operative field becomes filled with blood and such attempts at repair are unsuccessful. An autotransfusion may be used, but otherwise, in the absence of whole blood, plasma expanders will maintain the blood pressure at an acceptable level.

POST-OPERATIVE CARE

See ovarian cystectomy.

PSYCHOLOGICAL CARE

The psychological care required by a patient who has suffered an ectopic pregnancy must be entirely patient-led, determined by professional awareness of the patient's perception of her predicament.

The patient and her partner may be suffering the grief of loss of a much-wanted baby, compounded by the major crisis of emergency surgery. They may also be having to contemplate further surgery to repair any damage to the fallopian tubes, and must came to terms with the effects of this on their ability to produce a family.

Conversely, the patient and her partner may not have been aware of the existence of a pregnancy, nor may it have been wanted. They will be faced with the difficulties inherent in overcoming surgery that might have been avoided by a termination of pregnancy. The patient will probably spend 5 days in hospital, followed by a lengthy period away from work.

Myomectomy

This is removal of a benign tumour (fibroid) arising from the myometrium of the body of the uterus. It is usually performed only for those women who later wish to achieve a pregnancy, because there is a substantial risk of haemorrhage. In some cases, multiple fibroids distort the endometrial surface, making implantation difficult. When this is the case, the surgeon may attempt to remove as many as possible.

In the long term, myomectomy may improve the chances of pregnancy and will almost certainly reduce the amount of menstrual loss, although that may not be the end of the patient's problems. There is a risk of the fibroids recurring, at which point hysterectomy is inevitable.

PRE-OPERATIVE CARE

At least 4 units of blood must be cross-matched. Consent should be obtained for hysterectomy as well as for myomectomy. If haemorrhage becomes uncontrollable during operation, hysterectomy is a life-saving measure.

POST-OPERATIVE CARE

The observation of vaginal loss, verbal and non-verbal signs of pain and the symptoms associated with internal haemorrhage are all-important. A wound drainage system will be in use and must be closely observed for excessive blood loss. Any indication of haemorrhage must be reported immediately.

PSYCHOLOGICAL CARE

As in tubal surgery, the patient may nurture false or unrealistic hopes of becoming pregnant as a result of her surgery. She is likely to suffer more pain than she had anticipated, because of the handling of the uterus during surgery. If a hysterectomy was unavoidable, she will begin a grieving process for all her losses: of her ability to become pregnant, her perception of herself as a whole woman (body image), and, temporarily, her independence, work, etc.

Hysterectomy

The uterus can be removed by a variety of surgical approaches.

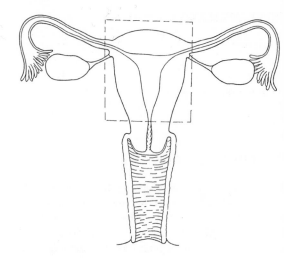

Figure 9.2 Subtotal hysterectomy

TYPES OF HYSTERECTOMY

Sub-total hysterectomy

Only the body of the uterus is removed (Fig. 9.2). This is now rarely performed because the remaining cervix is still at risk of malignant disease.

Total abdominal hysterectomy

In this procedure, the body of the uterus and the cervix are removed (Fig. 9.3). It is not only the most common form of hysterectomy, but is also estimated to be the surgery most commonly performed on women in the UK (Lewis and Chamberlain, 1990).

Total abdominal hysterectomy and bilateral salpingo-oophorectomy

The body of the uterus and the cervix are removed, together with one or both fallopian tubes and ovaries (Fig. 9.4). The decision to remove the ovaries is usually made at the time of operation, depending on whether they appear to be functioning. If they do not appear to be diseased, and if their retention will not exacerbate the progress of disease, they are left in place. Hormone-dependent diseases, such as endometriosis, furnish ample reason for the removal of functioning ovaries; if ovarian hormones continue to circulate, they will promote the extension of disease.

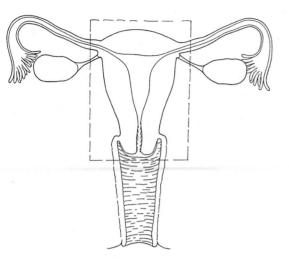

Figure 9.3 Total abdominal hysterectomy

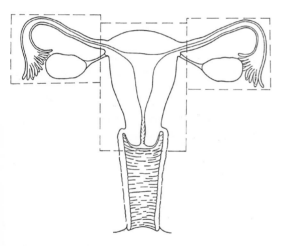

Figure 9.4 Total abdominal hysterectomy and bilateral salpingo-oophorectomy

Wertheims's radical hysterectomy

This extensive operation for cancer of the cervix involves removal of the uterus, cervix, fallopian tubes, ovaries, broad ligament, local lymph nodes and glands, and upper third of the vagina (Fig. 9.5). If caught at a sufficiently early stage, a cure may be effected (Lewis and Chamberlain, 1990). There are many reasons for hysterectomy, including:

- fibroids;
- menorrhagia;

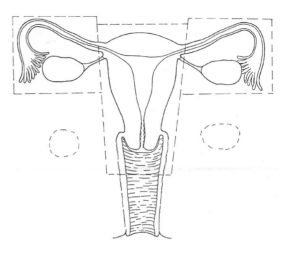

Figure 9.5 Wertheim's radical hysterectomy

- malignancy;
- uterine prolapse;
- endometriosis;
- pelvic inflammatory disease;
- ruptured uterus.

Explanations of these conditions are to be found in standard texts (*see* further reading).

> **STUDENT ACTIVITY**
>
> Think of what your reactions would be if you or your best friend were faced with the prospect of a hysterectomy. Ask several close female friends what their reactions would be.

PRE-OPERATIVE CARE

In addition to major surgical care, an ultrasound scan may be performed prior to surgery. The size of any fibroids present must be assessed.

POST-OPERATIVE CARE

The patient often feels weak for the first 2 post-operative days but thereafter generally recovers quite quickly. Flatulence may be a problem but is relieved by mobilization as the patient rapidly becomes self-caring.

Usual bowel and bladder care should be carried out. Sexual intercourse can be resumed after 4–5 weeks; women who have had radical hysterectomy must be fully aware of the effect of the surgery on this aspect of their lives, and both partners should be involved in discussions. A trained sexual counsellor may be of help, particularly if the patient experiences dyspareunia, a common complaint, causing great distress in this most intimate area of life and one for which the partners may have been unprepared. It occurs because the vagina is considerably shorter than before.

PSYCHOLOGICAL CARE

There are ambivalent reactions to this operation. On the one hand, the patient may experience relief that her original symptoms have disappeared.

> **Patient comment**
>
> 'I felt nothing but relief that there was an end to the heavy, messy bleeding, endlessly feeling tired and having to worry about contraception. For me, the hysterectomy was liberating. One year on, I feel terrific and am very glad I decided to have it done.'

On the other hand, she may experience disturbing feelings relating to loss of body image, loss of femininity, invasion of privacy and gross insult to her person. She will pass through a grieving process before she is completely healed (Broome and Wallace, 1984) and should be helped to do so.

The patient who has undergone this surgery for malignant disease will have her distress compounded by anxiety. No assurance can be given that it will not recur, although a cure may be achieved if it is performed early enough (Hernandez and Rosenshein, 1989).

Many women state that hysterectomy is as traumatic and painful as childbirth, but without the baby that makes it all worthwhile. They do not realize that the mechanism of pain perception obliterates the memory of some pains if the stimuli are not repeated; they remember only the pain most recently laid down in memory.

Some women see their role in life as producing and rearing children so may state that they feel 'less of a woman' and no longer 'useful to society'.

Hysterectomy thus presents a particular challenge to the nurse. All her communication and listening skills are needed each time. She must remember that each patient is different in her emotional response to what is happening. The nurse should also be able to recognize when another professional may be able to offer more skilled help, and refer appropriately.

Major vaginal surgery

Pre-operative care

Major vaginal and abdominal surgery do not differ in the admission procedure and preparation. Two additional points must, however, be noted: the patient will need to have an empty bowel, and she will need a vulval instead of a pubic shave.

An enema on the morning of operation may be necessary and should be offered to the patient, who should understand its importance. The vulval shave may need to be carried out by the nurse, because of the difficulty of reaching the area, especially if the patient is elderly or suffers from a musculoskeletal disorder preventing full mobility.

An important aim of all vaginal surgery is to achieve the desired result without impairing the patient's ability to enjoy sexual intercourse.

Major vaginal surgical procedures

Vaginal hysterectomy

The uterus is removed through the vagina instead of through the abdominal wall, the obvious advantages being that there is no division of the abdominal musculature and no abdominal scar. The patient can leave hospital earlier, providing there are no complications. Stress incontinence can also be relieved at the same time. The ovaries can be removed using this approach.

PRE-OPERATIVE CARE

A vaginal examination will determine the suitability of this approach, and an ultrasound scan will allow assessment of the size of the uterus. It must not be too large for removal by the vaginal route.

Blood loss is not usually great following a vaginal hysterectomy, so it is less urgent to have blood available, although the patient's blood type should be identified for more rapid cross-matching and supply.

POST-OPERATIVE CARE

As the wound site is inside the vagina, the patient may return from theatre with a vaginal pack to exert pressure on the vaginal walls. The patient should remain in bed until it is removed. The intravenous infusion, providing ready venous access, should continue until the risk of bleeding following removal of the pack has passed.

Vital signs should be recorded regularly prior to removal of the pack and on at least two occasions thereafter. Vaginal blood loss should be checked at these times; there should be no fresh loss.

If a pack is in place, it will cause pressure against the vaginal wall and on the urethra, so a urethral or a suprapubic catheter will be in place. A suprapubic catheter has the advantage that normal micturition can take place without its prior removal, while a urethral catheter needs to be removed and then replaced if the patient is unable to micturate.

Vaginal surgery does not involve division of the abdominal musculature so the patient is less likely to adopt a bent posture following abdominal incision. She will, however, be uncomfortable sitting down and may prefer to sit on a pillow.

Straining at stool should be avoided by the daily administration of a mild aperient to prevent tension on the suture line.

As there has been no handling of the gut, eating and drinking can be reinstated quickly. The patient may begin to take plain water whenever she feels ready and can progress to a full diet at her own pace, the only inhibiting factor being nausea resulting from the anaesthetic.

A daily bath rather than a shower will help to keep the operative site as clean as possible and is very soothing. Douching is only carried out if there is any suspicion of infection. Use of a bidet in hospital must be careful as it is often a vehicle for cross-infection (Simons, 1985), but one may be used at home if desired. Complaints of pain must be attended to as they arise; they may be fewer than after abdominal surgery. Discharge is planned for the third post-operative day, providing that this is at least 24 hours after removal of a urinary catheter and the patient is passing urine normally.

Discharge advice and long-term recovery rate are the same as for a patient undergoing abdominal surgery.

PSYCHOLOGICAL CARE

Hysterectomy provokes a deep feeling of loss in some patients and relief in others. The lack of a scar may cause problems because those around the patient quickly forget what has happened to her and expect too much. These demands, together with her inner turmoil, may cause her to feel very isolated. This can be offset to some extent by careful preparation of the patient, her partner and family before discharge. Discussions should take place together, so that all know the limitations imposed upon the patient. Advice should also be given in writing, as much of it will be forgotten. Although familiar to professional staff, the hospital is alien to the patient and her family, which inhibits concentration and clear communication.

Vulvectomy

This is removal of the vulval area and is therefore neither vaginal nor abdominal surgery. It is performed for malignant disease of the vulva and can take a simple or radical form. Cancer of the vulva is usually seen in patients over 60 years of age, accounting for about 5% of genital cancers in women (Lewis and Chamberlain, 1990).

In a simple vulvectomy, the labia majora, clitoris and fourchette are removed, while in the radical procedure the labia majora, labia minora, clitoris, perineal body, inguinal–femoral groin nodes, with their connecting lymphatics, and all surrounding tissues are excised. This is extremely mutilating surgery and is very stressful for the patient and her partner physically, psychologically and emotionally.

PRE-OPERATIVE CARE

Extensive investigations, including an ECG, radiological examination and ultrasound scan, are needed to determine the spread of the disease. An intravenous pyelogram can assess the extent of the tumour.

The whole of the pubic crown and the vulval area should be shaved thoroughly, and bowel preparation carried out in a similar way as for vaginal surgery.

POST-OPERATIVE CARE

Physical care is mainly concerned with the wound. With such a large amount of tissue loss, it is unlikely that the surgeon will have been able to juxtapose the wound edges for suturing. If he has, the suture line must be very carefully monitored to keep it intact. Usually, there will be no suture line but only a large wound, which must be allowed to granulate from the bottom, healing by secondary intention.

The large tissue loss necessitates continued bedrest for the first 5–6 days. The patient should be encouraged to exercise her feet and legs while in bed as much as possible, and the physiotherapist will see her at least twice daily to minimize post-operative complications resulting from immobility. Deep breathing exercises must be encouraged by the nurse and not simply left to the patient or physiotherapist.

The physiotherapist will supervise early mobilization, aiming to prevent stiffness of the wound. If the scar tissue becomes too tight, the patient may suffer from long-term walking problems.

A urethral catheter will be in position when the patient returns from theatre. This keeps the wound site free of contamination with urine and eliminates the need for frequent movement to use a bedpan. The catheter will normally remain in place for 10–12 days or at least until the patient is mobilizing well.

Resumption of normal dietary intake is left to the patient, but she should take a minimum of 1.5 L of fluid daily. There is no rationale for maintaining intravenous access after this operation as there is no great blood loss; the intravenous line may be removed as soon as a reasonable fluid intake is established.

Pain is not usually a marked post-operative feature, although any complaints must, of course, be taken seriously and attended to. The removal of sutures often causes the most pain, so nitrous oxide and air (Entonox) should be available.

The patient will need to stay in hospital until wound healing is complete, possibly as long as 4 weeks. Wounds are large, and, as the patients are older, healing may proceed more slowly. A diet that ensures enough calories, protein and vitamin C will promote effective healing.

On discharge, the patient should not go home to an empty house but should have somebody who can take care of her for at least a further 2 weeks. This protracted convalescence delays the outpatient consultation until about 8–10 weeks after operation. Advice, except on resumption of sexual intercourse, is the same as for vaginal surgery. Because the patient is often older, it must not be assumed she is no longer sexually active. If she and her partner require sexual counselling, it must be very sensitively given. Prior to surgery, it is necessary for a nurse to build up a good relationship with the patient, so that she is able to discuss these very intimate areas of her life. The patient should, before she gives consent, understand that this form of surgery is likely to impair the quality of her sexual activity or prevent it altogether, although, the surgeon will do all that is possible to avoid this.

PSYCHOLOGICAL CARE

Without doubt, this is the most challenging aspect of the care. An enormous degree of embarrassment is associated with the operation and the condition that necessitated it. The patient may initially have been very reluctant to see her GP, and it is often only because she can no longer hide the odour related to the lesion that she eventually visits him. A female doctor eases the embarrassment for some, but not all, women.

Patients in the age group most frequently affected by cancer of the vulva do not readily speak about their intimate concerns, so the nurse must exercise great discretion in how she frames

and times her questions on admission. It is essential to establish and maintain a good rapport with the patient. Everything should be carefully and honestly explained and all the patient's questions answered.

Post-operatively, the patient may find it difficult to look at her wound and may resent others seeing it. She may find it difficult to accept the reality of what has happened and will begin a grieving process, possibly for her life. The value of good communication and listening skills cannot be overemphasized.

In all respects, vulvectomy is a considerable ordeal for all those involved. It makes many emotional demands on the patient and the caring team. Recovery is slow and, at the same time, the patient is expected to come to terms simultaneously with her cancer and with mutilating surgery, which, even then, cannot promise a cure. This surgery carries a poor prognosis, with only a 15% survival rate. One-fifth of women do not survive the operation or the post-operative period (Hernandez and Rosenshein, 1989). The principal complications of surgery are wound infection and failure of the wound to heal.

Conclusions

Gynaecology is often perceived as a routine, undemanding speciality. It may be true that the physical nursing care is not particularly technical, but the same cannot be said of the emotional and psychological aspects, which are highly demand-

ing of the nurse's time, understanding and empathy. It is this aspect that is estimated to account for 75% of the nurse's working time (Broome and Wallace, 1984).

Summary

1 The principles of general surgery are applied to disorders of the female reproductive tract.

2 Physical care of these patients may be confined to a very short stay in hospital.

3 The psychological and emotional support needed by the patient and her partner, based

on accurate information, is therefore of paramount importance.

4 Advice on contraception and sexual activity is essential following many procedures.

5 Developments in equipment and techniques mean that patients may have quite major surgery with little external evidence.

CASE HISTORY

Mrs Hue, aged 45, has returned from theatre following an abdominal hysterectomy. She appears very pale and anxious. On checking her, you find that her respiratory rate is 25, her pulse 95 beats per minute her blood pressure 90/50 mm Hg and her vaginal loss very heavy. What immediate actions should you take and why?

Review Questions

1 Why does the patient complain of shoulder tip pain after laparoscopy? How would you explain it to her, and what suggestions would you make to help her to reduce the pain?

2 Why is the cervix at risk of infection after dilatation and during pregnancy?

3 What is the difference between endometrial ablation and transcervical resection of the endometrium?

4 How may the nurse ensure the patient's privacy and dignity during a vaginal examination?

5 What is the lithotomy position, and why should you check the mobility of the patient's hip and spine before positioning her?

6 Why is the gynaecological patient not placed in a head-down tilt if her blood pressure is low? What is done instead?

ACKNOWLEDGEMENT

Thanks must go to Wendy Jones, Macmillan Nurse Tutor, for her help in the compilation of this chapter; her grasp of the English language makes the chapter that much easier to read.

References

Broome, A. and Wallace L. 1984 *Psychology and gynaecological problems.* London: Tavistock.

Hernandez, E. and Rosenshein, N.B. 1989 *Manual of gynaecologic oncology.* Edinburgh: Churchill Livingstone.

Lewis, T.L.T. and Chamberlain, G.V.P. 1990 *Gynaecology by ten teachers,* 15th ed. London: Edward Arnold.

Menzies, A. 1990 Matter over mind. *Nursing Times* 86(24), 53.

Sadler, C. 1990 Womb service. *Nursing Times* 86(6), 16–17.

Sampson, C. 1982 *The neglected ethic – religious and cultural factors in the care of patients.* Maidenhead: McGraw-Hill.

Simons, W. 1985 *Learning to care on the gynaecology ward.* London: Edward Arnold.

Winfield, U. 1986 Too close a shave? . . . how safe is pre-operative shaving? *Nursing Times, Journal of Infection Control* 82(10), 64, 67–68.

Further reading

Barker, G.H. 1986 *The new fertility – a guide to modern medical treatment for childless couples*. Ely: Adamson Books.

Bevis, R. 1991 *Caring for women*, 4th ed. London: Baillière Tindall.

Breitkopf, L. and Bakoulis, M.G. 1988 *Coping with endometriosis*. Hemel Hempstead: Prentice Hall.

Carson, V. and Benner 1989, 'Spiritual Dimensions of Nursing Practice.' W.B. Saunders Co.: Philadelphia, USA.

Chadwick, R. and Tadd, W. 1992 *Ethics and nursing practice*. Basingstoke: Macmillan.

Chapman, C.R. and Turner, J.A. 1986 Psychological control of acute pain in medical settings. *Journal of Pain and Symptom Management* 1, 9–20.

Coyle, N. 1979 Analgesics at the bedside. *American Journal of Nursing* 79, 1554–7.

Dickson, A. 1983 *A woman in your own right – assertiveness and you*. London: Quartet Books.

Dickson, A. 1985 *The mirror within – a new look at sexuality*. London: Quartet Books.

Dyson, A. and Harris, J. 1990 *Experiments on embryos*. London: Routledge.

Haslett, S. and Jennings, M. 1988 *Hysterectomy and vaginal repair*. Beaconsfield: Beaconsfield Publishers.

Hawkridge, C. 1989 *Understanding endometriosis*. London: Macdonald Optima.

Henriques, N. and Dickson, A. 1986 *Women on hysterectomy, or how long before I can hang-glide?* London: Thorsons.

Keeri-Sauto, M. 1979 Drugs or drums – what relieves post-operative pain. *Pain* 6, 217–30.

Lee, S. 1986 *Law and morals – Warnock, Gillick and beyond*. Oxford: Oxford University Press.

Liu, D.T. and Lachelin, G.C.L. 1989 *Practical gynaecology*. London: Butterworths.

Potts, M., Diggory, P. and Peel, J. 1977 *Abortion*. Cambridge: Cambridge University Press.

Price, B. 1990 *Body image – nursing concepts and care*. Hemel Hempstead: Prentice Hall.

Reynolds, M. 1984 *Gynaecological nursing*. Oxford: Blackwell Scientific.

Roberts, H. 1992 *Women's health matters*. London: Routledge.

Scott, L.E. and Plum, G.A. 1984 Examining the interaction effects of coping styles and brief interventions. *Pain* 20, 79–91.

Taenzer, P., Melzack, R. and Jeans, M.E. 1986 Influence of psychological factors on post-operative pain, mood and analgesic requirements. *Pain* 24, 331–45.

Thompson, S.C. 1981 Will it hurt less if I can control it? – a complex answer to a simple question. *Psychological Bulletin* 90, 89–111.

Tindall, V.R. 1991 *Illustrated textbook – gynaecology*. London: Gower Medical Publishing.

Walters, W.A.W. 1991 *Clinical Obstetrics and Gynaecology* – Human reproduction: Current and future ethical issues. Eastbourne: Baillière Tindall.

Webb, C. 1986 *Feminist practice in women's health care*. Aylesbury: HM+M.

Webb, C. 1996 *Women's health – midwifery and gynaecological nursing*. London: Hodder & Stoughton.

Whitfield, C. 1990 *People who help*. London: Profile Productions.

Useful addresses

Cervical Stitch Network 15 Matcham Street, London E11 3LE. Tel: 0181-555 5248. Part of the Miscarriage Association, the network provides information, advice and local contacts for women who need, or might need, a cervical stitch during pregnancy.

Endometriosis Society 65 Holmdene Avenue, Herne Hill, London SE24 9LD. The Society's aims are: to foster self-help and mutual support among endometriosis suffers; to develop greater awareness of endometriosis among the medical profession and the general public; to encourage further research into better treatments for endometriosis and its associated infertility, and to assist where possible; to promote further research into the epidemiology of endometriosis; to improve the recognition of 'at-risk' groups; and to encourage earlier diagnosis. Approximately 100 local groups and contacts exist throughout the UK.

Hysterectomy Support Group 11 Henryson Road, Brockley, London SE4 1HL. Tel: 0181-690 5987. Formed to encourage self-help through the informal sharing of information and experiences about hysterectomy, pre- and post-operatively. Informal support is given by letter, over the telephone or through group meetings by a network of contact workers. It is totally voluntary.

Issue 318 Summer Lane, Birmingham B19 3RL. Tel: 0121-359 4887, 0121-359 3562. A nationwide self-help organization for people having impaired fertility and struggling to found a family, also assisting older childless couples and people feeling distressed by their childlessness. It provides a quarterly newsletter, a network of contacts for personal advice and assistance, some professional counselling, leaflets and information on infertility, its treatment and related matters, and regional and national conferences. Advice is available to couples seeking donor insemination and other controversial treatments. Issue campaigns for better facilities and priority for infertility treatment and for improved understanding of the problems involved, both medical and social. It also seeks greater awareness of the problems of childlessness and its advantages and opportunities for those who cannot found their family.

Miscarriage Association PO Box 24, Ossett, West Yorkshire WF5 9XG. Tel: (0924) 264579 (weekday mornings). Information and support for women and their families/friends who have suffered miscarriage or threaten to. It provides quarterly newsletter information sheets, local groups and contacts. They aim to inform health professionals and the lay public about all aspects of miscarriage and hope to influence them towards better understanding, care and treatment of miscarriage patients.

National Abortion Campaign Wesley House, 4 Wild Court, London WC2B 5AU. Tel: 0171-405 4801. Campaigns for the defence and extension of the 1967 Abortion Act, providing educational material for students and information about visual material. They also produce a range of AIDS material.

Women's Health Concern (WHC) PO Box 1629, London W8 6AU. Tel: 0171-602 6669. It exists to help women to become more knowledgeable about their cyclic health, especially the menopause and the proper use of hormone replacement therapy. Professional counselling, treatment and care for gynaecological conditions that have been commonly ignored or mistreated for generations are available. WHC offers courses for nurse counsellors and symposia for doctors and health professionals. Leaflets, books and booklets are available.

Women's Health and Reproductive Rights Information Centre 52 Featherstone Street, London EC1Y 8RT. Tel: 0171-251 6580, 0171-251 6332. A national information and resource centre for women's health. It operates an extensive library, answers health enquiries by post or telephone and publishes a newsletter and many leaflets on women's health. Women can be put in touch with health groups, support groups, voluntary organizations and individuals willing to offer help.

Women's National Cancer Control Campaign (WNCCC) 1 South Audley Street, London W1Y 5DQ. Tel: 0171-499 7532, screening helpline 0171-495 4995. A health education charity primarily concerned with the promotion of measures for the early detection and prevention of cancer in women. There are five mobile screening units used for workplace and public screening programmes. There is also a screening helpline and an information service. WNCCC produces literature in nine different languages and has audiovisual material for hire or purchase.

Urological surgery

Dominic Mawdsley

Introduction

The purpose of this chapter is to cover the most common procedures, investigations and surgical interventions relating to renal and urological surgery and its related nursing care.

Issues common to urological surgery

General pre-operative care

The patient will normally be admitted at least a day prior to surgery to allow adequate preparation for major surgery and general anaesthesia. Those patients undergoing minor surgery (such as check cystoscopy) may be admitted as day cases.

Urinalysis will be performed and a mid-stream specimen of urine (MSU) sent to exclude the possibility of urinary tract infection (UTI), which may require treatment prior to instrumentation. Bacteraemia is possible subsequent to any instrumentation of the urinary tract and may lead to life-threatening septicaemia if it is not detected and treated promptly and appropriately. Should malignancy be suspected, a urine specimen may be sent for cytology.

It is also important to ensure that the patient has an adequate bowel movement prior to surgery. In the case of transurethral resection of the prostate (TURP), post-operative constipation and straining may cause haemorrhage from the prostatic bed.

STUDENT ACTIVITY

Look up the procedure of taking an MSU. What is the rationale for this? Try the technique out for yourself.

Post-operative care

Some urological surgery (such as TURP) shows no evidence of surgical incision so it is tempting to assume that the patient has not undergone major surgery. This is not the case, and the principles of post-operative surgical care therefore apply.

The patient may return to the ward with an intravenous infusion and a urinary catheter. An intravenous infusion will replace blood or fluid lost both pre- and post-operatively. It will remain in situ until the patient can tolerate sufficient fluids orally. In the case of a paralytic ileus, the infusion remains in place until gut mobility has returned to normal and the patient is able to tolerate 1.5–2.0 L of fluid orally within a 24 hour period. This may take 3–4 days to achieve, and oral fluids should be gradually increased depending on the patient's tolerance and the presence or absence of bowel sounds.

Unless otherwise indicated, the urethral catheter may be removed as soon as the patient is mobile enough to void without undue discomfort. Early mobilization (within 2 days post-operatively) is important in the prevention of complications such as deep vein thrombosis. Anti-embolism stockings and/or subcutaneous anticoagulation therapy may be employed. Any wound drain present will be removed when output is minimal or has ceased.

Fluid balance

The monitoring of fluid balance is of paramount importance in urological nursing so a fluid balance chart should be accurately maintained. This will monitor deficiencies in urine output, fluid/irrigant overload and dehydration.

Catheter management

The principle underlying all aspects of catheter management is the prevention of nosocomial infection of the urinary tract resulting from catheterization. Crow *et al.* (1986) found that 10–12% of patients admitted to hospital require catheterization to relieve anatomical or physiological obstruction of the urinary tract, to facilitate post-operative repair and urine drainage or to measure urine output accurately.

Urinary catheterization may cause ascending infection of the urinary tract and inflammation with scarring or stricture of the urethra. The hazards may be reduced by choosing the right catheter for the patient's needs, ensuring that it is inserted using the cleanest technique possible and correct management of the drainage system. Thus a high standard of nursing care with regard to catheter management is fundamentally important providing the patient with a comfortable and uncomplicated hospital stay.

DRAINAGE SYSTEM

A 'closed system' of catheter drainage can reduce the incidence of nosocomial infection from over 80% to less than 10% (Wright, 1988). However, it has also been suggested that the risk of acquiring a UTI via the catheter increases linearly per day of catheterization; bacteria can contaminate the drainage bag and pass along the tubing into the bladder (Crow *et al.* 1986). Patients who have catheters in place long-term will usually acquire bacteria in their urine. Unless the patient develops symptoms of infection, bacterial presence has no significance, and a long-term catheter can remain in situ for as long as it continues to drain satisfactorily.

Overall, the choice of catheter, length of catheterization and its management are all factors affecting the chance of acquiring a urinary tract infection.

Urinary tract infections

A possible side-effect of any urological surgery is a urinary tract infection. Patients should be made aware of symptoms such as burning when passing urine, cloudy and smelly urine and a feeling of wanting to pass urine frequently and urgently. This may then lead to increased haematuria. Patients should be advised to increase their fluid intake and to visit their GP to give a urine sample and seek treatment. Patients should avoid becoming constipated as any straining may cause bleeding, a well-balanced, high-fibre diet should therefore be recommended.

Discharge planning and advice

Discharge planning should start on admission. An initial plan can have been made, determining the services that the patient will require on leav-

Points to consider when caring for a patient with a catheter:

- Observe the appropriate universal precautions at all times

- Clean gloves should be worn and a clean container used when emptying the drainage bag. Patients emptying their own bags need not wear gloves but should wash their hands both before and afterwards.

- The drainage bag should be positioned below the level of the patient's bladder at all times. This ensures a downward flow of urine and prevents urinary stasis

- Drainage bags will have to be disconnected from the catheter if they are damaged or blocked. Disconnection at any other time should be discouraged as this provides an extra portal for the introduction of infection

- Patients should be encouraged to drink 1.5–2.0 L of fluid daily, which helps to prevent the encrustation of the catheter and bacteria collecting in the urine.

- Meatal cleansing, using a clean disposable flannel and soap, should occur as part of the patient's daily hygiene routine. This may be done by the nurse or by the patient if he prefers.

ing hospital. These may include a continence advisor or district nurse to follow up the initial treatments and inpatient care.

There is no set period post-operatively when a patient is discharged, as recovery rates vary with the individual, and potential post-operative complications need to be taken into consideration. Generally speaking, however, it is relative to the scale of the surgery. Thus a patient having a cystoscopy may be discharged home the same day, a patient who has undergone a TURP may be discharged home 3 days post-operatively, and a patient having had a nephrectomy may be discharged 8 days after operation.

Discharge advice should be specific following urological surgery. Advice concerning the resumption of sexual activity should relate to activity prior to illness or admission to hospital. Some urological surgery may also result in a change in body image. Counselling for both the patient and partner may then be required and should be undertaken in as discreet a manner as possible.

Patients will usually require an outpatient appointment, and explanations should be given concerning any medications a patient may be required to take at home.

Cystoscopy and associated procedures

Cystoscopy

Cystoscopy is the insertion of a long, rigid telescope into the bladder. The cystoscope contains rod lenses for light transmission; illumination is achieved via a powerful light source. Different telescopes will offer different angles and views within the bladder, which is distended during the procedure with sterile water or 1% glycine. This or other types of irrigant may be used during surgery to reduce haemolysis occurring within the circulatory system during resection of the prostate or bladder tumour.

Cystoscopy can be both diagnostic and therapeutic, diagnosing bladder carcinoma, chronic and interstitial cystitis, inflammatory conditions, bladder stones and trauma strictures.

Admission and investigation

Depending on the fitness of the patient, the investigations required and the diagnosis, the patient can be admitted as a day case or on the day prior to cystoscopy.

It may be necessary to examine the upper urinary tract for abnormal masses or other lesions; this is best done with an intravenous urogram (IVU) or ultrasound.

Explanation prior to operation

The procedure is often undertaken under general anaesthesia, requiring the prior restriction of fluids and food. The procedure lasts between 10 and 30 minutes, depending on the need to resect

abnormalities. If extensive resection is required, a catheter may be introduced to facilitate urine drainage until the degree of haematuria is reduced to a rose colour (commonly 12–36 hours post-operatively).

This procedure may be performed using local anaesthesia, and a flexible cystoscope may also be used. This can only view the intravesicular wall; should resection be required, a rigid scope must be inserted under general anaesthesia and laser or electrodiathermy methods used.

Post-operative comfort may be assisted by ensuring that the patient is not constipated prior to the operation, particularly if resection is anticipated. Post-operative straining may increase bleeding from the site of resection.

The operation

The patient requiring a rigid cystoscopy will be positioned in the modified lithotomy position to allow the surgeon adequate access to the urethra and a view of all angles of the bladder wall. Flexible cystoscopy does not require this position. This latter method of cystoscopy is being increasingly used for long-term follow-up of bladder tumours on an outpatient basis.

The genital area is cleansed with an antiseptic lotion and the cystoscope introduced into the urethra via the meatus (lignocaine 1–2% may be used in flexible cystoscopy to aid lubrication and reduce discomfort). The urethra is viewed for abnormalities and the cystoscope passed into the bladder, which is distended with irrigating fluid. The interior of the bladder is examined and biopsies or resections made if required. The cystoscope is then removed.

Post-operatively

Following cystoscopy, if a catheter has not been left in situ, some localized discomfort may be experienced on the first and perhaps the second time of voiding. Intense dysuria may occur, but this will lessen after analgesic administration and drinking fluid to dilute the urine. Haematuria of varying degrees may also occur owing to the trauma of instrumentation. This will improve within 12–24 hours, and a normal fluid intake (30 ml/kg per 24 hours) should be encouraged to dilute the haematuria. The patient may also notice some bubbles in the urine immediately after cystoscopy; this is a result of air that is inevitably introduced into the bladder during the procedure. If a catheter has been inserted, it will probably remain in situ for 12–36 hours or until haematuria is reduced to a rose colour. The degree of haematuria is affected by the level of fluid intake, and this should be calculated accordingly. When the catheter is removed, the initial frequency of voiding is erratic. Fluid intake should be reduced to normal for that individual unless haematuria is present.

If a biopsy has been carried out during cystoscopy, the histology result is usually not available for about 7 days. The patient will usually be given an outpatient appointment for that time so that results and any recommended treatment can be discussed.

Transurethral resection of bladder tumour

Cystodiathermy and transurethral resection of a bladder tumour are carried out for the treatment of well-differentiated, non-infiltrating tumours via a resectoscope containing a diathermy loop. When an electrical current is applied, the loop is used to resect the tumour in sliced chippings. The resected tumour is then sent for histological assessment.

Discharge advice following bladder resection

The patient should not undertake any physical exercise of a strenuous nature (e.g. jogging, sex, hard manual labour, carrying heavy shopping or housework) for at least 1–2 weeks after a resection within the bladder. Undue exercise may cause haematuria, the usual source of bleeding being the area of operation. Commonly, the scabs from the healing tissue lift off the resection site about 10 days post-operatively, and a small amount of haematuria may then occur. Should this happen, the patient should be advised to decrease physical activity and increase fluid intake until it resolves, usually within 24 hours.

It is also necessary to stress the importance of keeping the outpatient appointment, where the results of any biopsies will be discussed and further treatment recommended. This may necessitate a return to hospital for regular check cystoscopies.

Cystodistension

This procedure is used principally for the treatment of interstitial cystitis in cases of bladder shrinkage. The bladder is distended by hydrostatic pressure to normal capacity or is overdistended under anaesthesia.

Urethral dilatation

Urethral dilatation may be undertaken for urethral stricture under either general or local anaesthesia depending on the severity of the stricture and the trauma involved in its dilatation. The stricture is stretched with the aid of different dilators graduated in Charrière or French gauge and often referred to as 'sounds' or 'bougies'. In the OPD, the patient lies flat, and once the penile meatus is cleansed, local anaesthetic (lignocaine gel 1–2%) is inserted into the urethra and left for 5–10 minutes to take effect. The dilators are carefully passed into the urethra, starting with the smallest and repeating the procedure with dilators of increasing size until the stricture has been dilated sufficiently to allow an adequate flow of urine.

Transurethral and retropubic prostatectomy

The prostate gland is present only in men and serves to provide a lubricant fluid that combines with the sperm to produce the total ejaculate. The gland is made up of a number of lobes that encircle the urethra just below the neck of the bladder, and is composed of an outer fibrous capsule and inner glandular tissue.

Benign prostatic hypertrophy is a common condition thought to affect 40% of white males over the age of 50 years (Sturdy, 1986), resulting in urinary outflow obstruction. It has been estimated that 1 in 10 men will require treatment for this at some time during their lives (Maxfield *et al.*, 1994). Symptoms include hesitancy, poor urinary flow, frequency and nocturia. The patient may also experience dysuria and haematuria, often due to infection resulting from urine retained in the bladder. In order to exclude neoplasm, any episode of haematuria should be investigated.

The patient may also experience a feeling of incomplete emptying following voiding, which may be the inability of the failing detrusor (bladder) muscle to maintain a high enough pressure to push all the urine past the outflow obstruction, leading eventually to chronic retention of urine. Some patients may also experience a sudden inability to void at all. This is termed acute retention of urine and is not usually related to chronic retention.

Another cause of prostatic enlargement is that of carcinoma of the prostate, which may be treated with hormone or local radiotherapy treatment.

A retropubic prostatectomy (RPP) is performed for a grossly enlarged gland that would otherwise require a lengthy transurethral resection. The need for RPP is usually determined on digital rectal examination and/or transrectal ultrasound, being confirmed on urethroscopy at the time of surgery.

Admission

The patient may be admitted the day prior to surgery to allow enough time for pre-operative preparation. Additionally, the patient may also have attended a pre-admission clinic to provide blood specimens and an MSU.

A urinary flow rate is obtained to establish the degree of obstruction. A normal flow rate is approximately 20–30 ml/sec; in cases of urethral obstruction by the prostate gland, this may diminish to as little as 5 ml/sec. The patient should void at least 150–200 ml in order to provide a flow rate accurately reflecting the degree of obstruction.

If prostatic enlargement has caused chronic urinary retention for some time, an IVU may be indicated to ascertain whether there is any hydronephrosis. Serum urea and electrolyte measurements are essential in cases where the patient has a degree of renal failure. Accurate fluid balance should be maintained; in cases of renal failure resulting from chronic outflow obstruction, prolonged diuresis may occur after relief of the obstruction. Daily weighing of the patient may be another method of calculating excessive fluid loss.

Additionally, an empty rectum and the prevention of constipation are preferable, thus reducing post-operative straining, which may cause bleeding from the prostatic bed. The surgeon may undertake a digital rectal examination at the time of surgery.

Prior to operation

Prior to operation, the patient will require psychological counselling about sexual activity and potency, i.e. the ability to attain and maintain an erection. Owing to the inevitable resection of the bladder neck mechanism, resistance to the ejaculate is reduced, possibly resulting in retrograde ejaculation. When this occurs, ejaculate enters the bladder, causing the urine to appear cloudy on first voiding after ejaculation. The patient should understand that, while he will remain potent, fertility will be reduced. Additionally, sensation on ejaculation may also be diminished. Should the patient intend to father children, the possibility of sperm banking should be considered and discussed with him and his partner.

Transurethral resection of the prostate

Prior to the commencement of surgery, the patient is placed in the lithotomy position.

The operation (which normally lasts approximately three-quarters of an hour) involves removal of the obstructing lobes of the prostate by chipping out the centre of the prostate using a resectoscope passed up the urethra while the patient is anaesthetized (either generally or locally). A small wire loop attachment is pulled through the sections of the prostate using a diathermy current to effect precise resection and coagulation of bleeding vessels on the prostatic

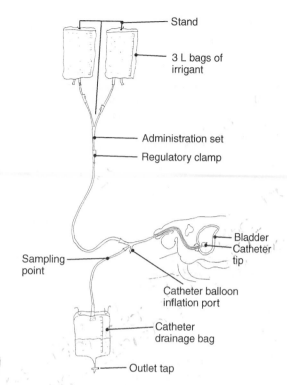

Figure 10.1 Three-way irrigating catheter and drainage system

bed. The prostatic chips are washed out of the bladder, and a satisfactory degree of haemostasis is achieved. During resection of the prostate, a non-electrolytic solution must be used to avoid dissipating the electrical diathermy current. Absorption of irrigation fluid (about 700 ml on average) occurs during TURP. Thus sterile glycine solution is used in the UK to make the irrigation fluid iso-osmotic with blood. Following surgery, 0.9% normal saline solution is used for irrigation via a three-way catheter, preventing obstruction to urine flow by clot formation (Fig. 10.1).

Retropubic prostatectomy

As late as possible prior to surgery, the lower abdominal and pubic hair will need to be removed. An RPP involves incising the prostatic capsule, shelling out the obstructing lobes and resuturing the capsule through a retropubic incision. As well as a urethral catheter, a suprapubic catheter may be inserted. Insertion of a wound drain facilitates healing without haematoma formation.

An intravenous infusion will replace fluid or blood lost during surgery until such time as the patient is able to tolerate sufficient oral fluid to maintain his own hydration. Patients who have undergone an RPP commonly develop a mild paralytic ileus and will only be able to drink and tolerate fluids in gradual but increasing amounts, built-up only as bowel sounds and peristalsis return, (usually within 24–36 hours). The remaining post-operative care is similar to that for any abdominal surgery.

Post-operative care

Following both types of surgery, the patient may experience pain, either from the site of the surgery or from the catheter. An adequate state of analgesia should be maintained.

The patient should sit up as soon as his vital signs stabilize. Deep breathing should be encouraged; if appropriate, the patient should hold and support the wound firmly if and when he wishes to cough.

The colour of the urine and the degree of blood loss should be noted. The nurse should promote the drinking of as much fluid as the patient can tolerate within the limitations set by the medical staff. It should be explained that the aim is to drink at least 10 glasses or 14 cups worth (2 L) a day to dilute the blood in the urine and prevent clot retention.

Some blood will probably ooze around the outside of the catheter and is to be expected. The meatus should be cleaned or the patient shown how to clean around the catheter at least twice a day or as necessary. Soap, water and a disposable flannel should be used.

The catheter may be quite large in size (22–26 Charrière/FG), and the large balloon may irritate the bladder, causing cramp-like spasms that the patient experiences as a sensation of acute urgency. He should be encouraged to relax the perineal and inner pelvic area when this happens. If this does not ease the discomfort, antispasmodic drugs may be administered. Commonly used are propantheline 15 mg three times daily or oxybutinin 5 mg twice daily.

Patient comment

'It feels like I want to pee but I know the tube is doing it for me.'

It should be explained to the patient that seepage of blood around the catheter and the degree of haematuria increase after straining to defaecate. A high-fibre diet and/or glycerine suppositories should prevent this.

The catheter is removed as soon as the urine has cleared to a light rose or yellow colour, usually 2–4 days post-operatively. The balloon at the end of the catheter is deflated by aspirating through the side arm of the catheter until all the water has been removed, and the catheter is then gently withdrawn. This can be uncomfortable and an analgesic may be required prior to the procedure. After an RPP, the catheter may be held inside the bladder by a suture. This secures the end of the catheter, which is held in place on the abdomen by a small zinc button. To remove the catheter, the suture is cut under the button and the catheter easily removed with minimal discomfort.

Patient comment

'It feels like peeing razor blades at first.'

It should also be explained that initial voiding may be erratic and occur without warning. It is important either to place a urinal close by or to prompt the patient to be near the toilet. The bladder has become unused to contracting without an obstruction and the bladder neck mechanism will have been removed, leaving only the distal sphincter mechanism to maintain continence. This may need retraining, and in order to achieve this, regular voiding, depending on the timing of the urge to void, will help to establish a satisfactory sociable micturition pattern. For example, if the desire to void and urge incontinence occur every hour, the patient should purposely void every three-quarters of an hour at first and then gradually lengthen the intervals. Patients can be taught pelvic floor exercises (while sitting on the bed or chair) to help them gain awareness of their external sphincter and where it is sited. These exercises will also tighten and strengthen the pelvic floor muscles, allowing them to cope with times when they fear they may be incontinent (Norton, 1986; Blandy and Moors, 1989). The exercises should be practised several times an hour and the exact muscles identified. For example, if the patient tries to stop the flow of urine during micturition, he may be able to feel tightening of the muscles he needs to exercise. Encouragement and explanation will motivate the patient to achieve full continence. A small pad or dribble pouch may be used to avoid soiling of the pyjamas or trousers. Avoidance of night sedation for 1–2 nights after catheter removal may allow the patient to wake enough to enable voiding. Likewise, advice on reducing or ceasing to drink after about 6 pm may assist in providing an undisturbed night. Advice on removal of the catheter and careful monitoring of the fluid balance may prevent potentially upsetting experiences. However, patients should be advised against restricting their fluids too severely in order to prevent urgency and urge incontinence.

Pelvic floor exercises

There are two basic pelvic floor exercises that the patient can incorporate into his daily routine to help prevent dribbling incontinence and improve flow:

- When voiding, the patient should be encouraged to stop midstream. In doing so, he will be contracting his pelvic floor muscles

- Whether lying or sitting, the patient should be encouraged to contract his pelvic floor muscles at least five times daily in order to strengthen them

The wound drain in cases of RPP is removed as soon as it ceases to collect haemoserous fluid (24–48 hours post-operatively). The sutures or clips can be removed once the skin has healed adequately, usually after 7–10 days.

Patients who have undergone TURP are discharged approximately 4 days post-operatively, while those who have undergone RPP can expect to be discharged after 6–10 days. Discharge depends on physical state, other medical conditions and convalescent requirements.

Post-operative complications

An MSU should be obtained at approximately 24 hours after catheter removal to ensure that the patient has not developed a UTI owing to instrumentation or catheterization (McCormack, 1977; Meers et al., 1981). A UTI may stimulate a secondary haemorrhage from the prostatic bed, which is a common complication, often resulting in clot retention and subsequent readmission.

Another serious complication following endoscopic resective surgery is perforation of the bladder. If the surgeon is aware that this has occurred, a catheter will be left in situ for up to 10 days post-operatively in order to allow the perforation to heal. However, the condition may remain undetected at operation, so careful observation of the in- and outflow volumes of irrigant should be maintained and accurately documented, noting any deficit of output as irrigant may leak extravesically, causing abdominal distension and discomfort. In severe cases, the patient may return to theatre for a laparotomy and insertion of wound drain, as well as the possible insertion of a suprapubic catheter in addition to the urethral catheter to facilitate urine drainage.

Another complication that occurs specifically in cases of prostatic resection is that of transurethral resection syndrome (TUR syndrome). This involves the absorption of large amounts of irrigant into the venous system via the resected vessels within the prostatic tissue, causing hyponatraemia and hypervolaemia. The patient may become hypertensive and confused, and coma may ensue.

Standard treatment is to stop intravenous and irrigation fluids and to administer diuretics. While most patients recover without ill-effect, heart failure may ensue as a result of the absorption of large amounts of irrigant, and death from cardiac arrest occasionally occurs (Thompson and Woodhouse, 1987).

Discharge advice following prostatectomy

The patient may experience varying degrees of haematuria for up to a fortnight following surgery.

He should be told to rest as much as possible, although staying in bed is unnecessary. Occasionally there is frank haematuria, which can usually be eliminated by increased fluid intake (up to 3 L over a 24 hour period). Should this not resolve the haematuria, the patient should contact his GP as a further hospital admission may be necessary for catheterization and bladder washout.

A normal convalescence may require the patient to be away from work for 4–6 weeks depending on the type of employment (office work or manual labour). Strenuous physical exercise should be avoided for the first 2–3 weeks as this may stimulate bleeding from the site of surgery. Patients who have undergone RPP should be advised to avoid heavy lifting for at least 6 months until the abdominal wound and underlying tissues have healed sufficiently to withstand the strain. The patient also needs to be taught a safe and correct lifting technique. Normal bathing or showering can take place, providing that the wound has healed.

Issues common to renal surgery

The general principles of pre- and post-operative care in renal surgery are similar to those of urological surgery. Specifically, however, the site of operation (the loin) may cause breathing to be uncomfortable post-operatively. Instruction regarding full lung expansion and deep breathing exercises is important but should be accompanied by reassurance that adequate analgesia will be maintained. This will aid exercise and facilitate early mobilization post-operatively.

Nephrectomy

The kidney may be removed for the following reasons:

- non-function;
- neoplasm;
- abnormalities, for example tuberculosis, outflow obstruction caused by a large staghorn calculus or scar tissue causing renal impairment.

Specific investigations prior to admission include an IVU to ensure that the other kidney is present and functioning adequately, and to contribute towards diagnosis.

A renogram may also be required to determine each individual kidney's function. An ultrasound is frequently performed, particularly if the patient is likely to experience an allergic reaction to the IVU contrast, and will determine whether a lesion is hydronephrotic or solid.

Admission

The operation site should be marked in indelible ink by the surgeon to ensure removal of the correct kidney.

Nephrectomy is usually performed under general anaesthesia, the patient being placed in the lateral position on the unaffected side on the theatre table, which is tipped down at both ends. This allows the loin to be stretched and the rib cage to be raised above the site of incision, which is usually parallel with the 12th rib.

The operation

The operation takes approximately 1.5 hours. The kidney is identified and mobilized, the renal artery and vein isolated and ligated, and the affected ureter ligated. The kidney is removed and sent to the pathology laboratory. In some cases (usually those involving transitional cell carcinoma), the ureter may be removed down to the bladder; this may entail a separate incision over the bladder.

Nephrectomy is an operation starting to be undertaken laparoscopically in cases in which the diagnosis is not that of suspected neoplasm. This operation currently takes several hours, and patients may suffer from complications such as respiratory distress and haemorrhage resulting from major surgery. A drain should be left in situ for 48-72 hours, allowing accurate monitoring should post-operative haemorrhage occur.

Post-operative nursing care

A state of adequate analgesia is particularly desirable to allow comfort and ease of movements, and to assist the patient to gain full lung expansion. Sitting the patient up as soon as vital signs and an unobstructed airway allow will help deep breathing, expanding the lung bases.

Discharge

This usually occurs 6–8 days post-operatively, depending on individual progress with regard to wound healing, gut motility and general mobility, as well as the social circumstances and plans for convalescence.

DISCHARGE ADVICE FOLLOWING NEPHRECTOMY, PYELOPLASTY AND LITHOTOMY

The patient is advised to convalesce for 4–6 weeks post-operatively depending on his occupation.

The incision site is a weakness in the muscle wall and will need time to heal adequately before being strained. The patient should therefore be advised not to lift anything heavier than a full kettle for the initial 4 weeks after surgery, gradually increasing the weight being lifted; this should be done with care.

Pyeloplasty

A pyeloplasty involves refashioning the pelvi-ureteric junction (PUJ) of a kidney that does not function properly and causes obstruction to urinary outflow from the kidney. This may be caused by scar tissue resulting from previous surgical intervention, infection, trauma or, most commonly, congenital abnormality.

Investigations prior to surgery

A common symptom of PUJ obstruction is acute colicky pain in the loin provoked by drinking large amounts of fluid, which indicates that an IVU is required for diagnosis. If this demonstrates the characteristic dilatation of the renal pelvis and strictured ureter below the PUJ, a renogram will often be performed to confirm the diagnosis and estimate the function of the affected kidney. An MSU should be sent for culture, and appropriate antibiotic treatment may be required peri-operatively.

Specific pre-operative preparation

The operation site must be marked with indelible ink by the surgeon to indicate the affected kidney. Some surgeons may prescribe anti-embolism stockings and/or subcutaneous anticoagulation therapy. Generally, however, such patients tend to be young and relatively fit and are thus able to mobilize quickly post-operatively. The patient should have had an adequate bowel action within 24 hours of surgery to prevent discomfort on post-operative straining. Constipation commonly occurs if the patient is sedentary, dehydrated, unable to eat or drink or receiving opiate analgesics.

The operation

The incision is usually above or below the 12th rib and will necessitate the patient being positioned on the unaffected side with the site for operation exposed uppermost. The theatre table is tipped down at either end so that the loin is stretched and the kidney becomes more accessible. Surgery takes approximately 1.5 hours. A loin approach is used, the kidney mobilized and the dilated renal pelvis incised. A flap of redundant renal pelvic tissue is then used to create a wider PUJ in one of a variety of ways.

Post-operatively

A Cummings nephrostomy tube or similar type of catheter (i.e. double J stent) may be left in situ as a splinting catheter to drain the urine and allow the anastomosis to heal. A wound drain is left in place to drain haemoserous fluid from the operation site and prevent the formation of a haematoma. The wound drain is removed when the output from the drain is minimal or has ceased. The nephrostomy tube is left for at least 8–10 days, at which point a nephrostogram is usually performed. This involves the injection of radio-opaque contrast medium down the nephrostomy tube in order to determine whether there is adequate drainage down the ureter and healing without extravasation from the anastomosis. Once this has been established, the nephrostomy tube may be clamped/spigotted for 24 hours and the patient observed for loin pain, pyrexia or leakage around the nephrostomy tube, which will occur if the ureter is obstructed, preventing urine draining to the bladder. If the ureter is unobstructed, the nephrostomy tube may be removed (after analgesics have been offered) by releasing the securing external suture and firmly pulling out the tube. The site may then be dressed with a dry dressing and secured with tape.

Discharge

This usually occurs approximately 12 days post-operatively, depending on wound healing and gut motility as well as social circumstances and plans for convalescence.

Surgery for renal calculi

There are various methods of stone removal and treatment, depending on the size, shape, density and position of the stone within the renal tract. Most stones are formed by the precipitation of crystals in the urine and are composed of calcium, oxalate, phosphate or urate.

Investigations

Investigations are undertaken in order to establish the exact location of the stone(s) and how they have affected the urinary tract (e.g. hydronephrosis owing to obstruction). This is best investigated by means of an IVU or ultrasound.

Although a plain abdominal X-ray of the kidneys, ureter and bladder may outline the majority of stones, it will not delineate their position with reference to the urinary tract. This may be appropriate in cases of allergy to IVU contrast, but an ultrasound scan of the kidneys will provide much more detailed diagnostic information.

An MSU is obtained for culture in order to detect any infection prior to instrumentation of the urinary tract.

Other factors that contribute to the precipitation of these stones are

- Working in an environment that causes excessive perspiration, dehydration and therefore concentrated urine (e.g. those people living and working in the tropics or working in an engine room)

- Foreign bodies such as those forming the core of a stone and causing a snowball effect (e.g. dissolvable sutures, prostatic chips, necrosed renal papilla or fragments of catheters)

- Stones also form for metabolic reasons such as hyperparathyroidism, which causes calcium to be extracted from the bones and be taken up into the circulation, leading to high urinary concentrations

- Stones can also form in areas where urine is stagnant, such as in the bladder, secondary to prostatic obstruction

- Cystine stones form as a result of the condition cystinuria, whereby the renal tubules have a congenital inability to reabsorb a certain group of amino acids from the glomerular filtrate

- Uric acid stones, associated with a high level of serum uric acid and gout, tend to precipitate in urine infected by *Proteus mirabilis* and some other bacteria that alkanalize the urine.

The most significant complication of obstruction and infection is that renal function may be compromised. For this reason, the patient's temperature must be monitored carefully as it may be the first indication of bacteraemia. In this circumstance, a nephrostomy tube may be placed in the affected kidney to relieve the obstruction; this may be done under a local anaesthetic.

Metabolic disorders may result in certain types of stone. The relevant substances, such as uric acid and cystine, may be measured in urine and serum specimens. Calcium and uric acid levels can be measured in a 24 hour urine collection, while cystine requires a random urine sample of approximately 50–100 ml.

Stones may occur anywhere in the urinary tract. If in the kidney, symptoms may include loin pain, repeated urinary tract infections and haematuria. The stones can become so enlarged that they adopt the shape of the kidney calyces – termed staghorn calculi. They may be so large and insidious in their growth that they slowly impair renal function until very little remains and the kidney serves only as a focus for infection.

Small renal stones can become dislodged and move down the pelvis to the PUJ and ureter. This causes excruciating pain of sudden onset, often resulting in vomiting, sweating and abdominal distension.

Patient comment

'I've never felt anything like it. The pain was excruciating and nothing would make it go away.'

For those patients who have a stone lodged high in the urinary tract, pain starts in the loin and gradually moves down, radiating to the front of the abdominal wall as the stone moves down the ureter. Stone movement is accompanied by peristaltic movements of the ureter. Haematuria may be caused by trauma to the urothelium.

The majority of ureteric stones will be passed into the bladder if they are less than 4 mm in diameter. The urine should be sieved to obtain the stones for analysis, which may direct subsequent investigations and treatments.

Stone surgery strategies include:

- Open nephrolithotomy – removal of a stone from within the renal caliceal system

- Pyelolithotomy – stone removal from the pelvis of the kidney

- Ureterolithotomy – removal of a stone from the ureter

- Cystolithotomy – removal of a large bladder stone via an abdominal incision

- Lithopaxy – crushing of a bladder stone endoscopically using a lithotrite (an instrument with jaws to crush the stone) and washing out the remaining grit

- Percutaneous nephrolithotomy – removal of a stone, via a tube inserted through a small skin puncture in the loin, under X-ray screening while the patient is anaesthetized

Another method of treating stones without surgical intervention is that of extracorporeal shock wave lithotripsy (ESWL). This is a non-invasive intervention that uses shock waves to disintegrate the stone into grit-sized particles, which may be extracted per urethram. It is sometimes performed under general anaesthetic, although this is to a certain extent determined by the type of lithotripter available.

Admission

The patient is usually admitted a day prior to surgery to allow adequate preparation. A full explanation of the surgery and post-operative expectations is important. The affected side is marked in indelible ink by a medical officer.

Pre-operative care

Specific investigations include an IVU and, immediately prior to surgery, a kidney, ureter and bladder X-ray. These provide an image of the exact position of the stone and demonstrate any recent movement. The IVU will also establish whether there is obstruction within the upper urinary tract caused by the stone. Ultrasound is also being increasingly used to delineate stones in the urinary tract (Campion *et al.*, 1994).

The site of operation on the loin or lower abdomen can cause breathing to be uncomfortable post-operatively. Explanation of full lung expansion and deep breathing exercises is important, as is advice concerning adequate analgesia prior to chest physiotherapy to facilitate exercise and early post-operative mobilization.

The operation

The operation site depends upon the position of the stone – a loin approach for nephro-, pyelo- and upper ureterolithotomy, and an abdominal approach for uretero- or cystolithotomy. The operation usually lasts 1.0–1.5 hours but may be longer. If stones are removed during nephrolithotomy, an X-ray of the kidney is undertaken per-operatively using small kidney-sized plates placed underneath the kidney to ensure that all the stones have been removed prior to closing the skin. Wound drains may be left in situ post-operatively to facilitate adequate drainage of haemoserous fluid and ensure effective wound healing.

A ureteric splinting catheter is usually positioned by the surgeon to facilitate urine drainage until the ureteric oedema has reduced sufficiently to allow an unobstructed urinary flow to the bladder. A urethral catheter may be left in situ to facilitate urine drainage while post-operative pain prevents the patient moving into a position to pass urine.

Post-operative nursing care

A blood transfusion or intravenous infusion is administered to replace blood loss per- and post-operatively and to maintain hydration and fluid balance until the patient is able to drink a sufficient amount of fluid – 1.5–2 L of fluid orally within a 24 hour period. This may take 3–4 days to achieve, and oral fluids should be gradually increased depending upon the patient's fluid tolerance and bowel sounds.

The splinting ureteric catheter may be removed following an X-ray used to outline the patient's ureter with radio-opaque contrast medium approximately 10 days post-operatively. The wound may be closed with clips or nylon/silk sutures, which are removed 6–8 days post-operatively.

Discharge

This usually occurs 8–10 days post-operatively, although this depends entirely on the individual's progress with regard to wound healing, gut motility and mobility, and the social circumstances and plans for convalescence.

Percutaneous nephrolithotomy

This involves a combination of resources, including an endoscopic approach and surgical technique under the guidance of an image intensifier. Thus the multidisciplinary skills of a radiologist, radiographer, anaesthetist, urologist and scrub nurse are merged in one procedure.

Admission

The patient is usually admitted the day prior to surgery, having undergone the necessary investigations. The affected side is marked in indelible ink by a medical officer. The procedure usually takes 1.0–1.5 hours under general anaesthetic.

Cystoscopy and retrograde catheterization of the affected ureter are performed. The prone oblique position is preferred to facilitate easy access to the loin. Contrast medium is injected via the ureteric catheter in order to identify the exact positioning of the stone (Fig. 10.2).

The appropriate renal calyx is punctured percutaneously, and, once the collecting system has been entered, a guidewire is manipulated down the tract. Serial dilators are passed over the guidewire up to 26 or 30 Charrière/FG in size. The urologist can then pass a nephroscope via an Amplatz tube placed in the tract to maintain the passage (Fig. 10.3). Irrigation of the tract is ach-

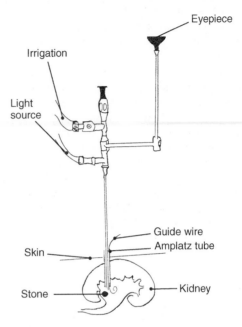

Figure 10.3 Nephroscope viewing a stone within the kidney

ieved via a channel in the nephroscope, facilitating viewing the stone by distending the renal pelvis. Forceps can be used to remove the stone if it is small enough, or an ultrasonic or electrohydraulic probe can be used to shatter the stone into manageable fragments for removal.

A nephrostomy tube is left in situ to drain urine and blood from the renal pelvis while tissue oedema settles post-procedure, also allowing further access to the renal pelvis for nephrostograms or subsequent attempts to remove any remaining stones. The nephrostomy tube may also act to tamponade any bleeding from the renal tissue.

Post-operatively

Occasionally, haemorrhage from the kidney occurs which is not resolved by tamponade and which may then require open surgical intervention. Clots of blood from the renal pelvis may also

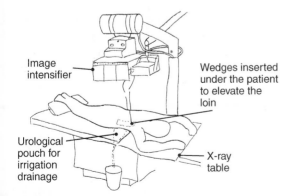

Figure 10.2 Position of the patient undergoing percutaneous nephrolithotomy

be present, causing ureteric colic that may require a fast-acting analgesic.

Once awake, the patient may eat and drink as he wishes. An adequate fluid intake of at least 1.5–2 L within a 24 hour period should be promoted. This will assist in reducing the patient's haematuria.

The nephrostomy tube should be firmly secured to the skin, ensuring that it does not pull at the sutures or fall out. It is removed at the surgeon's discretion following a nephrostogram that should demonstrate an unobstructed ureter and total clearance of stones. The small incision from which the nephrostomy tube is removed may leak urine for a short time. This usually resolves within an hour or so but may require a stoma bag to collect the drainage; it will eventually heal within 2–3 days. A dry dressing should be applied, and the patient can be discharged. A 6 week follow-up appointment should be given.

Discharge advice

The patient may be able to return to work within 2–3 weeks depending on his employment.

Some blood in the urine may be experienced about 10 days following surgery. It is usually a small amount, which will stop within 24 hours. Should this occur, the patient should be advised to drink 1–2 L of fluid within 2–3 hours so that the urine is diluted. If bleeding persists and becomes heavily blood stained (dark red urine with clots), the patient should visit his GP or attend an A&E department.

Urinary diversion – ileal conduit

This elective surgery involves the implantation of the ureters into a segment of the ileum, which has been formed into a stoma in the abdominal wall. Depending on the reason for surgery, for example carcinoma of the bladder, cystectomy may be performed at the same time. Common reasons for this surgery are damage or disease of the bladder, chronic incontinence or retention of urine, congenital abnormality, trauma to the pelvis and interstitial cystitis.

Admission

This takes place 3–4 days prior to surgery. Psychological preparation, involving both doctor and stomatherapist, should have commenced in the OPD or during a previous admission.

A good rapport between the patient and nurse is essential so that trust is established and any fears can be explored. A level of understanding must first be established; more information can then gradually be introduced by the nurse/ stomatherapist, using aids and diagrams. It is important to note the patient's reaction at this time as an indication of acceptance of the forthcoming operation and its potential implications. Literature can be made available for the patient to read at leisure, and the opportunity should be given to meet an ex-patient who has undergone the same surgery.

Assessment of the patient's general capabilities (manual dexterity, sight, sensation) are essential. Enquiries should also be made into the patient's living conditions to establish whether there may be any potential problems, for example sharing a bathroom with many other people.

If possible, it may be beneficial for the patient to involve someone else, such as a partner, especially if the patient loses independence and is unable to care for the stoma. The subject of sex should also be discussed and the patient reassured that normal sexual relationships can continue following discharge, except perhaps in the case of a man having a cystectomy as the nerve supplying the penis may be damaged, leading to impotence. In this situation, it may be appropriate to involve a sex therapist or psychosexual counsellor.

Pre-operatively

Specific investigations are IVU or ultrasound to confirm normal upper urinary tracts, and a full blood count to establish haemoglobin level, which may be low in those patients with a history of haematuria.

Careful consideration is given before siting the stoma. The nurse/stomatherapist should discuss the type of clothing worn, for example waistline and braces and the normal range of movements (particularly relevant to wheelchair-bound patients). The stoma should be sited within the rectus muscle, avoiding skin creases, bony prominences, scars and the umbilicus. The chosen site should then be marked with an indelible pen and checked carefully as the patient moves about. The patient should be shown some of the equipment and encouraged to wear a bag in order to experience the sensation and detect any potential problems with positioning.

STUDENT ACTIVITY

Stick a urostomy bag containing 250 ml of water on to your abdomen, get dressed and try to follow your normal daily activities.

Pre-operative bowel preparation is required to empty the bowel of any waste products and reduce the spillage of faecal matter, which may cause septic complications. Prophylactic antibiotics may also be prescribed, to be given with pre-medication and on induction.

The operation

Surgery involves the isolation of a segment of ileum, complete with its own mesenteric blood supply, via an abdominal incision. A stoma is formed on the surface of the skin, from which a small spout of ileum extends. The ureters are implanted in the distal end of the segment, which is otherwise closed. The urine drains continuously through the stoma into a collecting appliance via ureteric splints inserted during surgery to prevent obstruction caused by post-operative oedema.

Post-operative nursing care

It is essential for the stoma to be viewed easily so a clear drainable stoma bag should be applied. This should be observed on a half-hourly basis, lessening as the patient's condition stabilizes.

Observations should include assessment of:

- Colour of the stoma. This should be pink and shiny. Any discolouration (e.g. mauve, blue or black) may indicate a diminished blood supply. If any alteration in the colour occurs, the bag and flange should be changed for a larger size in case the stoma has swollen post-operatively. If no improvement occurs, medical staff must be contacted.

- Bleeding from the stoma. A small amount is to be expected, but this should be monitored.

- Oedema. This is to be expected but should be monitored.

- Ureteric splints. Ensure that these are correctly placed so that the stoma can drain.

- Urine output. Urine will initially drain down the ureteric catheters through the urostomy into a catheter bag to prevent urine collecting in the urostomy bag, backtracking up the ureteric catheters and causing infection. At first, the urine may be blood stained, and there may be some mucus secreted by the ileal segment. The nurse will carefully measure and record the fluid output, aiming to detect any signs of ureteric obstruction or dehydration.

An intravenous infusion will be in progress to maintain hydration while the patient is nil by mouth during the paralytic ileus phase. A nasogastric tube may be in place; free drainage into a bag should prevent nausea and vomiting. When bowel sounds recommence, the tube can be clamped and small measured amounts of oral fluids commenced. If the patient tolerates this, the nasogastric tube can be removed. Once the patient is tolerating adequate amounts of fluid to maintain hydration, the intravenous infusion can be discontinued, normally at 3–5 days post-operatively. The patient can then graduate to a normal diet.

The wound drain remains in situ until drainage is minimal, usually at 48–72 hours post-surgery. The wound will be dressed as necessary, and the sutures remain in place for 7–10 days. The sutures around the stoma are usually dissolvable. The ureteric splints are normally removed after 10–12 days.

The stoma may need cleaning during the first few days, which can usually be carried out without removing the flange, using gauze and normal saline; it is a socially clean procedure. The stoma may be swollen and unsightly at this early stage, and it is important that the nurse reassures the patient that it will shrink over the next few days. The first complete flange and bag change normally takes place after 2–3 days. If the patient is apprehensive, it is not necessary for him to watch on this occasion. The patient should be introduced gradually to the procedure and be encouraged to participate more actively each time. Supervision will be required until the patient is competent with the entire procedure. For those with a distended abdomen, a mirror may be helpful for viewing the stoma.

Discharge advice

The patient is discharged about 2 weeks after operation when members of the multidisciplinary team are satisfied with progress and the patient and his family feel able to cope.

The stomatherapist will ensure that the patient has supplies of equipment adequate to last for 2–3 weeks. The patient will also be advised where to obtain further equipment, and the therapist will organize, through the GP, for the patient to be exempt from prescription charges.

Urethrosuspension for stress incontinence

This surgery is performed for stress incontinence in females. There are two main techniques:

- *colposuspension*, which is a technique involving open surgery to reposition the urethra by hitching up the surrounding tissue to reposition and support it;
- *the Stamey procedure*, whereby an endoscope is used to place stitches on either side of the urethra. These stitches are then made taut to reposition the urethra.

Admission

The patient is usually admitted 1–2 days prior to surgery. Careful assessment of incontinence is required, using time and amount charts and recording the number of incontinence pads used in a day. Techniques such as videocystography can assess bladder function and exclude bladder instability as a cause of incontinence. Pelvic floor exercises to promote continence should also be explained and the patient encouraged to carry these out.

The operation

Both procedures rely on repositioning part of the urethra within the intra-abdominal pressure zone, which prevents leakage of urine on coughing and sneezing. For the Stamey procedure, the lithotomy position is employed, and for colposuspension, the Lloyd Davies position. The operation takes approximately 1.0–1.5 hours.

Post-operative nursing care

On return to the ward, there will be an intra-venous infusion in situ, which will be removed once the patient can tolerate fluids orally without nausea. The patient may start eating as soon as she feels able. A vaginal pack is also in situ, being removed 24 hours post-operatively. The patient should be advised that there may be some dis-charge or bleeding for a few days afterwards.

After colposuspension, there will be an inci-sion just above the pubic hair line, and the sutures here are usually removed 5–7 days post-operatively. The Stamey procedure is carried out through two small incisions in the groin, the sutures of these also being removed on day 5–7.

The patient will have suprapubic and urethral urinary catheters in place, which should be mon-itored, recording the drainage accurately. The urethral catheter is normally removed about the third day post-operatively. Approximately 4–5 days after surgery, the suprapubic catheter is clamped and the patient encouraged to pass urine urethrally. Fluid intake should render the urine pale and plentiful/straw coloured or col-ourless, and the patient is advised to pass urine 2 hourly initially to strengthen bladder tone. As the patient becomes more confident, the intervals can be extended. Twice daily residual volumes will be measured to assess bladder function. After the patient has passed urine urethrally, the nurse unclamps the catheter and measures the residual volume in a jug. If the volume is less than 50 ml, the catheter is removed.

Discharge advice

As soon as the patient has returned to a fairly normal pattern of micturition, she will be dis-charged home. On average, this tends to be 10 days post-operatively.

The patient should be encouraged to conva-lesce for a minimum of 2 weeks at home and to avoid any lifting, returning to a normal routine and lifestyle. The patient should be advised to continue her pelvic floor exercises (*see* Part One).

An outpatient appointment will be arranged for 6 weeks post-discharge for the doctor to assess the patient's progress.

Repair of vesicovaginal fistula

This is performed to repair an abnormal tract between the bladder/urethra and vagina to pre-vent the drainage of urine via the vagina. The development of the fistula is usually the result of an accident, surgical trauma or trauma caused by radiotherapy to a pelvic organ.

Pre-operatively

The patient will be admitted 2–3 days prior to surgery. Specifically, she should be told that she will return to the ward with suprapubic and urethral catheters and a wound drain.

The patient may also require specific pre-operative investigations. These may include: an IVU to ensure that the upper urinary tracts are normal; a cystogram to identify the abnormal tract or fistula; a vaginal swab and an MSU to detect infection; and a full blood count to detect anaemia, which may be a result of radiotherapy.

The operation

A cystoscope is introduced via the urethra into the bladder, and the fistula is identified. A mid-line abdominal incision is then made and the fistula exposed. The edges of the fistula are excised, and the vaginal and bladder layers are repaired separately. Omentum is mobilized and placed into the vesicovaginal space to strengthen the repair.

The patient's position during the operation will depend on the position of the fistula, the duration of the operation depending on the difficulty of the surgery.

Post-operative nursing care

An intravenous infusion may be in progress for several days to maintain hydration; the patient may have a mild paralytic ileus as a result of manipulation of the bowel. Once the patient is no longer nauseated, she can commence small measured quantities of fluid. When she is able to maintain hydration independently, the infusion is discontinued. The patient can then graduate to a light diet when bowel sounds have occurred and flatus has been passed.

The patient will have a urethral catheter in situ for 10–14 days. There is a potential for infection owing to the site of the surgery and the presence of the catheter, so antibiotic cover will be given. Should there be any delay to healing, such as cystitis, the catheter will remain until it is resolved.

Vasectomy

This operation involves the division of the vasa deferentia, the tubes through which sperm is ejaculated from the epididymis to the urethra, under either general or local anaesthetic. This operation is intended to cause sterility. This should provide an effective and permanent method of contraception and requires a minimum of eight clear ejaculations post-operatively to ensure that there are no sperm remaining in the vas deferens.

Admission

This is usually on the day of surgery, and the patient will therefore be starved if having a general anaesthetic. Alternatively, the patient may undergo the procedure under local anaesthetic in the outpatient clinic. Both the patient and partner should undergo pre-operative counselling on the implications of sterilization.

Incisions are made either in the scrotum or inguinally to gain access to the vas deferens, which is located and then divided. The ends of the cut deferens are sometimes tied back on themselves to prevent them rejoining naturally.

Self-dissolving sutures are used for the external incisions, and small dressings are placed over the wounds and held in place.

Post-operative nursing care

A scrotal support and pad will protect the tender scrotum and can be worn for as long as the patient wishes. The patient may start to eat and drink as soon as he can without feeling nauseated.

Observations should be made of the wounds to detect a haematoma. It is thought that approximately 1% of patients develop a haematoma large enough to warrant surgical intervention (Fell, 1994).

A further complication is that of infection, which may be a result of bacteria already in the patient's semen. This can be treated with the appropriate antibiotics.

Discharge advice

The patient and his partner should be advised that he will not be completely sterile until after at least 6–8 ejaculations and should therefore take other contraceptive precautions until that time. Sterility is confirmed after two sperm counts 1–2 months later. The patient should refrain from sexual activity until scrotal tenderness has eased and he feels comfortable.

The patient should convalesce for approximately a week before returning to work and avoid unnecessary exertion and friction to the scrotum, such as that from riding a bicycle.

Circumcision

Circumcision involves excision of the penile foreskin. It may be undertaken for:

- phimosis
- paraphimosis
- injury

Admission

The patient is often admitted on the day of surgery provided that he is fit for anaesthesia and has fasted; the operation normally lasts 15–20 minutes.

The operation

Following cleansing of the site with antiseptic, the foreskin is removed and self-dissolving sutures are used to sew over the cut skin at the base of the glans. This is then covered with an appropriate dressing. Circumcision may be performed on children and young infants using a device called a 'plastibell', the foreskin being tied tightly to the device. This causes it to necrose at the site of the sutures and fall away naturally within a few days.

Post-operative nursing care

The patient may eat and drink as soon after the operation as he wishes without experiencing nausea.

Given the proximity of the dorsal vein and frenular arteries, haemorrhage is a potential postoperative complication. This must be taken seriously in young infants, in whom the blood loss of an apparently insignificant amount may represent a large part of the circulatory volume. The patient's vital signs should therefore be monitored on a regular basis and medical help sought if necessary. The wound should also be inspected regularly (1–2 hourly) to detect any significant haematoma.

The following morning, the dressing may be soaked off in the bath or shower. The wound site should be observed by a nurse; it will appear sore and inflamed. A sterile pad should be applied, supported by net pants in order to protect against the abrasiveness of the patient's clothing rather than for reasons of asepsis. Daily baths or showers followed by thorough but gentle drying with a soft towel are recommended for at least a week in order to maintain wound cleanliness.

Discharge advice

The patient is discharged home if the wound is satisfactory and the sutures are intact. This may be 24 hours following surgery. The patient can return to work after approximately 2–3 days convalescence. The patient is advised to wear loose, non-constricting trousers and supportive underwear for at least a week. The patient is also advised to refrain from sexual activity until the wound is no longer sore and inflamed.

Developments in urological surgery

Much work has recently been done on alternatives to prostatectomy. There may be situations in which patients present with outflow obstruction owing to an enlarged prostate but are not suitable candidates for standard surgical intervention. This may be because they are unfit for general anaesthetic or, in younger patients, are unwilling to risk retrograde ejaculation or impotence. Alternatives must therefore be considered.

There are several options, two of which are balloon dilatation of the prostate gland and insertion of a prostatic stent. Both involve re-establishing a patent prostatic urethra, the former through inserting a balloon and dilating it for 10–15 minutes, the latter by inserting a permanent stent over which epithelium forms over a 6–8 month period. Both procedures meet with a varied degree of success, they are described by Maxfield *et al.* (1994). Additional references can be found in the further reading section below.

Summary

1 All patients have urinalysis and an MSU to exclude problems before surgery.

2 Fluid balance records must be meticulous.

3 The selection, insertion and management of urinary catheters is outlined.

4 Specific preparation, per-operative considerations and advice on discharge are covered for the most commonly performed urological operations.

CASE HISTORY

Mr Liakos, aged 57, has had a urinary catheter in place for 5 days and has developed a urinary tract infection. Identify and explain how this may have been acquired. How could it have been prevented?

Review Questions

1 How do you work out the patient's fluid requirements?

2 Draw a diagram of a three-way catheter to explain how it works to a patient.

3 How is hyperparathyroidism associated with renal calculi?

4 What does lithotripsy do?

5 List the observations to be made on a patient with a newly formed ileal conduit stoma.

6 List seven major sources of fibre in the diet.

ACKNOWLEDGEMENTS

With acknowledgements to Elizabeth Wright and Clare Beattie, the original chapter material.

References

Blandy, J. and Moors, J. 1989 *Urology for nurses.* Oxford: Blackwell Scientific.

Campion, J., Lockett, R.M. and Rainsbury, S.E. 1994 Urinary tract stones. In: Laker, C. (ed.) *Urological nursing.* London: Scutari Press.

Crow, R., Mulhall, A. and Chapman, R.G. 1986 Indwelling catheterisation and related nursing practice. *Journal of Advanced Nursing,* **13**, 489–95.

Fell, S. 1994 Scrotal disorders. In: Laker, C. (ed.) *Urological nursing,* London: Scutari Press.

McCormack, R.C. 1977 In Hook, E.W. (ed.) *Current concepts of infectious diseases.* New York: John Wiley & Sons.

Maxfield, J., Dennison, K. and Forristal, H. 1994 Prostatic problems. In: Laker, C. (ed.) *Urological nursing.* London: Scutari Press.

Meers, P.D., Ayliffe, G.A.J., Emmerson, A.M. *et al.* 1981 Report on the national survey on infection in hospitals. *Journal of Hospital Infection* **2**(suppl.), 1–39.

Norton, C. 1996 *Nursing for continence* 2nd edn. Beaconsfield: Beaconsfield Publishers.

Sturdy, D.E. 1986 *An outline of urology.* Bristol: IOP Publishing.

Thompson, F.D. and Woodhouse, C.R.J. 1987 *Disorders of the kidney and urinary tract.* London: Edward Arnold.

Wright, E.S. 1988 Catheter care: the risk of infection. *Professional Nurse* **3**(12), 487–90.

Further reading

Blandy, J.P. 1989 *Lecture notes on urology,* 4th edn. Oxford: Blackwell Scientific.

Booth, J. 1983 *Handbook of investigations.* London: Harper & Row.

Bullock, N., Sibley, G. and Whitaker, R. 1989 *Essential urology.* London: Churchill Livingstone.

Burkitt, D. & Randall, J. 1987 Catheterisation: urethral trauma. *Nursing Times* **83**(43), 59–60, 63.

Burkitt, D. & Randall, J. 1987 Safe procedures. *Nursing Times* **83**(43), 65–6.

Chappell, C.R., Milroy, J.G. and Rickards, D. 1990 Permanently implanted urethral stent for prostatic obstruction in the unfit patient. *British Journal of Urology* **66**, 58–65.

Dickson, C. 1995 Operatic procedures for benign prostatic hypertrophy. *Nursing Times* **91**(38), 34–5.

Getliffe, K.A. 1995 Long term catheter use in the community. *Nursing Standard* **9**(31), 25–7.

Kohler-Ockmore, J. 1993 Catheter concerns. *Nursing Times* **10**(1), 25–31.

Laker, C. (ed.) 1994 *Urological nursing.* London: Scutari Press.

McLonghlin, J. and Williams, G. 1990 Prostatic stents and balloon dilatation. *British Journal of Hospital Medicine* **43**, 422–6.

Pomfret, I. 1991 The catheter debate. *Nursing Times* **87**(37), 67–8.

Pomfret, I. 1994 An unsuitable job for a woman? *Nursing Times* **90**(22), 46, 48.

Roe, B. 1990 Do we need to clamp catheters? *Nursing Times* **86**(43), 66–7.

Roe, B. 1991 Looking at the evidence. *Nursing Times* **87**(37), 72–4.

Rogers, J. 1991 Pass the cranberry juice. *Nursing Times* **87**(48), 36–7.

Wheeler, V. 1990 A new kind of loving. *Professional Nurse* **5**(9), 492.

Willis, V. 1995 Catheters: urinary tract infection. *Nursing Times* **87**(37), 72–4.

Winn, C. and Thompson, J. 1996 Catheterisation: extending the scope of practice. *Nursing Standard* **10**(52), 49–53.

Wright, E.S. 1987 Percutaneous nephrolithotomy. *Professional Nurse* **3**(3), 76–9.

Wright, E.S. 1988 Extra-corporeal shock wave lithotripsy. *Professional Nurse* **3**(4), 121–3.

Vascular surgery

Penelope Simpson

Introduction

This rapidly evolving field is increasingly being dealt with by separate specialist units rather than by general surgeons. This chapter deals mainly with reconstructive vascular surgery, needed because diseases such as atherosclerosis are associated with diminished blood supply. *See* Chapter 7 for the cardiothoracic effects of atheroma.

Patients who present for vascular surgery are likely to have widespread systemic disease and certain features in common with each other.

Issues common to most vascular surgical procedures

Smoking is a major risk factor associated with vascular disease, so some surgeons refuse to operate on those continuing to smoke as it reduces the chances of success. For example, the saphenous vein is often used for femorodistal arterial bypass grafting. It can be damaged by smoking, which is associated with endothelial dysfunction of the femoral arteries and saphenous veins. All patients undergoing bypass graft surgery are advised not to smoke, and vein graft patency is improved in those who give up (Higman et al., 1994). The nurse's role is to educate patients in how smoking affects their disease process and to support their attempts to cut down or give up.

Pulse volume monitoring

Peripheral pulse volumes need to be recorded regularly to identify the patency or otherwise of vessels and grafts. A method of scoring, based on a scale from 0–4 (adapted from Brunner and Suddarth, 1989), can be useful:

0	Not palpable – absent pulsation
+1	Thready, weak, fades in and out – marked impairment of pulsation
+2	Difficult to palpate, stronger than +1 – moderate impairment
+3	Easily palpable, not easily obliterated with pressure – slight impairment
+4	Strong and bounding, normal pulsation – no impairment

Pulses monitored include the dorsalis pedis, posterior tibial, femoral and popliteal. The colour, temperature and sensation of limbs are also recorded.

Constriction of vessels

Patients are advised against wearing tight, constricting clothes such as girdles, corsets, garters,

belts, jeans and tight stockings, all of which restrict blood flow to the extremities.

Anticoagulant therapy

To prevent platelet aggregation and the formation of emboli, most post-operative patients are prescribed aspirin 75 mg daily for the rest of their lives. Patients taking warfarin will need a teaching programme to ensure that they understand their therapy and the need for follow-up (Wyness, 1990; Tritschler, 1994).

Diabetic patients

Patients will be closely monitored to ensure that their blood glucose level remains well controlled, as poor metabolic control is associated with atherosclerosis. Approximately 50% of UK diabetic hospital admissions are for foot problems. Lumley (1994) argues for a team approach, combining chiropodists, orthotists, physicians and surgeons to ensure optimum treatment of the diabetic patient and his associated risk factors. A diabetic nurse specialist is essential.

Infection

Infection of prosthetic vascular grafts, although relatively uncommon, (1–6%) is associated with high amputation and mortality rates (Stansby *et al.*, 1994). Short- and medium-term infections are thought to result from implantation of organisms at the time of surgery, so intravenous antibiotics are usually given prophylactically during surgery. In some cases, however, graft infection may be delayed for months or even years. Stansby *et al.* (1994) postulate that late vascular graft infections are the result of dental procedures in those with peridontal disease or dental infection. For this reason, they suggest that patients be educated about the importance of dental care and given a card or booklet to show their dentist before treatment so that appropriate antibiotic prophylaxis may be employed.

Infections are most prominent in patients with groin incisions, the most common organism being *Staphylococcus*, arising from the patient's skin. If one of the graft anastomoses is involved in the septic process, presentation may be by massive bleeding. If the graft but not the anastomosis is involved, the presentation will be one of vague malaise and fever. Once the diagnosis has been confirmed, treatment includes removal of the infected graft with if possible, reconstruction of the vascular system (Harris, 1992).

Carotid endarterectomy

Surgery is necessary if 70% of the carotid artery lumen is stenosed. The patient will usually have a history of transient ischaemic attacks (TIAs) and transient loss of vision. He is likely to have hypertension, which must be stabilized before admission.

Detection and treatment (endarterectomy) of asymptomatic carotid stenosis can reduce the incidence of stroke (Towne and Hobson, 1994) and TIAs (Strandness, 1993).

Patients being considered for carotid endarterectomy may undergo four-vessel carotid contrast arteriography to delineate the nature and extent of arterial pathology. Non-invasive testing, consisting of duplex ultrasonographic scanning plus sound spectrum analysis, is suggested to be an alternative method for accurately evaluating the carotid bifurcation (Ballard *et al.*, 1994 Horn *et al.*, 1994).

Admission and assessment

The patient is usually admitted on the day before surgery unless he has attended a pre-admission clinic, in which case he can arrive on the day of operation.

Pre-operative care

Usually, one side at a time is dealt with. If bilateral surgery is proposed, a pre-operative vocal cord check is performed in ENT outpatients.

The patient must not go to theatre unless his blood pressure is under control, so a series of baseline vital sign observations may be necessary.

The operation

Operation includes clamping of the carotid artery to allow access, with carotid shunting in those patients with poor cerebral reserve (Palombo *et al.*, 1994). The technique may include patch angioplasty to increase the diameter of the vessel; this may be of particular relevance to women and smokers (Gelabert *et al.*, 1994). It reduces the number of immediate post-operative complications and significantly lowers vessel restenosis and occlusion rates 1 year after surgery (Ranaboldo *et al.*, 1993). Some patients undergo local anaesthesia in the form of regional cervical block for part of the procedure (Shah *et al.*, 1994).

Post-operative care

As there is a risk of debris entering the cerebral circulation, the patient will be closely monitored, for some considerable time, in the recovery area for evidence of cerebral emboli and may need to be returned to ITU or a high-dependency area. The patient's vital signs and neurological observations are monitored in case of a cerebral bleed causing stroke.

The small, modified vertical incision at the side of the neck will be closed with a subcuticular stitch or clips and covered by a dressing. A suction drain may be in situ, monitored for excess blood loss and usually removed at about 24 hours post-surgery. To check for facial nerve damage, the patient is asked to smile and the face observed for lack of symmetry. TIAs may occur.

The blood pressure will probably fall postoperatively so antihypertensive medication will be reviewed (Kumar, 1994).

Providing steady progress is achieved, the patient may go home about 3–4 days after surgery.

Discharge advice

The patient may notice numbness in the anterior portion of the neck, caused by division of branches of the cervical plexus.

Hypertension may resolve spontaneously with improved cerebral blood-flow. If it does not, compliance with antihypertensive medication and monitoring will be encouraged, as will compliance with anticoagulant medication and monitoring.

Advice on alcohol reduction may be necessary.

Complications

These include:

- stroke;
- vocal cord damage;
- facial nerve damage;
- acute laryngeal oedema (Holdsworth and McCollum, 1994);
- TIAs or cerebrovascular accident;
- haemorrhage;
- thrombosis or occlusion;
- restenosis – more likely in women (De Letter et al., 1994) and smokers (Gelabert et al., 1994);
- death, the procedure having a 3% mortality rate (Kumar, 1994).

Successful surgery reduces the incidence of TIA and stroke by 75% (Kumar, 1994). In future, developments in percutaneous transluminal angioplasty may allow this to become the preferred therapy in carotid artery stenosis (Kachel, 1994).

Aortic aneurysm

The aorta is the main arterial blood vessel. An aneurysm in this vessel is a weak ballooning part of the abdominal aorta which is at risk of rupturing and therefore needs surgical treatment. Nearly 10 000 patients die from ruptured aortic aneurysm in England and Wales each year (Yusuf et al., 1994b), many before they reach hospital, and mortality after emergency surgical repair remains nearly 50% (Bergqvist and Bengtsson, 1992). It is linked to atherosclerosis, is more common in smokers and can run in families (Baird et al., 1995) owing to a genetic defect, increasing the risk fivefold. Morris et al., (1994) suggest that 6% of all men over 65 and 1% of women of the same age have an aortic aneurysm.

The patient may present with abdominal or back pain, or complain that his 'heart has dropped', exhibiting a pulsating abdominal swelling. The signs and symptoms of aortoiliac occlusive disease may include intermittent claudication,

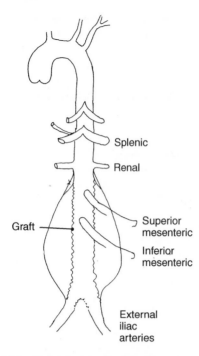

Splenic

Renal

Graft

Superior
mesenteric

Inferior
mesenteric

External
iliac
arteries

Figure 11.1   Abdominal aortic aneurism

diminished femoral pulses and impotence in males (Robinson, 1992). The patient with a leaking aneurysm complains of abdominal and back pain, and often presents collapsed or in shock.

The most common site of aortic aneurysm is the abdominal aorta between the renal arteries and the aortic bifurcation (Fig. 11.1).

The condition may be diagnosed by ultrasound, X-ray or CAT scanning. In a screening programme, simple ultrasound is used to identify any aortic swelling. Large swellings (over 5.5 cm) in otherwise healthy patients are scheduled for surgery before they rupture (a risk of 20%), and smaller ones (less than 4 cm) are monitored as their risk of rupture is less than 1% per annum (Scott, cited by Stuttaford, 1994). Scott *et al.* (1993) further propose that surgery is an unnecessary risk for abdominal aortic swellings less than 6 cm in diameter.

It is suggested that asymptomatic aortic aneurysm, successfully repaired surgically, can return life expectancy to near normal (Stonebridge *et al.*, 1993). Patients with aortic aneurysm often have generalized arterial disease, leading to a high risk

of post-operative morbidity and mortality (Yusuf *et al.*, 1994a).

Prosthetic graft aortic replacement is the currently effective treatment, although further developments include placing an intraluminal stent-anchored, Dacron prosthetic graft using retrograde cannulation of the common femoral artery under local or regional (Parodi *et al.*, 1994) or general anaesthesia (Yusuf *et al.*, 1994a).

Admission and assessment

Pre-operatively, further Doppler studies and angiography may be necessary to determine the dimensions of the aneurysm and the extent of distal disease and occlusion. If complications or open surgery is anticipated, the patient will be nursed in ITU for 24 hours post-operatively, so a pre-operative visit may be helpful. There is a risk of respiratory failure requiring mechanical ventilation for more than 24 hours in those patients with the longest history of smoking, lower pre-operative arterial partial pressure of oxygen and a large intra-operative blood loss (Jayr *et al.*, 1993).

A pre-operative translumbar aortogram may have to be performed under general anaesthetic, in which case the patient is prepared as for theatre. A radio-opaque dye is injected into the aorta in the lumbar region past the lumbar vertebrae to outline the arterial tree and show the extent of the problem. The patient will need to be on 24 hour bedrest after this, with frequent observations of the (undressed) puncture site for bleeding at the same time as vital signs and neurovascular observations are made (Table 11.1).

Table 11.1   Neurovascular observations of the affected limb(s)

- Colour – pink, pale, white, cyanosed, dusky, brown, black, yellow, grey
- Temperature – hot, warm, cool, cold
- Sensation – normal, hypersensitive, pins and needles, painful, numb
- Pulses – present, strong, weak, absent

See Pulse volume monitoring above

An ECG will be performed as the patient may have coronary artery atheroma. A chest X-ray will show calcification in the artery, and the aneurysm will show up as a calcified mass. A fasting blood glucose check may also be made.

If the patient is taking anticoagulants, these may be stopped 24 hours before surgery. Clotting times will be checked.

Pre-operative care

Having established the extent of the proposed surgery, the patient is prepared as in Part One for major surgery. This may include some form of bowel preparation (see Chapter 8) in case an abdominal approach is required, as the bowel is moved aside during this operation. Heparin and antibiotics may be prescribed, and blood will be grouped and cross-matched. Intra-operative salvage may be used to transfuse the patient's own blood, lost during surgery. The shed blood is suctioned away from the site, isolated in a reservoir and washed ready for transfusion.

Types of operation

1 Laparotomy and aortic clamping are still used.

2 Endovascular repair – elective involving open surgery with a 5% mortality rate and a 10 day stay:

*   Straight aorto-aortic (Parodi et al., 1992). Small aneurysms can be treated with a femoral incision, allowing a stent (tube) to be inserted (while still compressed) into the femoral artery in the groin and up into the aorta, where it can be expanded against the weakened patch in the vessel wall (Stuttaford, 1994).

*   Bifurcated aorto-iliac (Yusuf et al., 1994a). Minimally invasive (keyhole) surgery can be used to insert an artificial 'inner tube' into the artery to prevent it bursting. One small incision is made in the right groin,

through which a trouser-shaped graft is inserted into the aorta, where it bifurcates. This can be used in men at risk who may not be fit enough for conventional 'open' surgery. The patient can normally leave hospital in a couple of days.

*   Straight aorto-iliac (May et al., 1992) replacement.

3 Emergency endovascular repair of leaking aortic aneurysm (Yusuf et al., 1994b) is undertaken via a common femoral arteriotomy. A stent is used to support the graft and maintain patency. If either common iliac artery is occluded with embolism coils, a femorofemoral Dracon bypass graft is inserted to restore blood flow to the occluded side.

Leaking/ruptured aneurysm

Diagnosis is by ultrasound and CT scan. An intravenous infusion is started immediately to render the patient haemodynamically stable. Blood is taken for urgent group and cross-matching as 10 units will be needed. The patient is closely monitored for vital signs as shock is a risk, and girth measurements may be ordered to detect abdominal distension due to haemorrhage.

Post-operative care

With open surgery, patients need post-operative management in ITU. The aim of post-operative nursing care is to ensure haemodynamic stability and observe for signs of graft patency. Care will include:

*   intermittent positive pressure ventilation;
*   an ECG, as the patient is likely to have coronary artery disease;
*   continuous arterial blood pressure monitoring, as hypertension may threaten the suture line;
*   monitoring of central venous pressure;
*   measures to minimize stress, such as keeping the patient fully informed and comfortable;
*   observation of peripheral circulation – increasing toe temperature indicates good blood supply to the feet, and pedal pulses (which may

need to be located with Doppler ultrasound in the cold patient) indicate pulse patency;

- hourly monitoring of urine output – prolonged hypertension due to rupture, operative procedure or involvement of the renal arteries may cause renal tubular necrosis. Renal failure is treated by haemodialysis as there is a risk of graft infection with peritoneal dialysis;
- pain relief using opiate infusions or epidurals;
- pressure relief at regular intervals;
- abdominal girth monitoring, as an increase may indicate a leaking suture line, although a major leak will show up earlier as a rising pulse and falling blood pressure;
- a nasogastric tube placed on free drainage, with 4 hourly aspiration;
- monitoring for paralytic ileus, characterized by:

  - abdominal tenderness and distension;
  - no bowel sounds or flatus;
  - nausea and vomiting.

  There may also be:
  - fever;
  - decreased urinary output;
  - electrolyte imbalance;
  - dehydration;
  - respiratory distress.

The condition is managed by fasting, intravenous fluids and the insertion of a nasogastric tube on intermittent suction to monitor the drainage. If ileus is prolonged, parenteral feeding should be instituted.

The patient is gradually mobilized and freed from support equipment as it is no longer needed. Physiotherapy and nursing care will be directed towards prevention of chest infection and other complications of major surgery and bedrest. Thus most patients will be mobilizing by 48 hours post-operatively,

See Part One for principles of wound care, removal of drains, clips, stitches, etc.

Once normal bowel sounds are heard and the patient is freely passing flatus, he may graduate from restricted fluids to free fluids and then a light diet, as he is able. Dietary advice on salt restriction and, if necessary, keeping blood lipid levels normal are needed for when a full diet is resumed.

Those undergoing endoluminal repair have a shorter hospital stay and earlier resumption of normal activities (Yusuf *et al.*, 1994a).

Patient comment

'After four days I felt well enough to ask if I could go home. I was riding my bicycle again within four weeks.'

Discharge advice

Encouragement and support to give up smoking is essential.

A diet sheet and/or time with a dietitian may help the patient to adopt a more healthy diet for convalescence.

STUDENT ACTIVITY

Look up the role of cholesterol in the deposition of atheroma. Identify the functions of the two types of cholesterol and the dietary/lifestyle influences on these.

Siblings should be advised to undergo ultrasound screening for aortic aneurysm as their risk is enhanced (Baird *et al.*, 1995). Emerton *et al.*, (1994) suggest that a single ultrasound scan at the age of 65 can safely be used to exclude over 90% of those examined from future risk of significant dilatation of the aorta.

Complications

1 *Short term*:
  - infection (greater following rupture than elective surgery);
  - leaks or haemorrhage;
  - occlusion;
  - paralytic ileus;
  - cardiac complications such as peri- or post-operative myocardial infarction;
  - deep vein thrombosis;
  - pulmonary embolism;
  - colorectal ischaemia (Shigematsu *et al.*, 1994);
  - acute renal failure (Schepens *et al.*, 1994).

2 *Long term*:

- cardiac-related deaths (Johnston, 1994);
- occlusion;
- infection;

- thrombosis or embolism;
- fistula to bowel (aorto–enteric fistula);
- false aneurysm;
- anastomotic stenosis;
- ureteric obstruction.

Peripheral vascular disease

The onset of peripheral vascular disease is characterized by gradual occlusion of arteries in the lower extremities by atheroma. There will therefore be signs and symptoms such as progressive ischaemia, ulceration of the digits and intermittent claudication. Surgery to reconstruct or bypass the affected artery can only be palliative: it cannot cure the disease or prevent its progression (Ronayne, 1985).

The risk factors are often combined, thus increasing the risk.

Factors predisposing to peripheral vascular disease

- Atherosclerosis
- Diabetes
- Smoking
- Hypertension
- Hyperlipidaemia
- Obesity
- Ageing – patients over 80 years of age with critical ischaemia should not be denied the opportunity of vascular reconstruction, argue O'Brien *et al.* (1993). It may be cost-effective as the patient may be able to maintain independence

Care of the ischaemic limb

Acute ischaemia

This causes a limb to be:

- painful – large doses of morphine are often needed, although diabetics may have reduced pain sensation;
- pallid;
- pulseless;
- paralysed;
- affected by paraesthesia (pins and needles);
- perishing cold;
- a priority for urgent treatment to salvage the limb.

Monitoring takes place throughout the patient's stay.

Chronic ischaemia

The patient is likely to be suffering from pain at rest, unlike that of intermittent claudication characterizing the earlier stages of arterial insufficiency. It is therefore essential to keep the limb as comfortable as possible by reducing the demands made upon the inadequate blood supply, so the affected leg is kept dependant, cool and dry.

STUDENT ACTIVITY

Look at your toes to see whether they have hair on them, indicating a good blood supply. If not, do you have any of the risk factors for peripheral vascular disease?

Care of the ischaemic limb

1 Gravity maximizes the flow of blood to the tissues – elevating the leg may further compromise the limb

2 A cool limb demands less in the way of oxygen and nutrients from the already poor blood supply

3 The ischaemic limb is susceptible to infection and necrosis, and moisture may support bacterial growth, especially in the tissues of the foot

4 The patient is checked to exclude diabetes

5 Any arterial ulcers on the affected leg are dressed, according to local policy, aiming for comfort and freedom from infection. Trauma to the legs and feet must be avoided. Nail-cutting should be performed by a chiropodist. The legs are unlikely to be very hairy owing to the lack of blood supply, and the skin may look pale and shiny

6 Analgesics and antibiotics are usually prescribed after a swab has been taken for microbiological culture and sensitivity

7 The head of the patient's bed may be elevated to aid circulation to the lower limbs, a pressure-reducing mattress provided and a bed cradle placed to keep the weight of the bedclothes off the patient's legs (McCallum, 1984)

8 Femoral and pedal pulses may need to be monitored on a 4 hourly basis, manually or by Doppler ultrasound

Transfemoral arteriography

Angiography, such as a transfemoral arteriogram, will identify the extent of stenosis: mild, moderate or severe. It is a necessary diagnostic investigation prior to embolectomy, angioplasty or surgery. The patient is prepared as for theatre. The opposite groin may be used for access of the arterial catheter, once an intravenous anxiolytic hypnotic has been given, if needed. As the dye goes in the patient will feel: 'hot, flushed and nauseated'. No dressing or adhesive is applied to the wound so that observation for bleeding can be made with the initial half-hourly vital signs observations and foot pulses if requested. Bedrest may be indicated for up to 24 hours, the patient steadily sitting up more and more, and rolling from side to side.

Percutaneous transluminal/balloon angioplasty

This procedure is used to treat short lengths of atherosclerotic stenosis in the severely ischaemic leg to achieve ulcer healing (Ray *et al.* 1995). The International Normalized Ratio of clotting time and activated partial thromboplastintime ratio must be checked beforehand to ensure that clotting times are within the normal range.

Using local anaesthetic, this technique is usually performed by radiologists, but in some units vascular surgeons undertake it (Becquemin *et al.*, 1994). The patient is prepared as for theatre. The arterial catheter is advanced over a guidewire through stenosed and occluded arteries (Gordon *et al.*, 1994). A controlled injury is inflicted by the inflation of the built-in balloon, stretching the vessel wall, followed by division of the intima (innermost wall) and media (middle layer). The disrupted arterial layers heal by medial fibrosis and intimal regeneration. The plaque is presumably compressed and re-moulded by the catheter (Payne, 1992). A laser may be used to recanalize the artery (Tyagi et al., 1994; Giuntini et al., 1994).

Atherectomy

This is the controlled, transluminal removal of atheromatous tissue from the arterial wall via arteriotomy or percutaneous insertion. An ather-ectomy device may drill, pulverize or shave the plaque (Payne, 1992).

Post-angioplasty/atherectomy care

The patient is usually placed on bedrest for 6–24 hours, depending on the size of catheter used. Vital signs are monitored frequently, watching for trends such as hypotension and tachycardia that may indicate haemorrhage. The neurovascular status of the affected limb is monitored by check-ing colour, temperature, sensation and pulses (see Table 11.1 (p. 246) and pulse volume monitoring, above), and comparing results with the other limb. The observations are designed to detect signs of occlusion or improved circulation.

Compartment syndrome may be caused by:

1 Decreased compartmental size:

- closure of facial defect
- tight dressings
- localized external pressure

2 Increased compartmental content:

- bleeding
- increased capillary permeability
- increased capillary pressure, e.g. venous obstruction

The puncture site will be checked for bleeding, haematoma discolouration and swelling. Com-partment syndrome may occur, resulting from increased pressure in the closed compartments of the upper or lower extremities (Mravic and Massey, 1992).

Some patients react to the contrast medium with urticaria, itching, dyspnoea or anaphylactic shock. An indwelling catheter may be necessary while the patient is on bedrest. Pain relief will be given and the patient placed comfortably, with regular changes of position to relieve pressure. Antiplatelet and thrombolytic drugs may be pre-scribed, and laboratory monitoring will include prothrombin time and platelet count (Payne, 1992).

Other complications may include

- post-catheterization pseudoaneurysms (Cox et al., 1994);
- restenosis (Treiman et al. 1994);
  and of atherectomy with the rotablator:
- early thromboemboli, occlusions and poor late patency (CRAG, 1994).

Major vascular bypass surgery

This type of surgery is needed by patients with peripheral vascular disease resulting in disabling claudication, critical limb ischaemia or gangrene. Many of these patients are likely to have diabetes mellitus, and may smoke or have given up after vascular damage has occurred.

Admission and assessment

Resting Doppler indices of both limbs may be ordered to check blood flow. Clotting times (APTR and INR) will be checked. Angiography, such as a transfemoral arteriogram, will determine the extent and severity of the disease. Other screening may be indicated for cardiac lesions, diabetes, etc.

Conservative treatment needs to be continued right up to the moment of surgery to avoid further gangrene (McCallum, 1984).

> **Patient comment**
>
> 'The pain in my foot was so bad that I was glad to have the operation [femoro-popliteal bypass graft].'

Pre-operative care

A chest X-ray, full blood count, blood grouping, cross-matching and saving, ECG, and fasting blood glucose may also be required. It may be helpful to ensure that the patient has had a bowel action prior to surgery.

Two hours before surgery, 2500–5000 i.u. of low molecular weight heparin may be given subcutaneously (Edmondson *et al.*, 1994), or it may be administered per-operatively when the clamps are in position. Prophylactic antibiotics may be given with the premedication or on induction.

A catheter may be inserted into the bladder at operation.

Types of operation

Three types of graft material are used:

1 autograft/autologous/autogenous vein (normally the long saphenous vein, dissected out, venous tributaries ligated, divided and dilated with heparinized saline);
2 dacron;
3 polytetrafluoroethylene (PTFE).

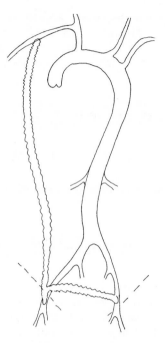

Figure 11.2 Axillofemoral bypass graft

AXILLOFEMORAL BYPASS GRAFT

Preparation and prophylaxis are as for aortic aneurysm surgery.

According to Schneider and Golan (1994), it may be characterized as a haemodynamically inferior reconstruction that should only be performed in high-risk patients. It may take place under general or a combination of epidural and local anaesthetic. An incision is made below the clavicle and a subcutaneous tunnel formed, deep to the pectoralis minor muscle along the lateral chest wall and medial to the anterior iliac spine. Two femoral incisions are made, as well as a tunnel to connect the two just above the pubic bone. The prosthesis is anastomosed to the axillary artery and the femoral arteries (Fig. 11.2).

AORTOFEMORAL (AORTOBIFEMORAL) BYPASS GRAFT

Preparation and prophylaxis are as for aortic aneurysm surgery. An abdominal incision and vertically placed infringuinal incisions are made. The graft is positioned from high on the aorta,

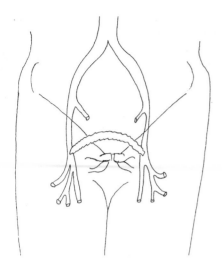

Figure 11.3 Femorofemoral graft

placed carefully through a retroperitoneal tunnel and attached to the appropriate branches of the femoral arteries.

FEMOROFEMORAL CROSS-OVER GRAFT

Vertical incisions in both groins are required to expose the femoral vessels, and a suprapubic tunnel connecting them is made to carry the graft (Fig. 11.3). Transfemoral cross-over bypass can be performed with an externally supported PTFE graft for unilateral occlusion of the iliac artery (Kambayashi *et al.*, 1993) in patients aged over 70 with disabling leg ischaemia.

FEMOROPOPLITEAL ARTERY BYPASS GRAFT

This may be performed under general or epidural anaesthetic.

Incisions are made in the groin, medial side of the leg, just below the knee and medial aspect of the thigh (Fig. 11.4). The graft is anastomosed from the femoral artery to the popliteal artery by means of a tunnel under the muscle layer, ensuring that there are no kinks in the graft (McCallum, 1984). Angioscopy may be used to inspect valve cusps and identify side branches of a vein graft (Hoskin, 1994). The vein graft may be reversed or used in situ (Sasaiima *et al.*, 1993).

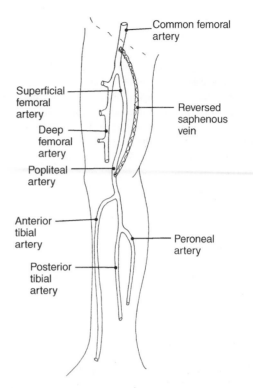

Figure 11.4 Femoropopliteal bypass

Post-operative care

Vital signs and neurovascular observations (*see* Table 11.1, p. 246) are initially recorded half-hourly, tapering off to 4 hourly as the patient progresses. The affected and unaffected limbs are compared, and wound sites are checked at the same time. If necessary, a window is left in the dressings to allow limb pulse monitoring.

Continuous oxygen is usually given for 24 hours, sometimes for longer after epidural anasthesia, often via nasal cannulae.

The leg(s) will be kept slightly flexed at an angle to reduce tension on the graft and stitch line. Particular care must be taken to relieve pressure on the heels. A bed cradle may be placed to keep bedclothes off the legs and allow easy access for monitoring graft patency.

Suction drains may be inserted to both knee and groin incisions. Their output is monitored, and, if it has reduced sufficiently, the drains are removed about 24 hours post-operatively.

The patient will be on bedrest for at least 24 hours post-operatively and then mobilized to encourage blood flow. Moving from bed to chair, he will progress to walking at about 48 hours post-operatively.

An intravenous infusion will be retained until the patient is drinking adequately, and acts to secure intravenous access for drugs such as insulin, heparin and antibiotics.

Subcutaneous low molecular weight heparin 5000 i.u. may be given daily for the next 7 days or until the patient is discharged. A daily dose of aspirin 75 mg will be started for maintenance anticoagulation.

Graft pulses are monitored meticulously, and Doppler studies will be performed before discharge.

The wound(s) are checked daily. Clips or stitches will be removed when healing is sufficiently advanced, at about 8–10 days post-operatively. If the patient needs crutches for mobilization following axillofemoral bypass grafting, these must be elbow rather than axillary crutches to avoid pressure on the graft. For the same reason, tight waistbands are to be avoided (Rook *et al.*, 1989), and the patient should not lie on the affected side.

When sitting in a chair, the patient should elevate his legs and avoid any pressure on the calves. Graduated compression stockings may be prescribed.

Discharge advice

The patient will be discharged to the care of the district or practice nurse if appropriate, as early as is practical.

The important time for adapting to chronic illness is the early convalescent phase after leaving hospital. There is likely to be a difference in the attitudes of those having first-time and repeat surgery, which will be reflected in their compliance with discharge advice. Patient teaching can be focused by using printed material on self-care that the patient can take home; this should have been acquired fairly early post-operatively so that individual concerns can be discussed and explored (Ronayne, 1985).

The convalescent diet needs to contain reduced amounts of fat and salt, and the patient needs gradually to increase the amount of exercise to maintain collateral circulation. Diabetics must make sure that blood glucose levels are tightly controlled.

If support stockings have been prescribed, the patient must be able to put them on and take them off unaided or use a device provided by the occupational therapist to do so. Foot care remains of great importance, as does a daily exercise programme.

Patients will be encouraged to reduce or give up smoking, and both active and passive smoking should be avoided as far as possible.

Following axillofemoral bypass graft, any compression of the graft must be avoided.

Complications

- Pulmonary embolism.
- Cardiac complications, such as peri- or post-operative myocardial infarction.
- Bleeding at the anastomosis site, or wound haematoma.
- Deep vein thrombosis – warfarin will be prescribed, to be continued once the patient returns home.
- Thrombosis of an axillofemoral bypass graft, the risk of which is increased by any sort of compression, such as gardening for long periods. It is treated by admission and heparin infusion.
- Occlusion, causing loss of graft patency, is minimized by antiplatelet therapy. Edmondson *et al.* (1994) have demonstrated the advantages of low molecular weight heparin over aspirin and dipyridamole; it possesses anti-thromboembolitic and antiproliferative effects. It is given by subcutaneous injection daily for 3 months, and patients are taught to administer it themselves.
- Urinary retention.
- Intimal hyperplasia, needing antiproliferation therapy.
- Stroke.
- Infection (*see* above).
- Chest infection.

- Pressure sores.
- Acute disruption of PTFE grafts adjacent to axillary anastomoses, a complication of axillo-femoral grafting (Taylor *et al.*, 1994). Graft breakdown can lead to sudden and fatal haemorrhage.
- Stenosis can occur from 2 days to 316 (median 15 months) months post-surgery (Nehler *et al.*, 1994), producing a recurrence of symptoms.

- Anastomotic aneurysms (Gawenda *et al.*, 1994).
- Groin lymphatic complications such as lymphocutaneous fistula or lymphocoele (Tyndall *et al.*, 1994).

Long-term graft limb complications occur, so patients require lifetime surveillance (Littooy *et al.*, 1994).

Leg amputation

A patient may need a partial or complete amputation of a leg for:

- trauma;
- malignancy;
- arterial insufficiency as a result of atheroma, which can be complicated by diabetes; causing
- gangrene;
- chronic infection;
- intractable pain and
- muscle necrosis caused by sudden ischaemia;
- failed arterial surgery.

Admission

The patient will usually be admitted 1–3 days pre-operatively for assessment and preparation. All patients threatened with amputation must be evaluated to see whether salvage by vascular reconstruction is possible (Linholt *et al.*, 1994). The most likely candidate for amputation is a male who smokes and has a history of previous vascular surgery.

The site chosen by the surgeon may be above, through or below the knee, depending on where an effective blood supply is found. Doppler ultrasound (Keachie, 1992) or arteriogram studies will be made to determine what is best for the individual. The operation removes the diseased part of the leg high enough to ensure proper healing of the resulting rounded stump made of healthy skin.

Care of the ischaemic limb

(*see* box on p. 250)

Keep the limb low, cool and dry, except in the case of a patient with calf and knee oedema facing a below-knee amputation. He may have the limb elevated, if he can tolerate it with very strong analgesics, or at least neutral.

Pre-operative care

Specific preparation for surgery helps the patient to focus on replacing a painful, useless limb with a prosthesis that will increase mobility and may thus improve general health. Discussions will include the possibility of post-operative phantom limb pain. Arranging a meeting with a successful amputee may be helpful. The patient needs time to adjust to a major change in body image, is likely to need to talk about this at some length and may exhibit the stages of grieving as he adjusts to the idea of his loss. Bargaining, depression, anger and denial are likely to feature in his response.

Patient comment

'I was born with two legs and expected to die with two legs.' (Broadhurst, 1989)

As the patient will be relying more than is normal, on his other leg and arm muscles for mobility a programme of arm and leg strengthening exercises will be set up with the physiotherapist. A set of springs may be attached to the patient's bedhead, and he must be encouraged to make regular use of them. The sound leg will also be exercised to strengthen it, and balance work with the trunk is necessary, especially for bilateral amputees. If possible, gait analysis will be performed. In order to be able to bear weight on his replacement leg, the patient must be able to straighten his hip and avoid hip flexion deformity; the relevant exercises must be done regularly, both pre- and post-operatively. The patient will be taught exercises including prone-lying, free exercises, side-lying and standing, to increase the range of hip and/or knee movement.

The patient will be assessed for the safest walking and to minimize the risk of falling, depending on age, motor strength and balance. He must be taught how to walk with crutches or a frame, and how to use a wheelchair.

Social and family worries will have to be addressed, carefully establishing the patient's home circumstances and support system in order to maximize the chances of success. Planning for discharge begins on admission. Two to three weeks is the likely minimum length of stay for a young, relatively fit patient with no particular problems, rising to 3 or more months for an elderly person who encounters complications such as infection. Depending on local arrangements with the limb-fitting centre, the patient may be kept in hospital until the replacement limb is satisfactory. Other centres send the patient home in a wheelchair or on crutches with a temporary prosthesis to attend the limb-fitting centre as an outpatient. A pre-operative visit may give the patient some idea of the range of prostheses available. Home alterations such as bath handles and ramps, or even rehousing, may have to be organized, so early referral to other agencies such as occupational therapy and social services is essential.

If arterial insufficiency is caused by atheroma, it is likely to affect the patient's blood supply to his other leg, and also to his coronary and carotid arteries, rendering him at risk of the complications of surgery and anaesthesia. The aim is therefore to minimize the physiological impact as far as possible by keeping:

- the patient as active as possible prior to surgery;
- the patient well-hydrated, avoiding prolonged bouts of fasting that tend to be for administrative reasons rather than of direct benefit to the patient;
- the diabetic patient in good balance by regular monitoring of blood glucose levels;
- other disease processes stable, maintaining any necessary drug regimens.

The remaining leg must be protected, the aim of health promotion being to slow down the progression of atheroma as much as possible. If the patient smokes, a careful information and education programme must be established, with the aim of cutting right down or stopping altogether. Psychological support is essential.

The affected leg will be marked with indelible pen by the surgeon. Local policy will determine any specialized skin preparation. Shaving should be avoided to reduce the risk of skin nicks becoming infected.

Types of operation

1 Amputation of the toes or part of the foot may be sufficient for the diabetic patient in whom the disease is highly localized.

2 Below knee amputation is the preferred option as long as at least 14 cm of stump can be preserved for walking prosthesis fitting, providing the knee is not contracted more than 15°.

3 Through-knee amputation has a poor cosmetic result but is a comparatively quick and bloodless operation for those who are ill at the time of surgery.

4 Above-knee amputation. The best results for fitting a walking prosthesis can be achieved with a stump 10–12 cm above the opposite kneeline, as long as there is no significant hip flexion deformity.

5 Hip disarticulation or hindquarter amputation is usually performed for malignancy or extensive ischaemia or gangrene.

Spinal or general anaesthetic is used.

Post-operative care

If the patient has been identified as being at high risk of pressure sores, a pressure-reducing mattress should be placed on his bed before he returns from surgery. A trapeze or 'monkey pole' will be fitted to his bedhead, as will a rope ladder to the foot of the bed to help him move about in bed. An intravenous infusion will be in progress on his return from theatre, and a urinary catheter may have been inserted.

Exercising the stump will reduce the risk of hip or knee flexion deformity. The muscles take a while to adapt to the loss of the weight of the leg, the stump tending to be held high. It should never be elevated on a pillow, as that accentuates hip flexion. The wound will have a padded dressing applied with a firm bandage and may have some form of drainage device. The patient is encouraged actively to move the affected leg.

The patient is likely to still be able to 'feel' his toes.

Patient comment

'I feel really stupid saying this, but I have an excruciating pain in my foot which isn't even there.'

He will also be experiencing pain in the stump, so regular analgesia will be necessary. Pain makes the patient draw the stump up towards his abdomen and must be avoided.

Patient comment

'The pain was quite different from what I felt before the operation. This was a hot, clean sort of pain.'

He will be frightened of moving for fear of increasing the pain or damaging the stump, so effective pain relief is needed to reduce the hazards of immobility. The aim is to get him moving initially around the bed and changing his own position regularly, which is likely to increase his confidence when mobilizing out of bed. Patient-controlled analgesia can be very helpful (Warwick, 1992).

The first time of getting out of bed is a very frightening. The patient's co-operation has to be gained by increasing his confidence.

Patient comment

'I was terrified that I would fall over and bash the stump or that the nurses would drop me.'

At least two nurses are needed, the most experienced one being on the same side as the patient's stump. The first stage is to get the patient sitting on the edge of the bed, preferably with the intact leg closer to an armchair with a cushioned seat. Once he has adjusted to this position, the patient needs to be helped to stand briefly on his intact leg, then swivel on it in order to sit on the armchair. For safety, he will be advised not to sit down until he can feel the edge of the chairseat on the back of his leg and his arms are holding the arms of the chair. He is then safe to lower himself with assistance and get comfortable. Always support the below-knee stump in extension when the patient is sitting in a chair. A stump board is fitted to the wheelchair for this reason. After bilateral amputation, the base of the wheelchair will have to be weighted to prevent tipping over until the wheels can be set back to counterbalance the chair.

On returning to bed, the stages are reversed. Each time the patient stands up, he can be encouraged to swing the stump backwards as far as it will go, contributing to his ability to weight-bear effectively, i.e. vertically down through his hip. At no stage should the stump be elevated on pillows or pads. By realistically planning for success at each stage, the patient will gain confidence and look forward to the next stage. This is important as the estimated cost of treatment per amputee is over £80 000. Eighty per cent of patients are provided with a replacement limb, but only about half of these end up actually using them (W.G. Prout, personal communication, 1989).

The patient's pain pattern will be monitored, as an increase in severity may signal infection, stump necrosis or formation of a large haematoma. The wound must be inspected and vital signs monitored for indicators of infection.

Patient comment

'The pain felt sort of throbbing and dirty, so I knew something was going wrong.'

The physiotherapist will plan a full exercise programme; weightbearing on the sound limb is started as soon as possible on the first or second post-operative day. Maintaining and improving balance while standing is vital. The mobility aid will be chosen by the physiotherapist, who will help the patient to use parallel bars in the early stages. Standing is kept to a minimum in the first week in order not to increase stump oedema. The pneumatic limb may be applied from about the seventh post-operative day, depending on healing.

When to start the patient walking, and on what, is a team decision, depending on the patient's general progress. Patients usually feel able to embark on this at about 3 days post-operation, and it can be a great boost to morale to get moving again. The patient will only be allowed to mobilize alone when it is judged safe. Most patients start getting around in a wheelchair. Transfers to and from wheelchair are taught by the physiotherapist, occupational therapist and nursing staff. Before the patient goes home, he will be taught how to transfer from wheelchair to car and vice versa. Ideally, he will be able to negotiate stairs safely on crutches before returning home.

The theatre dressing will be left intact and is only redressed if it is essential. The final shape of the stump owes more to the operative technique than to external pressure. It has been suggested that using a semirigid dressing for patients with below-knee amputations may reduce the time until the stump is ready for prosthesis-fitting (MacLean and Fick 1994). A soft, tubular elastic support is applied to control oedema, maintaining a steady, even pressure without constriction. At about 14 days post-operatively, a firm, elasticated 'stump shrinker' is applied to reduce the remaining oedema. Owing to the underlying condition, sutures or staples will be left in for at least a fortnight, and the rate of healing will be carefully assessed at the time of planned removal. If there is any doubt, they will be left in for longer, and self-adhesive skin strips will be applied to support the wound edges.

A changed body image can be incorporated into the patient's mental framework more successfully by giving him responsibility for elements of his care. He will find looking at the stump without dressings very distressing and will be the best judge of when he wishes to do this.

Patient comment

'I'm sorry, I know I'm a big baby, but I'm not ready to look at it just yet, maybe tomorrow.'

Any wound is an ugly sight to the recipient and takes a lot of getting used to.

Patient comment
(male, aged 66, diabetic)

'Oh! It's not as bad as I thought it would be. I imagined it [forefoot amputation] to be all open, and bones sticking out, but it looks quite tidy.'

The whole area of the body looks and feels different and vulnerable. The patient can be encouraged to wash the wound area in the bath or shower once the dressings have been removed.

Patient comment

'I don't know what is worse – the depression or the anger' (Broadhurst, 1989).

The family or carers will need time and help to adjust to the altered body image, and their active involvement in patient care and rehabilitation is vital to success.

Once the stump has healed sufficiently, which may be from 7 to 14 or more days, a pneumatic mobility aid ('airbag') may be applied over the dressing to start the patient's standing balance and gait training. The airbag is applied first to cushion the stump and does not require very precise fitting. The support frame ends in a simple rocker at the lower end. The 'mushy' sensations will take time to get used to, as the feeling of the foot hitting the ground is lost. While using the aid, the patient is supervised by the physiotherapist. The time spent walking is gradually increased as patient tolerance increases.

An initial prosthesis is ordered and fitted as early as the stump condition allows, at around 15–20 days post-operatively. The weight of the prosthesis will approximate to that of the lost leg. It is needed for about 6–12 weeks until the patient has adjusted to its use and his stump has matured and taken on a stable shape and volume. At this stage, the definitive limb is prescribed. As soon as the patient is using a prosthesis, gait training should begin in the physiotherapy department.

If the patient suffers from phantom limb, sensations may develop from 24 hours to 1 week after surgery (Lyth, 1995). The range of sensations is very wide; some get worse in the first few weeks and then occur only occasionally or even disappear.

Phantom limb sensations

- Tingling
- Numbness
- Itching
- Warmth
- Coldness
- Heaviness
- Lightness
- Fixed joint(s)
- Distortion
- 'Normal' feeling of the limb being present

The higher the level of amputation, the more likely phantom pain, in its many manifestations, is to occur.

Phantom pain descriptions

- Pins and needles in the toes
- Continuous, or intermittent
- Sharp
- Stabbing or shooting (Roberts, 1988)
- Jabbing
- Strong electrical currents
- Burning
- Knife-like
- Pressure
- Cramps
- Crushing
- Throbbing
- Tearing (Lyth, 1995)

The severity of the pain relates to the amount of pre-operative pain (Houghton *et al.*, 1994). Experiences vary considerably between patients, but pain appears to worsen at night and after a change in the weather (Roberts, 1988). Attacks seen to decrease in frequency over the years (Houghton *et al.*, 1994).

It can be helpful to tap the stump to distract the nerve endings. A transcutaneous nerve stimulator may be prescribed to avoid large doses of analgesics.

A home assessment visit will usually take place before the patient is discharged, especially if he is elderly and/or a bilateral amputee. The assessment will include the occupational therapist, physiotherapist and members of other support agencies that may be needed. The district nurse may be involved or informed by letter or telephone of the findings. Weekend home visits are sometimes helpful to enable the patient and his family or carers gradually to adjust to the change. The home assessment visit is a very important part of the discharge plan, the patient and family trying out activities that have only been rehearsed in hospital. It may reduce anxieties and clarify misconceptions about how to manage in the future.

Complications

These may include:

- haemorrhage;
- wound infection;
- flexion and joint contractures;
- depression;
- severe phantom pain;
- social difficulties;
- problems with family acceptance;
- problems with mobility;
- inability to accept an altered body image;
- work difficulties.

Discharge advice

The patient is likely to feel very tired when he first goes home and for a month or more afterwards. A gradual improvement is to be expected (Raper, 1992; Reid, 1992; Smith, 1992).

The patient needs to persist with the exercises he has been taught by the physiotherapist. Resuming driving will depend on how well he adapts to his artificial limb. He may be able to drive an automatic or a modified car. Once the wound has healed, the patient can resume sexual activity. Heavy manual work or hobbies may be contraindicated, so job retraining may be needed.

Follow-up care related to the prosthesis will be handled by the limb-fitting centre. For some patients, wheelchair independence is the best result that can be expected. If persistent phantom limb pain is a problem, despite analgesic drugs, referral to a pain clinic may be arranged (Roberts, 1988).

The patient must take very good care of his health to preserve his remaining leg, as many lose their second leg within 2 years. Dietary advice is necessary for diabetics and those with raised cholesterol levels. Arterial bypass surgery may be undergone to salvage the opposite leg.

Future trends in vascular surgery

The innovative multidisciplinary field of endovascular surgery applies the techniques of angioscopy, intraluminal ultrasound, balloon angioplasty, lasers, mechanical atherectomy and stents. The area can be defined as a diagnostic and therapeutic discipline that treats vascular disease with catheter-based systems and rapidly evolving technology and techniques. The current problem is the high rate of restenosis (Becker et al., 1991; Eton and Ahn, 1991). Pell et al. (1994), for example, report that the increased use of PTA was not associated with a reduction in the number of vascular operations. Rutherford (1994) deplores the replacement of aortobifemoral bypass with percutaneous transluminal angioplasty, stents and extra-anatomic bypass, suggesting that outcome assessment and risk benefit analysis may support its reinstatement. Michaels et al. (1994) argue for the development of vascular surgery as a separate specialty to cope with vascular emergencies, which are a substantial component of the workload.

Varicose veins

The surgical treatment of dilated and elongated saphenous veins with incompetent valves is necessary:

- if there are progressively advancing varicosities;
- in the presence of stasis ulceration;
- for cosmetic reasons.

The most common operation is tying off the main feeder to the varicose vein at the groin and below the knee, and then stripping it out, or removing it through tiny incisions down the length of the leg. If necessary, another feeder vein may be tied off behind the knee. The long and short saphenous veins are those most commonly involved.

Admission and assessment

The patient may be able to go home on the day of operation or possibly the next day, so a careful assessment is made to see whether her home circumstances are suitable for early discharge. The most suitable patient is one who has been caring for herself successfully before coming into hospital (Sutherland, 1991). There needs to be a competent person with her for the first night. Some units offer hotel-type accommodation to patients who have had day case surgery.

Pre-operative care

While the patient stands in a good light, the varicose veins will be marked on the leg with a skin pencil by the medical staff. The patient is encouraged to identify which veins are troublesome so that the correct ones can be dealt with. Doppler studies may be carried out.

The nursing staff will ensure that the patient understands what will happen to her while she is in hospital and what will be expected of her when she goes home. An information leaflet may also be provided.

The groin and leg may be shaved, and the patient will be asked to have a bath or shower. Check that she has had her bowels open within the last 24 hours.

Surgery will be performed under general or epidural anaesthetic.

Post-operative care

The patient will return from theatre with toe-to-groin crêpe bandages. The foot of the bed may be elevated 20–30° to prevent oedema. As part of the post-operative monitoring, the circulation to the toes will be checked by assessing colour, warmth and sensation. At the same time, the dressing over the groin wound will be checked for excessive bleeding. Other incisions on the leg may exhibit strike-through bleeding.

The anaesthetist may prescribe oxygen via a facemask for a few hours. Pain control must be effective enough to allow the patient to get out of bed on the day of surgery providing her blood pressure is sustainable, or, if this is not possible, the next day. She is encouraged to spend most of the day out of bed, either walking slowly or sitting with the legs elevated to encourage good blood flow. Standing is discouraged, as it is uncomfortable and puts undue pressure on the ligatures.

The crêpe bandages are replaced with elastic stocking(s), which need to be worn day and night until the leg sutures are removed. The leg wounds are sometimes secured with skin closure strips rather than stitches. The groin dressing may have to be replaced.

Before the patient is allowed home, she must have stable blood pressure, have passed urine and have drunk without undue nausea. She must be able to walk far enough, including steps and stairs, to be safe at home. The day, time and location of suture removal will have been arranged; usually, the district or practice nurse deals with these approximately 10 days after operation.

Haemorrhage and haematoma must be monitored.

Discharge advice

Pain will gradually decrease throughout the first week.

> **Patient comment**
>
> 'The pain was like sort of burning under the skin.'

Bruising will fade away in a few weeks, as will ankle swelling. Occasional painful lumps under the skin where the veins have been removed will settle down during convalescence. An elastic stocking will need to be worn until the leg is comfortable, which may be 2–4 weeks. It can be removed while the patient is washing and then replaced.

The most important activity is walking. The patient is strongly advised to increase her distance by an extra 50 m daily, aiming to achieve 4–5 km each day. If her leg hurts, she is doing too much. When resting, she needs to elevate her legs above waist level. When standing, she will be uncomfortable if she stays still.

Patient comment

'I had to shift from foot to foot, even when I cleaned my teeth.'

Heavy lifting is to be avoided (*see* Part One), as is straining at stool. By about 1 month, the patient should be able to cope with the level of activity and weightlifting normal for her before the operation.

It can be helpful to compare the post-surgery patient's lifestyle with that of an athlete who takes a break from a training schedule. She will need to regain her fitness and performance through a graduated return to the regular routine (Reid, 1992). There may even be scope for further improving her fitness.

She may resume driving when she can make an emergency stop without pain in the wound, and her sex life when she feels like it.

Patient comment

'The groin wound was bit of a turn-off, especially while it was purple, yellow and bristly, and I did feel more tired than I expected.'

The scars will need moisturising, and sunblock should be applied for the first 18 months to those scars that will be exposed to sunlight.

Return to work should be negotiated (Raper, 1992), depending on how the patient feels and what the job entails, both mentally and physically. Light work may be resumed after 2–7 days, heavy work within 2–4 weeks.

Complications

Patchy numbness of the skin around the areas operated upon is very common. It usually resolves within a year. Aches and twinges gradually settle. Wound infections may cause discharge and are treated with antibiotics.

Varicosities may recur, so the patient needs to continue the conservative measures instituted pre-operatively. These include the avoidance of tight garters or girdles, sitting or standing for long periods of time, crossing the legs when sitting down, injuring the legs and excess weight gain. The patient should elevate the foot of her bed at night, perhaps by putting pillows under the foot of the mattress, and may continue to wear elastic stockings, putting them on in the morning before getting up.

Summary

1 Patients needing reconstructive vascular surgery are likely to have widespread systemic disease, so continued protective care is necessary.

2 The principles of care of the ischaemic limb can be condensed to 'keep it cool, keep it down, keep it dry'.

3 The major investigations carry risks of their own, so specific monitoring is indicated.

4 The range of graft material is outlined and long-term care and complications spelt out.

5 The trend of future developments is predicted.

CASE HISTORY

Mr White is 55 years old and has taken early retirement from his job as a motor mechanic owing to ill-health. He is a diabetic and has been admitted for above-knee amputation of his right leg.

What preparations can you make to enhance his chances of successful limb replacement?

Review Questions

1 Why is a central venous pressure reading a more accurate determinant of the patient's haemodynamic status than an arterial blood pressure measurement?

2 What are the principles of care for a chronic ischaemic limb? Give reasons for each.

3 What effect does smoking have on arteries?

4 What seven pieces of dietary advice are given to someone who has atheroma?

5 Why is the leg not shaved prior to vascular surgery?

6 List the key features that distinguish an arterial from a venous ulcer.

7 Why is diabetes a risk factor for atheroma?

ACKNOWLEDGEMENTS

With grateful thanks to Claire Bownass, Debbie Lewin, Pam Bailey, Karen Lane and Pip Kerr for information, surgery to drafts, reviewing and general encouragement – I could not have done it without you! Also much gratitude to Adrian Marston, a patient teacher and mentor.

References

Baird, P.A., Sadovnick, A.D., Yee, I.M., Cole, C.W. and Cole, L. 1995 Sibling risks of abdominal aortic aneurysm. *Lancet* **346**, 601–4.

Ballard, J.L., Fleig, K., De Lange, M. and Killeen, J.D. 1994 The diagnostic accuracy of duplex ultrasonography for evaluating carotid bifurcation. *American Journal of Surgery* **168**(2), 123–6.

Becker, G.J., Martin, E.C., White, R.A. and Whittemore, A.D. 1991 High-tech option for leg ischemia. *Patient Care* **25**(11), 61–64, 65, 68.

Becquemin, J.P., Cavillon, A. and Haiduc, F. 1994 Surgical transluminal femoropopliteal angioplasty: multivariate analysis outcome. *Journal of Vascular Surgery* **19**(3), 495–502.

Bergqvist, D. and Bengtsson H. 1992 Ruptured abdominal aortic aneurysm: who should be operated upon? In: Greenhalgh, R.M. (ed.) *Emergency vascular surgery.* London: WB Saunders.

Broadhurst, C. 1989 Adjusting to amputation. *Nursing Times* **85**(43), 55–7.

Brunner, L.S. and Suddarth, D.S. 1989 *The Lippincott manual of medical-surgical nursing* 2nd edn, adapted for the UK. London: Harper & Row.

Cox, G.S., Young, J.R., Gray, B.R., Grubb, M.W. and Hertzer, N.R. 1994 *Journal of Vascular Surgery* **19**(4), 683–6.

CRAG 1994 Peripheral atherectomy with the rotablator: a multicenter report. The Collaborative Rotablator Atherectomy Group (CRAG). *Journal of Vascular Surgery* **19**(3), 509–15.

De Letter, J.A., Moll, F.L., Welten, R.J. *et al.* 1994 Benefits of carotid patching: a prospective randomized study with long term follow-up. *Annals of Vascular Surgery* **8**(1), 54–8.

Edmondson, R.A., Cohen, A.T., Das, K.D., Wagner, M.B. and Kakkar, V.V. 1994 Low molecular weight heparin versus aspirin and dipyridamole after femoropopliteal bypass grafting. *Lancet* **344**, 914–18.

Emerton, M.E., Shaw, E., Poskitt, K. and Heather, P.B. 1994 Screening for abdominal aortic aneurysm: a single scan is enough. *British Journal of Surgery* **81**, 1112–13.

Eton, D. and Ahn, S.S. 1991 Trends in endovascular surgery. *Critical Care Nursing Clinics of North America* **3**(3), 535–49.

Gawenda, M., Prokop, A., Sorgatz, S. Walter, M. and Erasmi, H. 1994 Anastomotic aneurysms following aortofemoral vascular replacement. *Thoracic and Cardiovascular Surgeon* **42**(1), 51–4.

Gelabert, H.A., el Massry, S. and Moore, W.S. 1994 Carotid endarterectomy with primary closure does not adversely affect the rate of recurrent stenosis. *Archives of Surgery* **129**(6), 648–54.

Giuntini, G., Midiri, M., Bentivegna, E. *et al.* 1994 [Laser-assisted angioplast in chronic obliterative arteriopathies of the lower limbs. The authors' personal experience.] *Radiologica Medica (Torin)* **88**(3), 277–84.

Gordon, I.J., Conroy, R.M., Tobis, J.M., Kohl, C. and Wilson, S.E. 1994 Determinants of patency after percutaneous angioplasty and atherectomy occluded superficial femoral arteries. *American Journal of Surgery* **168**(2), 115–19.

Harris, K.A. 1992 Graft infections. *Journal of Vascular Nursing* **10**(1), 13–17.

Higman, D.J., Strachan, A.M.J. and Powell, J.T. 1994 Reversibility of smoking-induced endothelial dysfunction. *British Journal of Surgery* **81**, 977–8.

Holdsworth, R.J. and McCollum, P.T. 1994 Acute laryngeal oedema following carotid endarterectomy. *Journal of Cardiovascular Surgery (Torino)* **35**(3), 249–51.

Horn, M., Michelini, M., Greisler, H.P., Littooy, F.N. and Baker, W.H. 1994 Carotid endarterectomy without arteriography: the preeminent role of the vascular laboratory. *Annals of Vascular Surgery* **8**(3), 221–4.

Hoskin, D. 1994 Angioscopy in femoral popliteal bypass graft. *British Journal of Theatre Nursing* **3**(12), 16–17.

Houghton, A.D., Nicholls, G., Houghton, A.L., Saadah, E. and McColl, L. 1994 Phantom pain: natural history and association with rehabilitation. *Annals of the Royal College of Surgeons of England* **76**(1), 22–5.

Jayr, C., Matthay, M.A., Goldstone, J. and Wiener-Kronish, J.P. 1993 Preoperative and intraoperative factors associated with prolonged mechanical ventilation: a study in patients following major abdominal vascular surgery. *Chest* **103**(4), 1231–6.

Johnston, K.W. 1994 Nonruptured abdominal aortic aneurysm: six-year follow-up results from the multicenter prospective Canadian aneurysm study. Canadian Society for Vascular Surgery Aneurysm Study Group. *Journal of Vascular Surgery* **20**(2), 163–70.

Kachel, R. 1994 PTA of carotid, vertebral, and subclavial artery stenoses. An alternative to vascular surgery? *International Angiology* **13**(1), 48–51.

Kambayashi, J.I., Kawasaki, T., Ouii, Y. and Mori, T. 1993 Revascularisation of the occluded donor artery of a femoro-femoral crossover by axillary bypass. *Cardiovascular Surgery* **1**(2), 138–42.

Keachie, J. 1992 Making sense of Doppler ultrasound. *Nursing Times* **88**(10), 54–6.

Kumar, P.J. and Clarke, M.L. 1994 *Clinical medicine: textbook for medical student and doctors.* London: Baillière Tindall.

Linholt, J.S., Bovling, S., Fasting, H. and Henneberg, E.W. 1994 Vascular surgery reduces the frequency of lower limb major amputations. *European Journal of Vascular Surgery* **8**(1), 31–5.

Littooy, F.N., Steffan, G., Steinam, S., Saletta, C. and Greisler, H.P. 1994. An 11-year experience with aortofemoral bypass grafting. *Cardiovascular Surgery* **1**(3), 232–8.

Lumley, J.S. 1994 Vascular management of the diabetic foot: a British view. *Annals of the Academy of Medicine Singapore* **22**(6), 912–16.

Lyth, H. 1995 Invisible problem. *Nursing Times* **91**(19), 38–40.

McCallum, C. 1984: Femoro-popliteal bypass graft. *Nursing Times* Theatre Nursing Supplement Oct 3, 10–12.

MacLean, N. and Fick, G.H. 1994 The effect of semirigid dressings on below knee amputations. *Physical Therapy* **74**(7), 660–73.

May, J., White, G., Waugh, R. Yu, W. and Harris, J. 1994 Treatment of complex abdominal aortic aneurysms by a combination of endoluminal and extraluminal aorto-femoral grafts. *Journal of Vascular Surgery* **19**, 44–9.

Michaels, J.A., Galland, R.B. and Morris, P.J. 1994. Organisation of vascular surgical services: evolution or revolution? *British Medical Journal* **309**, 387–8.

Morris, P., Collin, J. and Hands, L. 1994 Lower abdominal aortic aneurysm: a review. *Practitioner* **238**, 427–30, 432–3.

Mravic, P.J. and Massey, D.M. 1992 Compartment syndrome. *Journal of Vascular Nursing* **10** 8–11.

Nehler, M.R., Moneta, G.L., Yeager, R.A., Edwards, J.M., Taylor, L.M. Jr and Porter, J.M. 1994 Surgical treatment of threatened reversed infrainguinal vein grafts. *Journal of Vascular Surgery* **20**(4), 558–63.

O'Brien, T.S., Lamont, P.M., Crow, A., Collin, J. and Morris, P.J. 1993 Lower limb ischaemia: is limb salvage surgery worthwhile? *Annals of the Royal College of Surgeons of England* **75**(6), 445–7.

Palombo, D., Porta, C., Peinetti, F. *et al.* 1994 Cerebral reserve and indications for shunting in carotid surgery. *Cardiovascular Surgery* **2**(1), 32–6.

Parodi, J.C., Palmaz, J.C. and Barone, H.D. 1992

Transfemoral intraluminal graft implantation for abdominal aortic aneurysms. *Annals of Vascular Surgery* 5, 491–9.

Payne, J.S. 1992 Alternatives for revascularisation: peripheral atherectomy devices. *Journal of Vascular Nursing* 10(1), 2–8.

Pecoraro, R.E., Reiber, G.E. and Burgess, E.M. 1992 Pathways to diabetic limb amputation: basis for prevention. *Diabetes Spectrum* 5(6), 329–34.

Pell, J.P., Whyman, M.R., Fowkes, F.G., Gillespie, I. and Ruckley, C.V. 1994 Trends in vascular surgery since the introduction of percutaneous transluminal angioplasty. *British Journal of Surgery* 81(6), 832–5.

Ranaboldo, C.I., Barros D'Sa, A.A., Bell, P.R., Chant, A.D. & Perry, P.M. 1993 Randomised controlled trial of patch angioplasty for carotid endarterectomy. The Joint Vascular Research Group. *British Journal of Surgery* 80(12), 1528–30.

Raper, J. 1992 Practised advice. *Nursing Times* 88(36), 26–7.

Ray, S.A., Minty, I. and Buckenham, T.M. 1995 Clinical outcome and restenosis following PTA for ischaemic rest pain or ulceration. *British Journal of Surgery* 82, 1217–21.

Reid, S. 1992 After the big sleep. *Nursing Times* 88(36), 28.

Roberts, A. 1988 Senior Systems of Life 26: Peripheral vascular disease 2 – Surgery. *Nursing Times* 84(23), 51–4.

Robinson, L.C. 1992 Atherosclerotic occlusive disease of the aorta. *Journal of Vascular Nursing* 10(4), 17–23.

Ronayne, R. 1985 Feelings and attitudes during early convalescence following vascular surgery. *Journal of Advanced Nursing* 10, 435–41.

Rook, J.E., Green, R.F., Purgliese, G.N. and Silane, M. 1989 Thrombosis of axillary-femoral bypass secondary to prosthesis suspension belt. *Archives of Physical Medicine and Rehabilitation* 70(7), 559–61.

Rutherford, R.B. 1994 Aortobifemoral bypass, the gold standard: technical considerations. *Seminars in Vascular Surgery* 7(1), 11–16.

Sasaiima, T., Kobuko, Y., Izumi, Y. and Inaba, M. 1993 Comparison of reversed and in situ saphenous vein grafts for infragenicular bypass: experience of two surgeons. *Cardiovascular Surgery* 1(1), 38–43.

Schepens, M.A., Defauw, J.J., Hamerlijnck, R.P. and Vermeulen, F.E. 1994 Risk assessment of acute renal failure after thoracoabdominal aortic aneurysm surgery. *Annals of Surgery* 219(4), 400–7.

Schneider, J.R. and Golan, J.F. 1994 The role of extra-anatomic bypass in the management of bilateral aortoiliac occlusive disease. *Seminars in Vascular Surgery* 7(1), 35–44.

Scott, R.A.P., Wilson, N.M., Ashton, H.A. and Kay D.N. 1993 Is surgery necessary for abdominal aortic aneurysm less than 6 cm in diameter? *Lancet* 342, 1395–6.

Shah, D.M., Darling, R.C. III, Chang, B.B., Bock, D.E., Paty, P.S. and Leather, R.P. 1994 Carotid endarterectomy in awake patients: its safety, acceptability and outcome. *Journal of Vascular Surgery* 19(6), 1015–19.

Shigematsu, H., Nunokawa, M., Hatakeyama, T. et al. 1994 Inferior mesenteric and hypogastric artery reconstruction to prevent colonic ischaemia following aortic aneurysmectomy. *Cardiovascular Surgery* 1, 13–18.

Smith, S. 1992 Tiresome healing. *Nursing Times* 88(36), 24–6.

Stansby, G., Byrne, M.T.L. and Hamilton, G. 1994 Dental infection in vascular surgical patients. *British Journal of Surgery* 81, 1119–20.

Stonebridge, P.A., Callam. M.J., Bradbury, A.W., Murie, J.A., Jenkins, A.M. and Ruckley, C.V. 1993 Comparison of long term survival after successful repair of ruptured and non-ruptured abdominal aortic aneurysm. *British Journal of Surgery* 80, 585–6.

Strandness, D.E. Jr 1993 Carotid endarterectomy: current status and effects of clinical trials. *Cardiovascular Surgery* 1(4), 311–16.

Stuttaford, T. 1994 Medical briefing: patching up a weak spot. *The Times* Jun 9, p.17.

Sutherland 1991 Day surgery: all in a day's work. *Nursing Times* 87(11), 26–30.

Taylor, L.M. Jr, Park, T.C., Edwards, J.M. et al. 1994 Acute disruption of polytetrafluoroethylene grafts adjacent to axillary anastomoses: a complication of axillofemoral grafting. *Journal of Vascular Surgery* 20(4), 520–6.

Towne, J.B. and Hobson, R.W. II 1994 Current status of operative treatment for asymptomatic carotid stenosis. *Canadian Journal of Surgery* 37(2), 128–34.

Treiman, G.S., Ichikawa, L. Treiman, R.L. et al. 1994 Treatment of recurrent femoral or popliteal artery stenosis after percutaneous transluminal angioplasty. *Journal of Vascular Surgery* 20(4), 577–85, discussion 585–7.

Tritschler, I. 1994 Anticoagulation therapy. *Nursing Standard* 8(49), 54–5.

Tyagi, S., Satsangi, D.K. and Khalikullah, M. 1994 Laser assisted balloon angioplasty in lower extremity occlusive disease. *Indian Heart Journal* 46(1), 25–30.

Tyndall, S.H., Shepard, A.D., Wilczewski, J.M., Reddy, D.J., Elliott, J.P. and Ernst, C.B. 1994 Groin lymphatic complications after arterial reconstruction. *Journal of Vascular Surgery* 19(5), 858–63, discussion 863–4.

Warwick, P. 1992 Making sense of the principles of patient controlled analgesia. *Nursing Times* 88(41), 38–40.

Wyness, M.A. 1990 Evaluation of an educational programme for patients taking warfarin. *Journal of Advanced Nursing* 15(9), 1052–63.

Yusuf, S.W., Baker, D.M., Chuter, T.A.M., Whittaker, S.C., Wenham, P.W. and Hopkinson, B.R. 1994a Transfemoral endoluminal repair of abdominal aortic aneurysm with bifurcated graft. *Lancet* 344, 650–1.

Yusuf, S.W., Whittaker, S.C., Chuter, T.A.M., Wenham, P.W. and Hopkinson, B.R. 1994b Emergency endovascular repair of leaking aortic aneurysm. *Lancet* 344, 1645.

Further reading

Cameron, J. 1994 Arterial leg ulcers. *Nursing Standard* 10(26), 50–5.

Carpenter, J.P., Baum, R.A., Holland, G.A. and Barker C.F. 1994 Peripheral vascular surgery with magnetic resonance angiography as the sole preoperative imaging modality. *Journal of Vascular Surgery* 20(6), 861–9.

Davies, A.H., Magee, T.R., Hayward, J.K., Baird, R.N. and Horrocks, M. 1994 Prediction of long saphenous vein graft adaptation. *European Journal of Vascular Surgery* 8(4), 478–81.

Fogarty, A.M. 1991 Angioscopy: new developments in vascular surgery. *AORN Journal* 53(3), 725–8.

Harward, T.R., Govastis, D.M., Rosenthal, G.J., Carlton, L.M., Flynn, T.C. and Seeger, J.M. 1994: Impact of angioscopy on infrainguinal graft patency. *American Journal of Surgery* 168(2), 107–110.

Holzenbein, T.J., Miller, A. Tannenbaum, B.A. *et al.* 1994 Role of angioscopy in reoperation for the failing or failed infringuinal vein bypass graft. *Annals of Vascular Surgery* 8(1), 74–91.

Kiely, T.M.A. 1989 Laura's story. *Nursing Times* 85(34), 35–8.

Milne, C. 1988 Varicose veins. *Nursing Standard* 2(28), 26.

Naylor A.R., Whyman, M.R., Wildsmith, J.A. *et al.* 1993. Factors influencing the hyperaemic response after carotid endarterectomy. *British Journal of Surgery* 80(12), 1523–7.

Pinzur, M.S. 1993 Gait analysis in peripheral vascular insufficiency through-knee amputation. *Journal of Rehabilitation Research and Development* 30(4), 388–92.

Stubbing, N. 1996 Using non-invasive methods to perform vascular assessment. *Nursing Standard* 10(45), 49–50.

Orthopaedic surgery

12

Mark Collier

Introduction

The term 'orthopaedic' derives from two Greek words: *orthos* = straight and *paedios* = of a child (Roaf and Hodkinson, 1980). Taken literally, the word implies the 'straightening of a child'. However, patients with orthopaedic conditions or requiring orthopaedic surgery span the full age continuum – from newborn to those in later years.

Orthopaedics is concerned with the musculo-skeletal system and all that facilitates its movement – bones, joints, muscles, nerves and tendons. For the detailed anatomy (Fig. 12.1) and physiology of bone and joints, the reader is referred to such textbooks as Tortora and Agnostakos (1987).

Identifying the needs of the orthopaedic patients begin with the systematic gathering of information from the patient's history, the physical examination, X-ray appearances and any appropriate special investigations such as arthroscopy, an endoscopic procedure performed in the operating theatre, which permits inspection and exploration of a joint (Apley and Solomon, 1988). Much of the diagnostic process will have been undertaken prior to the patient's admission to hospital, and, as a result, a set of medical notes will have been generated. It is, however, important to remember that the condition is only a part of the patient's total well-being, and all subsequent care should be planned in an holistic manner.

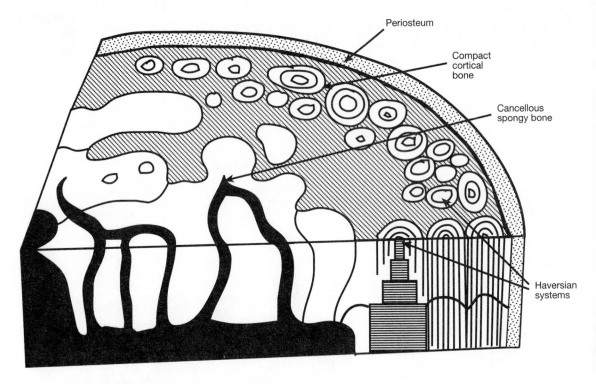

Section of a shaft of a long bone

Figure 12.1 Microscopic structure of bone (Haversian) systems

Patients admitted to hospital for orthopaedic surgery are usually experiencing some loss of function and/or restricted mobility, stiffness, pain and possibly some altered sensation of the affected body part, all of which affects normal activities of living.

As soon as the patient is admitted for surgery, the rehabilitative phase of care should begin, the aim of which is to create conditions enabling patients to readjust both mentally and physically and come to terms with their changed circumstances. Rehabilitation is then both a treatment and a socialization process, the main aims of which could be identified as:

- preventing further impairment;
- maintaining existing function;
- restoring maximal functioning of an affected body part.

Patient education is an essential part of the rehabilitative process, not only better to inform patients but also to help them participate more fully in their own care.

All health-care workers functioning in the orthopaedic setting have both a caring and rehabilitative role and act as essential members of the multidisciplinary team. The team may be composed in part of medical and nursing staff, physiotherapists, occupational therapists, speech therapists and orthotists (those qualified to measure and fit all types of orthoses, an orthosis being a device applied directly and externally to the patient's body with the object of supporting, correcting or compensating for a skeletal deformity or weakness, however caused).

In summary, the principles governing the actions of all health-care workers involved with the care of orthopaedic patients can be identified as:

- restoring and/or maintaining the function of affected body parts;

- promoting independence;
- preventing deformity;
- correcting any existing deformity;
- developing the powers of compensation and patient adaption if any loss of function is permanent or deformity is inevitable.

The majority of orthopaedic operations performed in hospitals – of both a general and a specialist nature – are elective, and therefore, for the purposes of this publication, the focus will be on the principles of care relating to patients following surgery to the knee, hip, spine and lower limb.

Orthopaedic conditions often requiring surgical intervention

It has been reported that one in seven people in the UK is significantly affected by arthritic disease (Hill, 1991), and this may result in patients being admitted to hospital for major orthopaedic surgery such as joint replacement (arthroplasty), fusion of affected joints in order to reduce the patient's pain (arthrodesis), surgical fracturing of a bone to correct deformities (osteotomy) and soft tissue interventions.

Osteoarthritis

Osteoarthritis is a degenerative wear-and-tear process occurring in joints that are impaired by:

- age;
- congenital defects (Perthe's disease/slipped upper femoral epiphysis);
- vascular insufficiency;
- previous disease or traumatic injury;
- obesity and malalignment of the involved joint.

Any joint may be affected, although it is commonly those of the lower (hips, knees and ankles) rather than the upper limb. The patient's occupation will have a bearing on the determination of the joints affected.

Clinical features

Most patients are past middle age. Onset is gradual, pain having increased over the years, with movements of the affected joint becoming more limited over time. Complaints of pain and stiff-

ness are usually more evident in the morning, after resting and in wet weather. Associated stiffness may decrease after an individual has been up for a few hours. Constant pain lowers the patient's morale (Hayward, 1975) and may lead to depression. As a result, interpersonal relationships are often adversely affected.

Aim of surgical intervention

This is to improve the patient's quality of life post-operatively.

Rheumatoid arthritis

Rheumatoid arthritis is an inflammatory condition, a subacute or chronic symmetrical polyarthritis (noted in more than one anatomical site) usually affecting the more peripheral joints, such as those of the hand. If unchecked, it will pursue a course of deterioration, with exacerbations and remissions over many years, accompanied by a general systemic disturbance such as malaise. This disease is characterized by swelling of the synovial membrane and peri-articular cartilages, subchondral osteoporosis, erosion of cartilage and bone, and associated wasting of muscle bulk.

The cause of rheumatoid arthritis is still unknown, but what is certain is that it affects more women than men. Patients may initially complain of malaise, tiredness, loss of weight and/or generalized muscle pains. Joint symptoms soon follow – pain and stiffness (especially after rest) swelling and deformity – affecting small joints first, especially those of the wrists, fingers and toes.

The main prognostic features of rheumatoid arthritis are:

- *Good*:
  - when seen in the male population;
  - if the age of onset is below 30 years;
  - if the duration of the disease process is less than 1 year;
  - if it is noted as occurring suddenly.
- *Poor*:
  - if the onset is insidious;
  - if early nodules are seen or vasculitis is diagnosed;
  - when scleritis is noted;

- if early progression of the disease is shown on radiological examination;
- if serology identifies the presence of rheumatoid factor.

Groups of anti-rheumatic drugs commonly in regular patient use are:

- simple analgesics, e.g. soluble aspirin;
- non-steroidal anti-inflammatory drugs, e.g. indomethacin;
- second-line drugs, e.g. Myocrisin (gold); these drugs being used to arrest the disease process as well as its syptomatology;
- corticosteroids, e.g. prednisolone.

Beware of multiple drug therapy: observe for unanticipated drug interactions and the use of long-term corticosteroids as there is the risk of patients suffering a steroid crisis.

Elective admission

This may be for:

- early active disease;
- disease progression;
- emergencies and complications;
- exacerbations and trauma;
- permanent joint impairment for surgical correction.

General principles of care

The majority of patients with musculoskeletal problems will be both anxious and in some degree of pain at the time of admission. All members of the multidisciplinary team, especially nurses, must therefore be able to offer both patients and their relatives a full explanation of any investigations and proposed surgery. A relaxed and co-operative patient is more likely to participate fully with any treatment care regimen than is one who is tense and feels uninformed (Boore, 1978).

Assessment

The orthopaedic nurse should comprehensively assess the patient's physical condition on admission.

MOBILITY

It is the responsibility of the orthopaedic nurse to have an understanding of the normal range of movements of a limb or joint in order to assess the patient's mobility and plan for the post-operative period. Goals should be set *with* the patient. Whatever model of nursing is being used as an assessment framework, the patient's mobility will always be a major consideration. While sitting and talking to the patient, both at the time of admission and subsequently, nurses and health-care workers can ascertain how the patient's problems of mobility affect her on a day-to-day basis:

- Is the mobility problem getting worse?
- What exactly is it that stops the patient moving as she wishes?
- What mobility aids are required?
- How is the patient's mobility reported by both the patient and relatives?
- How does the patient visualize mobility being improved?

STUDENT ACTIVITY

Stand in front of a full-length mirror. Taking each joint in turn – hip, knee, wrist, ankle – identify its normal range of movement and compare this with values given in a table, such as that in Schoen (1986).

DIET

Good hydration is an important pre-operative nursing goal, as a reduction in mobility and periods of enforced bedrest have been shown to contribute to urinary stasis, associated bladder infections and the formation of renal calculi (Brunner and Suddarth, 1988).

Urine includes, among other things minerals such as calcium, phosphate, oxalate and xanthine. When a patient's mobility is greatly reduced, as in osteoarthritis of the hip, there is an increased loss of calcium from bone owing to a reduction of the collagen in which calcium is normally deposited. This results in higher than normal levels of blood calcium and a subsequent increase in urinary calcium. If this situation is not corrected, renal calculi may form, possibly large enough to damage the substance of the kidney and block the flow of urine the kidney via the ureter. As a consequence, bacteria may thrive in the stagnant urine and result in a kidney infection that will then have to be treated with aggressive antibiotic therapy, which may alter the patient's appetite.

Occasionally, obese patients will be asked to have a weight-reducing diet prior to their hip replacement in order to lessen excessive downward forces on the new joint, whereas patients assessed as being underweight may be given a high-protein diet pre-operatively in order to improve their healing potential following surgery.

PAIN

Assessment of the patient's reported pain can be assisted by the use of both descriptive and visual analogue scales, which have been shown to be effective (Hill, 1991). McCaffrey (1979) has stated that. 'Pain is what the patient says it is'. The critical features of pain have been identified as:

- type;
- location;
- severity;
- duration;
- precipitating factors.

Many nurses have remarked on their inability to differentiate objectively between words used by patients such as 'ache', 'hurt', 'crushing pain' and 'throbbing pain', to describe pain. The McGill pain questionnaire was developed to describe pain in an effort to measure the severity implied by these words (Melzack, 1975).

Pain observation charts can also be used throughout the patient's hospitalization to compare the effectiveness of any treatments given.

The severity of pain can be to some extent accounted for by the use of the measures previously discussed. Duration and frequency of pain may be assessed by the use of a pain chart divided into hourly intervals (Davies, 1985). In this way, it can be seen whether reported pain increases following a specific activity, such as mobilization or physiotherapy, or eases as the result of the administration of an appropriately prescribed medication.

Precipitating factors shown to affect pain assessments have previously been identified and listed by Gaston-Johansson and Asklund-Gustafsson (1985). These are:

- attitudes – both of patients and health-care professionals;
- education – especially in relation to patient information;

- the experience of health-care workers involved with the patient;
- the patient's age, sex and cultural background.

Closely associated with the orthopaedic patient's pain is a loss of limb function and/or a restriction in joint movement that may severely limit the patient's potential for mobility.

SKIN

The maintenance of skin integrity is of primary importance to a patient whose mobility is restricted. It is therefore essential that all patient assessments on admission incorporate the use of a relevant pressure sore/ulcer 'at-risk' scale, such as the Norton, Waterlow or Lowthian scale. All risk assessment tools (and there are many more) should be used systematically and not as a one-off patient experience.

The prevention and development of pressure sores or ulcers, the essentials of a prevention programme, the use of assessment scales as previously identified, and patient management (including the appropriate use of various patient aids) have been discussed in detail elsewhere (Collier, 1990a, 1995a).

Planning/implementing care

GENERAL

1 Mobility – Avoid sustained flexion of the neck, back and hips during bedrest. Use appropriate splints and physiotherapy techniques.

2 Diet – This must be balanced and regulated to account for any anaemia, weight gain or weight loss.

3 Skin – Assess and observe on a regular basis as the development of a pressure sore or ulcer is unfortunately an all too common complication of enforced bedrest, and orthopaedic patients have been identified as one of the groups most 'at risk'.

Treat any local infections (septic foci) as directed prior to surgery in order to reduce the risk of bone infection such as osteomyelitis.

MEDICATION

The objectives of medication are symptomatic relief and/or alteration of the disease process.

Individuals requiring steroid therapy for the treatment of rheumatoid arthritis or chronic obstructive airways disease, or who have recently ceased treatment with steroids, should be given a 'maintenance' dose as prescribed in order to reduce the risk of a steroid crisis.

Pre-operative preparation

Patients are generally admitted the day before surgery, having taken account of their domestic and occupational circumstances. However, in some specialist centres or if indicated because of another medical condition, the 'work-up' period may be as long as a week. This would be most appropriate for a patient who is to undergo primary corrective spinal surgery for scoliosis (lateral curvature of the spine). During this pre-operative phase, it is desirable for the patients to meet members of the multidisciplinary team caring for them during their hospital stay. The

surgeon should also be encouraged to explain the surgical procedure to the patient.

Anaesthesia

Most orthopaedic surgery is performed under general anaesthesia. If the patient's medical condition contraindicates this, the medical team may consider local anaesthesia. The latter is predominantly used for surgery involving the upper limbs, when local nerve blocks can be used t good effect. Major joint surgery (hip) will occasionally be performed under local anaesthesia, and in this situation the anaesthetic may take the form of a spinal epidural or acupuncture. Most centres will prepare all patients for general anaesthesia unless specifically told otherwise.

In addition to the standard pre-operative care for surgery, there are likely to be other decisions to be made, depending upon local policy, on appropriate skin preparation, prophylactic antibiotic therapy and post-operative wound management.

Skin preparation

Prior to skin preparation, it is imperative that the limb or joint on which the operation is to be performed is clearly marked – by the medical staff – with a large arrow using a non-water soluble marker.

The value of pre-operative shaving has been shown to be somewhat uncertain (Winfield, 1986). A number of studies have shown a lower wound infection rate if the patient is not shaved pre-operatively (Seropian and Reynolds, 1971; Cruse and Foord, 1973). If the surgeon insists that limb hair is a source of wound contamination, the use of depilatory cream should be discussed. The advantages of this are that:

- in most cases, the patient can apply the cream herself, thus saving nursing time;

- depilation has been reported as being preferred by patients (Winfield, 1986);
- there is no risk of minor skin grazes and cuts, potential sites for colonization by bacteria.

The efficacy of solutions used for cleansing limbs pre-operatively has been questioned (Thomas, 1990, Collier, 1995b). There is little evidence to suggest that skin preparation over a number of days is more effective than a single application of a suitable lotion, such as betadine, in theatre, providing the patient is known not to be allergic to it. It could therefore be argued that bathing the limb with soap and water (the day before or on the day of surgery itself) is more than adequate pre-operatively.

Antibiotic therapy

Prophylactic antibiotic therapy is sometimes required as cover for patients undergoing orthopaedic surgery, particularly when a prosthesis – a metal implant used to replace a joint, part of a joint, a bone or a complete limb – has become infected and is being removed, rather than when a primary prosthesis is being inserted. If prescribed by the medical staff, antibiotic cover will usually be commenced on the day of surgery, either on the ward or per-operatively. Any reactions to previous antibiotic therapy should be carefully noted by the admitting nurse and reported to the senior ward nurse and medical staff as soon as possible.

Per-operative care

Positioning the patient on the operating table is of prime importance, not only to facilitate the surgeon's approach to the surgical site, but also to reduce pressure between the patient's skin and any equipment used. Orthopaedic surgery, especially procedures involving the spine, can be prolonged, so every effort must be made to reduce the pressure on the patient's skin throughout the operative period, as the development of pressure ulcers has been traced back to 'interface' pressures experienced per-operatively (Collier, 1995a). Equipment that may be used for this purpose includes a fracture table, sandbags and pneumatic bean bags in conjunction with prophylactic padding of bony prominences (Fig. 12.2).

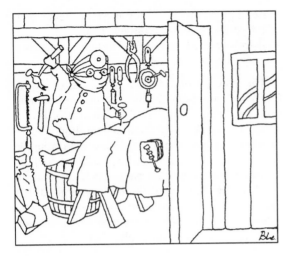

Figure 12.2 Per-operative phase

Use of tourniquets and diathermy

Tourniquets are frequently used if surgery is performed on the extremities (hand or foot) as this allows the surgeon to operate in a relatively bloodless field, enabling important structures such as nerves to be easily identified. While in use, manufacturer's instructions relating to inflation and deflation times must be adhered to, as a failure to follow these may lead to prolonged ischaemia or ultimately the loss of a limb as a result of gangrene.

When tourniquets are not practical, such as with hip and spinal surgery, electrical diathermy machines will be used to help control bleeding. Theatre nurses and technicians must ensure that all appropriate safety checks have been made prior to their use. Misuse can result in burns to the skin and other tissues.

X-rays in the operating theatre

X-ray equipment, for example the image intensifier, is often used in the orthopaedic theatre and, although this should only be used under the supervision of the radiographers, all staff have a responsibility to protect the patient and themselves when necessary. Care must be taken by the radiographer not to contaminate the operation field, and it is therefore essential that a climate of reciprocal assistance is created between all personnel involved. The maintenance of an aseptic operative field throughout the surgical procedure will help to reduce the incidence of both wound infection and bone infection such as osteomyelitis.

All personnel involved with the per-operative phase of patient care should act for and as the patient's advocate (Fig. 12.3).

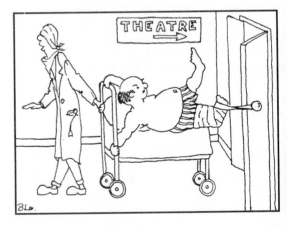

Figure 12.3 Acting for the patient

Post-operative care

Based on the patient's operation record and available assessment data, the main care considerations may include the following:

- tourniquet use during the operation?;

- pain – related to the surgical procedure and or immobilization;
- the potential for wound and other infections;
- the potential for loss of skin integrity owing to immobility;

- patient mobility – when and how much?;
- altered body image.

Tourniquets

If a tourniquet has been used, it must be removed as soon as the procedure is complete, and the relevant body part should be observed carefully for the restoration of normal circulation and, during the next 24–48 hours, for signs of neurological damage.

Pain

Surgery involving bones and joints can often be very painful.

> **Patient comment**
>
> **'How much more painful the removal of a bunion was when compared with previous abdominal surgery, of a major nature.'**

Assessment of the patient's pain can be undertaken utilizing a pain assessment tool. Post-operative analgesics should be given as prescribed and the effects closely monitored. Inadequate therapy may prolong patients' discomfort and ultimately affect their tolerance of any post-operative care, especially the planned mobilization programme.

Potential for wound and other infections

It is not uncommon in theatre for the surgeon to initiate a wound drainage system, possibly involving a vacuum, in an effort to reduce the large quantity of blood that is left stagnant and out of the circulation following major joint surgery (Roaf and Hodkinson, 1980). The wound itself is observed for bleeding and other discharge, and assessed as discussed elsewhere (Westaby, 1985; Collier, 1990b).

Bone infections cannot be detected as easily as wound infections; however, it should be stressed that careful observation of a patient's temperature

(pyrexia) and pulse (an increased rate) may elicit the first hint of the former.

Loss of skin integrity due to enforced bedrest

In 1988, Waterlow reported that the incidence of pressure ulcers in orthopaedic wards was 24.7%. It could therefore be argued that all health-care workers, with the patient's involvement, should decide how the patient will be moved periodically and regularly to prevent pressure sore development. It is generally accepted that a patient should not be left in the same position for more than 2 hours if lying on a normal hospital mattress and bed, or for the length of time as specified in literature relating to other specialist preventive equipment such as overlay mattresses.

A decision should be made, especially following spinal and hip surgery, on whether patients will be rolled or lifted (Overd, 1992), in order to facilitate assessment and care of the patient's skin during this initial post-operative phase.

Mobility

The general aim of any post-operative mobilization programme will be to return the patient to

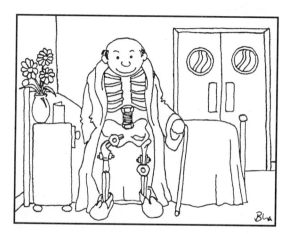

Figure 12.4 Mobilization

the highest level of function in the shortest period of time, bearing in mind the surgical procedure undertaken.

Bone does not mend as rapidly as other tissues (Brunner and Suddarth, 1988), which is especially important to remember following surgery to the lower limbs, as, in addition to facilitating 'normal' movement, bone must be able to bear the patient's body weight during ambulation, however slowly. Any exercise programme will be tailored to individual needs by the physiotherapist. The nurse should have a knowledge and understanding of this so that it can be continued and function maintained when the physiotherapist is not available. Mechanical devices such as continuous passive motion machines will occasionally be incorporated into the planned programme; they should not be used on a 24 hour basis and are only used until the patient is able to undertake active exercises utilizing his own muscle power.

There is sometimes a need for a traction system following orthopaedic surgery (*see* below). If so, a mobilization programme will be planned within the limits and constraints of the traction system.

Positioning

Following the immediate 'recovery' position, the majority of patients can be nursed effectively semi-recumbent. However, some may need to be nursed in the recumbent or supine positions, especially following spinal surgery. This creates problems should vomiting occur as there is the danger of the patient inhaling vomitus into the respiratory passages. Careful observation of the patient should avoid this.

If patients require prolonged nursing in the recumbent position, nursing care should pay particular attention to psychological well-being (preventing boredom), eating and drinking, and elimination needs, maintenance of patients' sleeping pattern as they may not be able to assume their normal sleeping position, how they will dress, being encouraged to change out of night attire during daylight hours, and their hygiene needs (skin, hair and teeth) for as long as is required. The occupational therapist or visitors may also be able to assist in the provision of suitable diversional therapy. For children, the continuation of educational activities is encouraged.

Principles of traction and orthopaedic bandaging

Traction

For a traction system to be effective, it must incorporate forces pulling against an object (traction) and forces pulling or thrusting in the opposite direction (countertraction). The two main forms of traction in common use are known as fixed, and balanced or sliding, traction.

Fixed traction is exerted on that part of a limb (body part) lying between two fixed points. For example, when a Thomas splint is in use, the leather-covered ring at the upper end which sits in the patient's groin region and the tapes tied to the distal end of the splint provide the two fixed points. The tapes exert the pull or traction force, while the pressure of the ring against the promin-

ent ischial tuberosity of the pelvis provides the opposing thrust, or countertraction.

Balanced (sliding) traction also encompasses two opposing forces, this time balanced or mobile. In order to balance one another, they must be separated by a raised structure – as with a see-saw. The most commonly used form of this traction found on the ward involves the foot of the patient's bed being raised – by the tilt mechanism or bed blocks – and weights being attached to the traction cord passing over a pulley on the bed end; these are in turn attached to the patient's limb. Because of the tilted position of the bed, the patient has a tendency to slide downwards towards the bedhead, so, for the system to be effective, the amount of weight exerting the traction must be 'balanced' against the patient's bodyweight (the countertraction).

WHY IS TRACTION USED?

There are four main reasons:

- to reduce pain following a fracture by helping to control muscle spasm;
- to correct or prevent deformity resulting from muscle spasm, soft tissue contracture or bone disease;
- to correct angulation and/or the overriding of fractures;
- as a post-operative fixation, for example to prevent dislocation of a hip prosthesis.

METHODS OF EXERTING TRACTION

The three main methods of exerting traction in common use are:

- skin traction;
- skeletal traction – often 'balanced';
- pulp traction – mainly used on the extremities.

Skin traction uses adhesive materials applied to the patient's skin (non-adhesive materials for patients with fragile skin), a pull then being exerted upon the fixed material. The pull is transmitted from the material and skin to the underlying tissues and bone. Because of the relative elasticity of the soft tissues, only a moderate amount of traction can be achieved. This type of traction may be used for either fixed or balanced traction and is generally not considered for prolonged periods of treatment. However, pelvic traction comes into this category and, in this situation, may be used for as long as 6 weeks for the treatment of low back pain.

Skeletal traction may look rather cruel as a metal pin, usually Steinmann or Denham, is placed through an area of strong bone (usually the lower end of the femur or upper end of the tibia), but this is, in fact, not only effective but also reported as being very comfortable.

Once the skeletal pin is in place, a metal hoop or stirrup is then attached, to which cords are tied. A weight is attached to the ends of these cords, which then pass freely over a pulley on the raised bed end. The pull is directed on the bone itself, so a greater amount of weight can be used for a longer period of time. A pull in this way is customarily applied as 'balanced' traction.

Pulp traction is considered when a prolonged and steady pull is to be applied to the fingers and toes but in reality is almost exclusively reserved for conditions affecting the thumb and great toe. The two previously mentioned forms of traction are not practicable.

A suture or wire is passed through the pulp of the digit(s) concerned and attached to some form of (usually custom-made) splint that encircles the thumb or foot. The traction force is gentle, primarily used to maintain the desired position of the digit while the healing progresses.

Orthopaedic bandaging

When the bones of an affected limb are fractured, either as a result of trauma or following surgical osteotomy, and left, the limb deformity is usually one of external rotation. In order to maintain any correction achieved by reduction or surgical intervention, bandages applied to the limb should be rolled onto the limb from the lateral towards the medial aspect, preferably in a 'figure-of-eight' fashion. This principle should be applied to all traction bandages and bandages used in the orthopaedic setting, as well during the application of plaster of Paris bandages in A&E and theatre (Collier, 1986).

Evaluating care/discharge

All patient care should be evaluated regularly and reported in the relevant hospital documentation. Any changes to a care plan should be noted. The resolution of patient's needs should be identified and signed off by a qualified nurse.

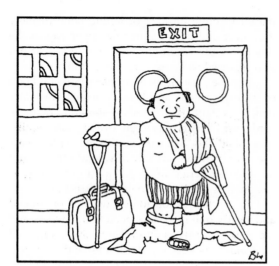

Figure 12.5 Discharge

As the patient is being prepared for discharge into a community setting, it may be necessary to liaise with the occupational therapist to organize a pre-discharge home visit, especially if the patient lives alone and has just been involved in major joint surgery or replacement. In addition, multidisciplinary case conferences may be arranged to identify appropriate support services required following discharge to help patients to live a relatively independent life. In some areas, community trusts have organized aftercare along the lines of the Community Orthopaedic Project of Essex (COPE).

Care in the A&E department

On arrival in the A&E department, the patient should be fully assessed using previously explained criteria (Bradley and Collier, 1994), the aims of which are to identify and correct any threat to the patient's survival, resuscitate the patient and stabilize the vital signs, determine the extent of other injuries and prepare the patient for definitive care, which may include transfer to another specialist centre.

A injury commonly seen in the A&E department requiring orthopaedic intervention is hip fracture. There is a high incidence of hip fracture among elderly people because their bones are more likely to be brittle as a result of osteoporosis and they are more at risk of falls. It has been reported that hip fractures are the most frequent cause of traumatic death in patients over the age of 75 (Brunner and Suddarth, 1988).

Hip and femoral fractures can also occur in younger patients following major trauma such as road traffic accidents. The clinical features of these injuries can include:

- swelling and discolouration in the hip or thigh region of the affected limb;

STUDENT ACTIVITY

Break open a honeycomb crunch bar. Osteoporotic bone looks like this.

Look up the risk factors of osteoporosis. Do any of them apply to you?

What changes could you make to reduce your risk?

- patient reluctance or inability to move or put weight on the affected leg;
- deformity at the fracture site or, in the case of a hip fracture, limb shortening with external rotation.

Crepitation may be heard on gentle palpation.

Observation of vital signs

Pulse, blood pressure and respiration should be recorded at regular intervals to monitor the patient's general status and the severity of any blood loss. If blood loss is great enough to create a risk of hypovolaemic shock, an intravenous infusion of Ringer's or normal saline solution should be commenced. Supplemental oxygen therapy may also be prescribed. Assessment and monitoring of the patient's pain, both specific and general, should also be undertaken.

Radiological assessment

Confirmation of femoral fractures can be facilitated by the use of X-rays.

Surgical intervention

Intervention depends upon the fracture but, if required, is indicated as soon as possible after injury in order to aid the bone's natural healing (Fig. 12.6). The pre-operative objective is to ensure that the patient is in as favourable condition as possible. Priorities of care therefore include immobilization of the fracture, fluid replacement, prevention of the effects of shock and administration of appropriate analgesia.

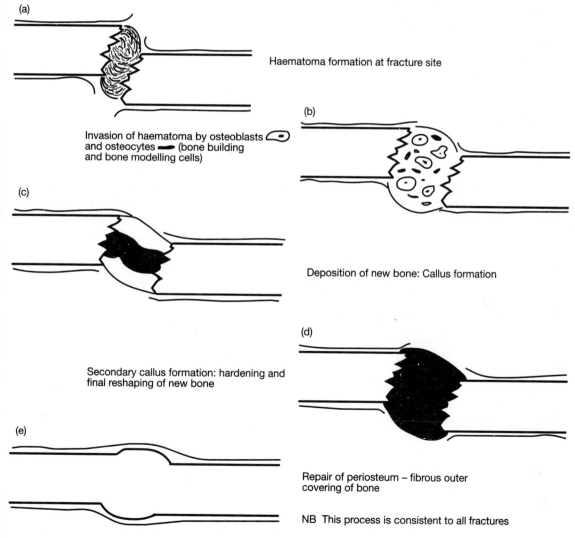

(a) Haematoma formation at fracture site

Invasion of haematoma by osteoblasts and osteocytes (bone building and bone modelling cells)

(b)

(c)

Deposition of new bone: Callus formation

(d)

Secondary callus formation: hardening and final reshaping of new bone

(e)

Repair of periosteum – fibrous outer covering of bone

NB This process is consistent to all fractures

Figure 12.6 Diagrammatic process of bone healing

Immobilization of the patient's fracture may include the use of traction (see above) or stabilization of the affected limb with a combination of pillows, sandbags and foam wedges in order to relieve painful muscle spasms and prevent further damage to tissues surrounding the fracture site.

Fluid replacement can be maintained by an intravenous line through which a variety of solutions, including blood, may be given, as prescribed and dictated by the patient's condition.

Pain relief can be administered intramuscularly, intravenously or via a facemask through which the patient breathes a mixture of gas and air (Entonox). If the patient is diagnosed as suffering from hypovolaemic shock, intramuscular analgesia may not be prescribed as it may not take effect until the patient's fluid level has been corrected; it may then take effect all at once, resulting in respiratory depression. Patients may be taken straight to theatre from the A&E department. If this is the case, all the usual pre-operative patient preparation should be undertaken as per local policy; however, the majority of patients will be admitted to a ward before being transferred to the theatre suite.

Elderly patients

This group of patients is more at risk of confusion, not only because of the stress of their trauma and unfamiliar surroundings, but also because of underlying systemic illness. They are thus more likely to be taking other medication, which will need to be identified, continued and monitored (*see* Chapter 2).

Chronic respiratory problems may also be present and contribute to the possible development of inadequate pulmonary ventilation or dictate when if at all, the patient is to operated upon.

Post-operative care following a hip or femoral fracture

Care is in many ways similar to that of elective hip surgery, illustrated in Table 12.2, p. 283.

SPECIFIC COMPLICATIONS RELATED TO FEMORAL AND HIP FRACTURES

One of the most serious complications of long bone fractures, in particular those affecting the diaphysis (shaft) of the femur, is that of fat embolus syndrome, which may occur 24–72 hours post-injury. It particularly affects young male patients and, if not detected, can lead to acute respiratory distress or sudden death.

Signs and symptoms to watch closely for if a patient is thought to be 'at risk' are:

- altered mental state – the patient may appear confused;
- complaints of chest pain on inspiration;
- (sudden) cardiovascular collapse;
- gradually increasing tachypnoea and tachycardia;
- petechiae (small red spots) over the patient's torso, in axillary folds and on the soft palate mucosa;
- localized muscle weakness or spasticity.

NURSING INTERVENTIONS

Administer fluids as directed to prevent shock and to dilute free fatty acids. Plasma expanders will often be given intravenously via continuous infusion. Administer drugs as prescribed to counteract the inflammatory response to free fatty acids and to increase the patient's cardiac output.

Reassure the patient as he may be very frightened and anxious as a result of hypoxaemia.

In summary, treat the symptomatology.

Delayed complications of hip fractures include protrusions of the chosen fixation device through the bone, causing pain, avascular necrosis of the femoral head owing to a compromised blood supply, non-union of the fracture and infection. Infection of the hip is suspected if the patient complains of moderate discomfort and has an associated elevated temperature – a subacute pyrexia.

Evaluation of care/patient discharge

Patients are usually discharged from hospital care approximately 14 days post-surgery, depending upon their general medical condition and whether they are able to mobilize safely and independently (refer to the previous discharge notes). Fracture braces may further protect a femoral fracture prior to the patient's discharge, mobilization being assisted by appropriate walking aids.

Patient comments

'With all this metalwork inside, will I set off

the security alarms at the airport when I next fly?'

'I am surprised how quickly and painlessly I have been able to mobilize in my fracture brace.'

The following section deals with elective orthopaedic surgery, including knee and hip procedures, giving additional notes regarding discharge considerations.

Care related to pin sites

Specific wound care may be indicated if an external fixation device has been used, with reference to care of the pin sites. Individual pin sites should be treated as individual wounds; the principles of care, can be summarized (Hoyt, 1986) as:

- promote the free drainage of any serous fluid;
- minimize local tissue damage.

Because of the local tissue's responses (redness, swelling, tenderness and discharge) to the presence of a foreign body, which is in this situation the skeletal pin, it is important frequently to observe the pin–skin interface. Serous drainage is produced when tissues slide over the pin and form a crust at this wound site/interface. As long as the fluid can drain freely, infection risks are reported to be minimal (Hoyt, 1986). In this author's opinion, this supports the view that pin site care should be performed on a daily basis and that, as long as the crust is not fixed to the pin, it should be left alone. If debridement is indicated (encrustation of the pin tract or increased skin tension is noted on assessment), this should be undertaken surgically in theatre, as the three most common vehicles for wound infec-

tion have been identified as hands, scissors and tape (Sproles, 1985).

If use of a cleansing solution is indicated, it could be argued that the solution of choice is normal saline. The efficacy of antiseptic solutions has been recently questioned by this author (Collier, 1995b) as well as others (Leaper *et al.*, 1987; Thomas, 1990).

The use of a dressing material to cover the pin tract has been widely debated (Mandzuk, 1991), but the most common of opinion prefers the use of a bulky, non-filamented gauze or non-adherent dressing in this area, the rationale being to reduce excess mobility of the pin across the tissues, which will facilitate the continued and further production of serous fluid. *Remember that the clear drainage of serous fluid is not in itself considered an adverse pin reaction or an early sign of infection (Sproles, 1985).*

In this author's opinion, the above protocol should be followed whether the patient is in a hospital or a community care setting and can be applied equally to the care of skeletal pins used to facilitate skeletal traction and of those associated with external fixation devices, whatever the anatomical site.

Table 12.1 Knee surgery

Anatomical region	Surgical example	Pre/per-operative considerations	Post-operative notes	Observations	Pain control
Knee	Prosthetic replacement	Operation is performed with the aid of a tourniquet	Large amounts of drainage are expected	Blood pressure, pulse, respiration and skin colour, both facial and of the extremity of the affected limb	Pain is assessed using an assessment tool and treated accordingly
			The patient is transferred onto the hospital bed with the aid of an easy slide	Assess for potential development of pressure ulcers, particularly around the foot of the affected limb	Continuous analgesic infusion is often administered via an IVAC, or epidural anaesthesia may be considered for a period of 24–48 hours
			The operation site is usually covered with a modified pressure dresing over a suitable primary dressing	Assess the wound for evidence of large amounts of oozing	After this period, intra-muscular pain relief is considered
			The affected limb will be positioned comfortably, avoiding extension of the knee	Neurovascular observations are performed on the extremity of the operated leg – colour, warmth and sensation. Frequency is dictated by the patient's condition	Anti-emetic drug therapy, such as stemetil or Maxolon, may also be required
			A bed cradle will be positioned to reduce the incidence of fixed plantar flexion (footdrop)	Blood loss is usually replaced if >500 mls	
			Anti-embolic stockings are *not* generally worn unless the patient has a history of previous deep vein thrombosis or has been identified as being 'at risk'	Note when the patient first passes urine	

Patient comment
'I was surprised how much I could move my knee following the operation – without severe pain!'

Table 12.2 Hip surgery: prosthetic replacement

Anatomical region	Surgical example	Pre/per-operative considerations	Post-operative notes	Observations	Pain control
Hip	Intravenous fluids are normally maintained for the first 24 hours

Fluids and diet may be reintroduced as the patient's condition allows, taking into account any reported nausea or vomiting | Wound drains will be removed as per criteria identified for prosthetic knee surgery (see Table 12.1)

Post-operative wound dressings will normally be taken down on the third day if there is no obvious oozing. Deep tension sutures, if used, will be removed on the fourth or fifth day, while skin sutures or clips will be removed between the seventh and tenth post-operative days, depending on assessment of the wound (Westaby, 1985) | Physiotherapy will be commenced at the earliest possible opportunity and will initially include plantar and dorsiflexion of both feet, static quadricep exercises and deep breathing

Mobilization will commence on the first or second post-operative day, assisted at first, keeping the affected limb extended at all times. Ambulatory aids will depend on the patient's age, balance and comfort

Patients are encouraged to get out of bed on the unaffected side and to return to bed on the opposite side, in order to maintain abduction of the operated hip, thereby further reducing the risk of hip dislocation | Patients must be educated in the importance of avoiding stooping and maintaining the hip in an abducted position. Patients can be encouraged to use a pillow at night at night to avoid crossing their legs. This information should be reinforced by all members of the multidisciplinary team

Patient discharge is anticipated between the fourteenth and twenty-first post-operative day and may be preceded by a home assessment with the occupational therapist (criteria as previously identified) | Dislocation of the hip prosthesis is due to joint 'laxity' caused by the division of muscle and other soft tissues at the time of operation. Stresses on the new hip should be kept to a minimum for between 3 and 6 months post-operatively. The patient should be encouraged at all times to sit in a 'high chair' that does not allow their hip to be flexed over 90°. Other preventive measures have been discussed in the text |

Table 12.3 Spinal surgery

Anatomical region	Surgical example	Pre/per-operative considerations	Post-operative notes	Observations	Pain control
Spine	Decompressions Laminectomy	Patients are usually admitted a few days prior to surgery for a period of traction to reduce any associated pain or other symptomatology During the pre-operative period, the patient will be guided in how activities of normal living will be performed in the post-operative phase of care The physiotherapist will instruct the patient on how to facilitate deep breathing exercises while lying in the recumbent position and how to log-roll on the bed when moving to an upright position All other pre-operative considerations are the same as for any other surgical procedure involving anaesthesia In theatre, surgeons may approach the spinal column either anteriorly or posteriorly. If anteriorly, the patient will be lying recumbent on the theatre table, but if posteriorly, the patient will be lying prone	Immediate post-operative recovery is as for knee surgery From theatre, the patient will be nursed in the recumbent position with both legs supported on pillows (heels free)	As for prosthetic knee surgery and include careful neurovascular observation of both lower extremities	Pain relief is usually administered via intra-muscular injections, although intravenous therapy is occasionally indicated following assessment. On the second or third post-operative day, oral drug therapy is usually reintroduced, remembering that the majority of these patients will have been on long-term analgesics pre-operatively. An objective of any prescribed pain relief should be to enable pain to be controlled by oral analgesia of a milder nature than was being taken pre-operatively

Table 12.3 Continued

Anatomical region	Surgical example	Pre/per-operative considerations	Post-operative notes	Observations	Pain control
		On return to the ward, the wound will be covered by a small dressing. One wound drain will usually be sited in order to decrease the risk of wound haematoma Wound drains are normally removed after 24 hours unless otherwise indicated Wound sutures/clips are removed between the fifth and seventh post-operative days, and a nobecutane spray dressing applied. The operation dressing is not usually removed before this time unless undue wound oozing has been noted or wound infection is suspected	A planned turning regimen will be commenced to reduce the risk of pressure ulcer development and to allow for assessment of the patient's skin and hygiene needs. For example, if the patient is being nursed on a Vaperm mattress (Scales, 1982) he may lie on his back for 4 hours before turning to one side for a further period of 2 hours. The lateral position may be alternated if tolerated. Patients lying on their side may feel more comfortable supported by pillows at the back and with a pillow between the knees Assisted standing and a few steps will be encouraged on the first post-operative day For 5 days, all patients will be encouraged either to stand upright or to lie flat on their bed, keeping the spinal column in as neutral a position as possible. After this period, sitting is allowed in a high-backed chair with the hip joints flexed. This regimen will be continued for approximately 4–6 weeks	On discharge, patients may require a walking aid, such as a stick, to assist continued mobilization Patient discharge is anticipated between the fifth and seventh post-operative day if the patient is mobilizing independently The occupational therapist will visit all patients to offer the use of aids, such as a 'helping hand' and long-handled shoe horn further to maintain the neutral position of their spine while performing activities of normal living All patients are encouraged to abstain from sexual intercourse for a period of at least 6 weeks post-operation because of the strain it places on the spine and the risk of haematoma development	Bleeding into the spinal canal or around the spinal column may cause pressure on the spinal nerves. In the case of a patient who has had surgery for the treatment of low back pain, this pressure might build up around the lumbar/sacral plexus, resulting in retention of urine and/or faeces and requiring additional nursing interventions

Patient comment
'Following my laminectomy, I was able to trust my back again and return to an almost normal lifestyle.'

Table 12.4 Surgical osteotomy

Anatomical region	Surgical example	Pre/per-operative considerations	Post-operative notes	Observations	Pain control
	Fluid and diet are reintroduced as tolerated by the patient	The wound is protected by a wool and crêpe dressing. One wound drain will normally be sited Wound drains are removed if the previously identified protocol has been observed The wound itself will be kept covered until the removal of skin sutures or clips between the fifth and tenth post-operative day Specific wound care may be indicated if an external fixator has been used	Physiotherapy exercises are commenced as soon after operation as possible. To assist 'active' exercises of the affected limb (patients using their own muscle power), a system of springs and slings is often set up on Balkham beams attached to the patient's bed A mobilization programme commences on the first post-operative day	Patient discharge is usually considered when new callus formation is noted on X-rays and the patient is able to mobilize independently and safely A home assessment visit may be needed depending upon individual circumstances	If an internal fixation device has been used to facilitate bony union, it is not usually removed unless it produces symptoms such as pain, local inflammation or an allergic reaction to the metallic alloy used

Primary indications for this surgical procedure are for correction of a skeletal deformity, be it an individual bone or joint as a result of trauma or the correction of a malunited fracture (Apley and Solomon, 1988). Once the relevant bone has been osteotomized, the principles for treatment are the same as for any other 'fracture' and may be summarized by the four R's: **R**ecognition, **R**eduction, **R**est and **R**ehabilitation. Whatever treatment is chosen, the primary objective will be to aid the normal healing process of bone (Fig. 12.6). Factors that can interrupt and delay bone healing are discussed elsewhere (Crawford Adams, 1972).

Summary

1 The specifics of elective surgical care for orthopaedic conditions are reviewed for a range of common operations.

2 The particular risks and complications of orthopaedic surgery and immobility are identified.

3 Programmes and principles of mobilization and rehabilitation are outlined.

4 Differences are drawn between elective and emergency care and conditions.

5 Operations representative of each main area are tabulated to illustrate the principles of care.

CASE HISTORY

Joe Bloggs, aged 19 and unemployed, suffered multiple fractures in a motorcycle accident. He is in traction in a bed, with both arms in plaster.

What are the hazards of immobility from which Joe is likely to suffer? How may the nurse anticipate and minimize these?

Review Questions

1 Describe the stages of bone healing, noting the factors that influence each stage.

2 What is the effect of weightbearing exercise upon bone?

3 List the activities, factors and dietary elements that protect against osteoporosis.

4 Why does the muscle go into spasm following a fracture?

5 What dietary advice is necessary for patients recovering from orthopaedic surgery?

6 List the strategies necessary to minimize the risk of dislocation after hip replacement.

ACKNOWLEDGEMENTS

With thanks to all my clinical colleagues at the Royal National Orthopaedic Hospital, Stanmore, Middlesex, especially Sister Pratt (Pre and Post Operative Ward).

References

Aggleton, P. and Chalmers, H. 1984 Models and theories. *Nursing Times* **87**(4), 33–5.

Apley, G. and Solomon, L. 1988 *Concise system of orthopaedics and fractures.* London: Butterworth.

Boore, J. 1978 *Prescription for recovery.* London: RCN.

Bradley, D. and Collier, M. 1994 *Principles of trauma and the treatment of traumatic wounds.* Educational leaflet 2(3). Northampton: Wound Care Society.

Brunner, L. and Suddarth, D. 1988 *Textbook of medical and surgical nursing,* 6th edn. Philadelphia: JB Lippincott.

Coffey, M. 1991 Total knee replacement.

Collier, M. 1986 *Welcome to your orthopaedic experience.* Kettering: Kettering Area Health Authority.

Collier, M. 1990a A sore point. *Community Outlook* Oct, 29–32.

Collier, M. 1990b Wound assessment: making informed choices. *Practice Nursing.*

Collier, M. 1995a *Pressure sore prevention and development.* Educational Paper, Vol. 3, No 1. Northampton: Wound Care Society.

Collier, M. 1995b Spells, potions and rituals – an enquiry to identify the major influences governing the use of wound cleansing solutions in clinical practice. *In*: Papadoparlas, I. and Lee, H. (eds) *Research for practice and education,* Vol. 2. London, North London College of Health Studies.

Crawford Adams, J. 1987 *Outline of fractures,* 9th edn. Edinburgh: Churchill Livingstone.

Cruse, P. and Foord, R. 1973 A five year prospective study of 23,649 surgical patients. *American Journal of Surgery* **121**(3), 251–2.

Davies, P. 1985 *Painful process of implementing research.* Stanmore: RNOH.

Gaston-Johansson, E. and Asklund-Gustafsson, M. 1985 A baseline for the development of an instrument for the assessment of pain. *Journal of Advanced Nursing* **10**, 539–46.

Hayward, J. 1975 *A prescription against pain.* London: RCN.

Hill, J. 1991 Assessing rheumatic disease. *Nursing Times* **87**(4), 33–5.

Hoyt, N. 1986 Infections following orthopaedic injury. *Orthopaedic Nursing* **5**(5), 15–22.

Leaper, D., Cameron, S., and Lancaster, J. 1987 Antiseptic solutions. *Nursing Times Community Outlook* **83**(14), 32–4.

McCaffrey, M. 1979 *Nursing management of the patient in pain.* Philadelphia: JB Lippincott.

Mandzuk, L. 1991 External pinsite care: a review. *CONA* **13**(1), 10–15.

Melzack, R. 1975 The McGill pain questionnaire. *Pain* **1**, 277–99.

Nickel, V. 1982 *Orthopaedic rehabilitation.* Edinburgh: Churchill Livingstone.

Overd, A. 1992 Should we lift or should we roll? *Professional Nurse,* Feb 311–19.

Roaf, R. and Hodkinson, L. 1980 *Textbook of orthopaedic nursing,* 3rd edn. Oxford: Blackwell.

Scales, J. 1982 Vaperm patient support system – a new general purpose hospital mattress. *Lancet* Nov 20, 1150–2.

Schoen, D. 1986 *The nursing process in orthopaedics.* Norwalk, CT: Appleton-Century-Crofts.

Seropian, R. and Reynolds, B.M. 1971 Wound infections after pre-operative depilation versus razor preparation. *American Journal of Surgery* **121**(3), 251–2.

Sproles, K. 1985 Nursing care of skeletal pin sites: a closer look. *Orthopaedic Nursing* **4**(1), 45–54.

Thomas, S. 1990 *Wound management and dressings.* London: Pharmaceutical Press.

Tortora, G.J. and Agnostakos, N.P. 1987 *Principles of anatomy and physiology,* 5th edn. London: Harper & Row.

Waterlow, J. 1988 Tissue viability – prevention is cheaper than cure. *Nursing Times* **84**(25), 69–70.

Westaby, S. (ed.) 1985 *Wound care.* London: Heinemann.

Winfield, V. 1986 Too close a shave? *Nursing Times Journal of Infection Control Nursing* Mar 5, 64–8.

Further reading

Bastiani, G. 1984 The treatment of fractures with a dynamic axial fixator. *Journal of Bone and Joint Surgery* **66B**(4), 538–45.

Bradley, D. 1980 *Accident and emergency nursing.* London: Baillière Tindall.

Crawford , Adams J. 1996 *Outline of orthopaedics,* 12th edn. Edinburgh: Churchill Livingstone.

Crow, J. 1977 The nursing process. *Nursing Times* **73**, 882–6.

Dandy, D.J. 1989 *Essential orthopaedics and trauma.* Edinburgh: Churchill Livingstone.

Gilchrist, B. 1992 *Textbook of adult nursing.* Revised by Brunner, L.S. and Suddarth, D.S. (eds). London: Chapman & Hall.

Kingman, S. 1988 Flexible clamp gives bones room to heal. *New Scientist* **120**(1638), 35.

Love, C. 1986 Do you roll or lift? *Nursing Times* **82**, 44–6.

McRae, R. 1983 *Clinical orthopaedic examination,* 2nd edn. Edinburgh: Churchill Livingstone.

McRae, R. 1989 *Practical fracture treatment,* 2nd edn. Edinburgh: Churchill Livingstone.

Mackinnon, P. and Morris, J. 1986 *Oxford textbook of functional anatomy,* Vol. 1, *Musculoskeletal system.* Oxford: Oxford University Press.

Manufacturers Profile 1990 The Orthofix Modulsystem. *Orthopaedic Product News* Dec 90/Feb 91.

Powell, M. 1982 *Orthopaedic nursing and rehabilitation,* 8th edn. Edinburgh: Churchill Livingstone.

Waterlow, J. 1985 A risk assessment card. *Nursing Times* **81**(48), 49–55.

Waterlow, J. 1988 Calculating the risk. *Nursing Times* **83**(39), 58–60.

Glossary

Activated partial thromboplastin time ratio (APTR) A measure of clotting time, the normal being 0.8–1.2.

Ablative dysrrythmia surgery Surgical removal of abnormal conduction pathways for dysrrythmias resistant to medical treatment.

Absorption Passage of a substance through a surface of the body into body fluids and tissues.

Activated clotting time (ACT) Qualitatively assesses the anticoagulant effect of heparin.

Adduction Movement of a joint towards or across the patient's midline (with reference to the normal 'skeletal' anatomical position).

Adult respiratory distress syndrome (ARDS) A respiratory disorder characterized by respiratory insufficiency and failure, usually occurring after aspiration of vomit or foreign body.

Afterload A term used to describe the forces opposing ventricular ejection, for example systemic vascular resistance.

Agglutination An antigen–antibody response in which cells become linked to one another to form a visible clump.

Anabolism A build-up of body protein, especially muscle; it is useful in convalescence.

Anastomosis Surgical joining of gut or blood vessels following resection so that they interconnect.

Angina pectoris Transient episodes of chest pain that may radiate down the left arm, often accompanied by a sensation of constriction about the heart. A symptom of myocardial ischaemia usually related to any activity increasing oxygen demand.

Angiography Injection of contrast medium via a catheter into the carotid, vertebral or femoral artery. As the contrast medium passes through the cerebral arteries, X-rays are taken which give clear images of the cerebral circulation.

Angioplasty A procedure to refashion blood vessels.

Angioscopy Looking into a blood vessel, using an ultra-thin, flexible, multibundle fibreoptic endoscope, the image being shown on a video screen monitor.

Ankle: arm index (AAI) Comparison of systolic pressure in the upper and lower extremities by Doppler ultrasonography. Ankle pressure is normally equal to, or slightly above, arm pressure. In occlusive arterial disease, ankle and lower leg pressures are lowered. Also known as ankle brachial pressure index (ABPI).

Anterior cervical spinal fusion Performed in order to release the spinal cord and nerve roots from pressure caused by narrowing of the intervertebral space and the diameter of the spinal canal. This usually occurs as a result of collapse of the intervertebral disc and the subsequent bony changes. Fusion is achieved by removing the intervertebral disc, thus encouraging the growth of fibrous tissue between the vertebrae or, in addition to removing the disc, by inserting a small piece of bone (usually taken from the patient's iliac crest) between the vertebrae.

Aortic aneurysm Dilatation of part of the aortic wall, producing a pulsating swelling.

Aortography/aortogram Injection of X-ray opaque dye via a catheter passed along the brachial or femoral artery, or direct translumbar injection, to demonstrate the aorta.

Aphakia Absence of the lens after cataract removal.

Aphasia Absence or impairment of the ability to communicate through speech, writing or signs, owing to dysfunction of the brain centres.

Aqueous Fluid contained in the anterior and posterior chambers of the eye.

Arteriography/angiography   Injection of an X-ray opaque substance into an artery to demonstrate the system. May also be performed using MRI.

Arteriosclerosis   Ageing and degenerative changes in the arterial system associated with thickening of the median layer of the vessel wall and some degree of atheroma. Loss of elasticity and calcification result in a decreased blood supply, especially to the cerebrum and lower extremities.

Arteriovenous malformation   A congenital abnormality characterized by abnormal collections of enlarged blood vessels.

Arthrodesis   Surgical fusion of a joint using either bone or 'metalwork'.

Arthroplasty   The operative procedure of reshaping or reconstructing a diseased joint to improve its function.

Aspiration   Drawing in or out as by suction, for example of cells from a lump to ascertain malignancy. Foreign bodies may also be aspirated into the nose, throat or lungs on inspiration.

Asthma   Paroxysmal constriction of the bronchial airways.

Astigmatism   Faulty vision caused by inequality of one or more refractive surfaces, usually corneal, preventing light rays from converging to a point on the retina.

Atelectasis   An abnormal condition characterized by the collapse of lung tissue distal to an obstruction by a plug of mucous, preventing the respiratory exchange of oxygen and carbon dioxide.

Atherectomy   Removal of atheroma from the arterial wall by means of a percutaneous transluminal approach, then drilling/pulverizing or shaving of the plaque with an atherectomy device.

Atheroma   Hard yellow fatty plaques deposited in the intima (lining) of arteries.

Atherosclerosis   Combination of arteriosclerosis and atheroma in large arteries, resulting in the reduction of blood supply or ischaemia.

Atrophy   A wasting or decrease in size of an organ or tissue.

Audiogram   Chart to measure the level of hearing in an individual.

Autogenous/autograft/autologous   Use of a person's own tissue, for example blood or vein graft.

Bacterial endocarditis   A bacterial infectious process of the endocardial surface of the heart.

Balloon angioplasty   *See* Percutaneous transluminal angioplasty.

Barium swallow   X-ray using an opaque medium, to detect abnormalities of the oesophagus to stomach.

Beta-blockers   Drugs inhibiting sympathetic activity, used in the treatment of dysrrythmias and hypertension.

Biometrist   A professional who carries out the procedure for measuring the length of the eye and the curve of the cornea by using 'biometry', an ultrasound scanner and keratometer. This is done to find the correct size and strength of intra-ocular lens implant prior to cataract surgery.

Biopsy   A small portion of tissue is removed under local or general anaesthesia for microscopic examination.

BIPP   Ribbon gauze impregnated with bismuth iodoform paraffin paste.

Bone scan   Imaging of the skeleton after injection of a radioactive isotope in order to detect bony secondary deposits (metastases).

Breast awareness   Women getting to know their breasts through everyday activities such as bathing, showering and dressing, in order to detect any changes.

Buerger's disease (thromboangiitis obliterans)   Occlusive small vessel disease occurring mainly in young male heavy smokers, some of whom may need grafts; it may even proceed to amputation of the digits, foot or leg.

Burr hole   A small hole made in the skull through which a biopsy may be taken, a haematoma or abcess drained or a CSF drain inserted.

Calcium-channel blockers   Drugs that slow the inflow of calcium into vascular smooth muscle fibres and reduce the workload of the heart.

Cardiac tamponade   A collection of blood between the heart and the anterior chest wall that is not removed by the chest drainage tubes and causes compression of the heart, leading to significantly impaired ventricular contractility and reduced venous return.

Cardiomyopathy   Disease of heart muscle.

Cardioplegia To ensure minimal myocardial damage during cardiac surgery, cardiac arrest needs to be achieved quickly. Cardioplegia involves injecting a cold fluid with a high potassium content into the root of the aorta or coronary ostia to cause rapid cardiac arrest and to cool and perfuse the coronary arteries.

Cardioversion Electrical conversion of a dysrrythmia by the application of a direct current shock synchronized with the patient's ECG.

Catabolism Breakdown of body protein, especially muscle, to liberate energy.

Cautery A heated metal instrument or caustic agent used for coagulation of tissue.

Central Nervous System (CNS) The brain and spinal cord.

Cerebral aneurysm A congenital or acquired weakness of part of the wall of a cerebral artery, commonly found on the circle of Willis (a circle of arteries at the base of the brain).

Cerebral oedema The presence of fluid in the cerebrum.

Cervix A 'necklike' structure, lying partly above and partly in the vagina, that keeps the uterus contents in.

Choledojejunostomy A surgical procedure in which the common bile duct is resited into the jejunum.

Cholesteatoma Expanding cyst made up of epithelial tissue that is trapped in the middle ear.

Claudication Leg weakness with cramplike pains in the calves, caused by poor blood supply, resulting in a limp, and thus decreasing walking distance.

Colloid Intravenous fluids containing non-diffusible particles of solutes that will not leak out of the capillaries, for example whole blood and plasma expanders. The osmotic effect exerted will help to maintain intravascular volume.

Colostomy The open end of the healthy colon brought to the surface of the abdomen to form an exit for waste matter.

Computerised axial tomography (CAT scanning) A method using X-rays to create an image of a thin cross-sectional 'slice' of the body. These X-rays are either absorbed or transmitted as a result of which the computer is able to calculate the differing densities of tissue within the cranium.

Cone biopsy Surgical removal of a cone-shaped segment of the cervix, including both epithelial and endocervical tissue, for microscopic examination to determine precise diagnosis.

Congestive heart failure Circulatory congestion caused by cardiac disorders.

Conservation Breast surgery involving removal of the tumour together with a margin of microscopically normal tissue.

Constrictive pericarditis Inflammation of the pericardium, causing pressure on the heart.

Craniectomy Operation performed in order to approach lesions affecting the cerebellar hemispheres and/or brain system. A hole is made in the cranium and enlarged by nibbling the bone away until the area is large enough to allow access to the lesion.

Craniotomy Operation performed in order to approach lesions affecting the cerebral hemispheres and/or adjacent structures. Burr holes are made; the bone is then cut in a circular fashion between these holes and the bone removed or turned back.

Crepitation Grating or crackling noise associated with the movement of fractured bone ends or arthritic joints, or with palpating soft tissue containing air.

Crystalloid Intravenous fluids given to maintain hydration and electrolyte concentrations.

Cyst A globular sac filled with fluid or semisolid material that develops, for example, in or on the ovary.

Cystectomy Surgical removal of the bladder, commonly performed for carcinoma of the bladder when more conservative interventions are no longer an option.

Cystodiathermy Commonly used in the treatment of carcinoma of the bladder. It involves removal of superficial new growths in the bladder by cauterization.

Cystogram A procedure to investigate bladder function, which measures bladder pressure on both filling and voiding.

Cystoscopy Procedure enabling the surgeon to view the inside of the bladder without making a surgical cut. A urethral approach is employed using either a rigid or a flexible cystoscope with a viewing lens and its own light source.

Dacron   Man-made knitted material used in grafts to replace or bypass faulty blood vesssels.

Decubitus ulcer   An ulcer, initially of the skin, resulting from prolonged pressure against skin areas of a person who remains in one position (lying or sitting) for any length of time.

Deep vein thrombosis   Formation or development of a blood clot within the deep veins of the legs.

Demineralization   Loss of mineral salts, especially from the bones.

Diabetes insipidus   A condition in which the patient produces large amounts of urine owing to an insufficiency of antidiuretic hormone (ADH).

Diabetes mellitus   A disorder of metabolism resulting from lack of insulin and predisposing to atherosclerosis.

Diffusion   The tendency of molecules of a substance (gaseous, liquid or solid) to move from a region of high concentration to one of lower concentration.

Digital subtraction angiography   A computer technique subtracting bone from angiography images so that blood vessels show up more clearly.

Dispensing optician   A professional who cannot test vision but can interpret prescriptions and dispense glasses or contact lenses.

Distal   Away from the point of origin, midline or central point.

Doppler ultrasonography   The use of high-frequency sounds to detect pressure, velocity and the location of blood flow in veins and arteries, indicating the extent of disease.

Dumping syndrome   A post-operative complication of gastric surgery that occurs during or after a meal. The patient may complain of weakness, a feeling of fullness, discomfort, nausea, sweating and diarrhoea.

Duplex ultrasonography   High resolution ultrasound imaging combined with pulse Doppler.

Dysarthria   Difficulty in articulating words, owing to weakness or lack of co-ordination of the muscles invoved in speaking.

Dyspareunia   Painful intercourse.

Dysphasia   Difficulty in swallowing owing to weakness or paralysis of the muscles involved.

Dysphasia   Difficulty in understanding the words spoken and/or difficulty in finding the right words. This is a disorder of language, usually resulting from injury to the speech area of the cerebral cortex.

Dyspnoea   Air hunger resulting in laboured or difficult breathing; sometimes accompanied by pain.

Dysrhythmia   An abnormal rhythm of the heart owing to an abnormal origin of impulse, or abnormal conduction through the heart.

Dysuria   Difficulty in passing urine or painful micturition. Causes, for example outflow obstruction (such as prostatic hypertrophy) or urinary tract infection, are various.

Ectomy   Removal of.

Ectopic   Something situated in an unusual place away from its normal location, for example an ectopic pregnancy being a pregnancy that occurs outside the uterus.

Effusion   The escape of fluid and its accumulation in tissues or a body cavity.

Ejection fraction   An assessment of cardiac function. It represents the ratio of stroke volume to end-diastolic volume and reflects the degree to which contraction abnormalities have compromised myocardial performance.

Electrocardiogram (ECG)   A recording of the electrical activity of the heart.

Electroencephalogram (EEG)   A recording of the electrical activity of the brain.

Embolectomy   Surgical removal of an embolism, usually using a fine (Fogarty) balloon catheter.

Embolus (pl. emboli)   A thrombus that circulates in the bloodstream until it becomes lodged in a vessel (= an **embolism**).

Endarterectomy   Surgery to remove an atheromatous core from an artery; also known as disobliteration or a rebore.

Endoluminal   Inside the vessel lumen.

Endometriosis   The ectopic growth and functioning of endometrial tissue.

Endometrium   The mucous membrane lining of the uterus, which changes thickness throughout the menstrual cycle. The upper layers shed at the time of the menstrual flow.

Endophthalmitis   Internal infection of the eye.

Endoscopic   Relates to endoscopy, the inspection of an internal cavity using an endoscope.

Enucleation   In this procedure, the extra-ocular muscles are cut, the optic nerve severed and the entire globe removed.

Erythema   Redness of tissues.

Eustachian tube   Narrow canal connecting the middle ear with the post-nasal space.

Evisceration   Procedure involving removal of the cornea and intra-ocular contents, leaving some sclera and the optic nerve.

Extra corporeal shock wave lithotripsy (ESWL)   An alternative treatment to invasive renal surgery for the removal of renal calculi, involving supporting and positioning the patient in water with the stones as the focus of converging shock waves. The shock waves pass through the water and disintegrate the stone, the fragments of which can then be passed *per urethram*.

Extravasation   Accumulation of fluid in the tissues owing to a cannula pulling out of the vein.

Extubation   Removal of an endotrachael tube following a period of ventilatory support.

Fallopian tubes   A pair of ducts that open at one end into the uterus and at the other into the peritoneal cavity near the ovary. Fertilization occurs in them and they carry the ovum from the ovary to the uterus. Also known as oviducts or uterine tubes.

Fat embolism   Obstruction of vessels by fat globules, usually as a consequence of fractures of long bones but also occurring in bones.

Fibreoptics   The process by which internal structures are visualized, using glass or plastic fibres to transmit light through a specially designed tube and reflect an enlarged image.

Fibroid   A benign tumour of fibrous connective tissue. Also known as a myoma.

Fibrosis   Formation of fibrous connective tissue as part of scarring and healing to replace lost tissue.

Fourchette   A tense band of mucous membrane at the posterior angle of the vagina connecting the posterior ends of the labia minora.

Free radical   A molecule containing an unpaired, unstable electron. It is usually converted to a stable molecule by the body's own defence system but can transfer from molecule to molecule, causing a chain reaction of oxidative damage.

Gastrectomy   An operation to remove all or part (partial gastrectomy) of the stomach.

Gastrojejunostomy   Surgical procedure to create an opening from the stomach into the duodenum.

Gastrostomy   Creation of an artificial opening into the stomach for the purposes of enteral feeding.

Gingivitis   Inflammation of the gums, characterized by redness, swelling and a tendency to bleed.

Glue ear   Thick effusion in the middle ear causing deafness.

Guttae   Drops.

Haematuria   The presence of blood in the urine, caused by lesions in the renal and urinary tract or by infection.

Haemodilution   The perfusate that circulates from the patient to the extracorporeal circuit during cardiac bypass. It consists of the patient's own blood and the oxygenator prime of a physiological solution such as 5% dextrose in lactated Ringer's with other additives.

Haemolysis   The destruction of red blood cells within the body, possibly leading to anaemia. Causes include infection and mismatched blood transfusions.

Halitosis   Unpleasantly smelling breath.

Hartmann's procedure   The diseased part of the bowel is resected and a stoma formed. The rectal stump is saved for later reconstructive surgery.

Hemiparesis   Weakness of the muscles of the upper and lower limbs and the trunk on one side of the body.

Hemiplegia   Paralysis of the muscles of the upper and lower limbs and trunk on one side of the body.

Hiatus hernia   Protrusion of the stomach upwards into the mediastinal cavity through the oesophageal hiatus of the diaphragm.

Histology   The science of dealing with the microscopic identification of cells and tissues.

Homeostasis   The state of equilibrium of the internal environment of the body.

Hydration   The addition of water to a substance or tissue.

Hyperkalaemia   An excess of potassium in the blood.

Hyperlipidaemia   An excess of lipids in the plasma, predisposing to atheroma.

Hypertension   Persistently elevated blood pressure exceeding 140/90 mmHg.

Hypervolaemia   An increase or excess of circulating blood volume. It may result in pulmonary oedema and cardiac arrythmia.

Hyphaema   Blood in the anterior chamber of the eye.

Hypokalaemia   A deficiency of potassium in the blood.

Hyponatraemia   An abnormally low level of sodium in the blood resulting in electrolyte imbalance.

Hypopyon   Pus in the anterior chamber of the eye.

Hypotension   A decrease in systolic and diastolic blood pressure to below normal.

Hypothermia   A body temperature below normal.

Hypoxaemia   A reduced oxygen concentration in the blood.

Hysterectomy   Surgical removal of the uterus.

Iatrogenic   Caused by treatment or diagnostic procedures.

Ileostomy   The open end of the healthy ileum is brought to the surface of the abdomen to form an exit for waste matter.

Immune system   The tissues, organs and physiological processes used by the body to identify a protein as abnormal and prevent it from harming the organism.

Impedance testing   A method of testing the mobility of the eardrum.

Incentive spirometry   A device used in postoperative chest physiotherapy that visually indicates the depth of the patient's inspiratory effort.

Induction of anaesthesia   The administration of the anaesthetic drugs.

Inotropic support   The use of drugs to increase myocardial contractility.

Institution   A place where individuals live together governed by one body that directs work, rest and play.

Intermittent claudication   Leg, commonly calf, pain on walking some distance, which is usually relieved by rest.

International normalized ratio (INR)   A standardization of prothrombin time (average value 0.8–1.2) used to measure the anticoagulant effect of warfarin.

Interstitial cystitis   A condition comprising dysuria, frequency, nocturia and tenderness or pain in the suprapubic area. Its cause is unclear but it may be diagnosed through cystoscopy, generalized reddening of the bladder mucosa being seen.

Intra-aortic balloon pump   A balloon device that reduces the workload of the heart and increases perfusion. It is positioned in the thoracic aorta, inflating during diastole and deflating just prior to and during systole.

Intravenous urogram (IVU)   A very common urological investigation in which the patient is given an intravenous injection of a radio-opaque contrast medium that will eventually be excreted in the urine. A series of X-rays is taken to indicate any abnormalities as the contrast passes through the renal and urinary tracts.

Intravesicular wall   The internal wall of the bladder (*vesico* bladder).

Intubated   Provided with an artificial airway using an orotracheal or nasotracheal tube.

Ischaemia   Deficiency of blood supply.

Keloid   Overgrowth of scar tissue that gets steadily worse, possibly leading to contraction of the area.

Kyphosis   Exaggeration of the normal posterior curve of the spine.

Labia majora   Two long lips of skin, one each side of the vaginal orifice outside the labia minora.

Labia minora   Two folds of skin between the labia majora, extending from the clitoris backwards on both sides of the vaginal orifice and ending between it and the labia majora.

Laminectomy Excision of the posterior arches and spinous processes of a vertebra to expose the intervertebral disc, the prolapsed disc and any bony fragments then being removed.

Laser Light Amplification by Stimulated Emission of Radiation. A source of intense radiation of the visible, ultraviolet or infrared portions of the spectrum. It is used to divide tissue, cause adhesions, destroy, or fix tissue in place.

Left atrial pressure Direct measurement of the pressure in the left atrium can help to assess intracardiac pathology and haemodynamic abnormality.

Limbus The corneal margin's outer rim, where the cornea ends and the conjunctiva begins.

Lithotomy position Position in which the patient lies supine with the thighs flexed upon the abdomen and the legs upon the thighs, which are abducted.

Lithotripsy Crushing of stones found in the renal and urinary system.

Liver ultrasonography Scanning to detect liver secondaries.

Locus of control Refers to an individual's sense of mastery of, or control over, events.

Lumbar puncture Procedure performed to gain access to the CSF. A needle is passed into the subarachnoid space via the gap between the vertebral spines at the lower end of the vertebral column, usually between L3 and L4 or L4 and L5, in order to avoid hitting the spinal cord.

Lumen The channel inside a tubular structure.

Lumpectomy Excision of a breast lump for examination.

Lymphoedema Excessive fluid in the tissues as a result of blockage or removal of lymph vessels/nodes.

Macular degeneration Deterioration of the area of clearest central vision.

Magnetic resonance imaging (MRI) Clear images of the body tissues are produced by monitoring the behaviour of hydrogen atoms when the head/body is passed through a magnetic field.

Malignancy A cancer, a virulent growth of cells.

Mammogram X-ray examination of the breast.

Breast screening by mammography is offered every 3 years to women aged 50–64.

Mastectomy Surgical removal of the whole breast.

Meninges Three membranes covering the brain and spinal cord: the pia, arachnoid and dura mater.

Meningitis Infection of the meninges.

Metabolism The sum of all physical and chemical changes taking place within an organism; energy and material transformations that occur within living cells.

Miosed Constricted, as in the pupil of the eye.

Miotic A drug to constrict the pupil.

Morbidity rate The number of sick persons, or cases, of disease in relation to a specific population.

Mortality data The date, rate and ratio of numbers of deaths in a given population.

Mydriatic A drug to dilate the pupil.

Myelography/Radiculography Contrast medium is introduced via a lumbar puncture into the subarachnoid space and X-rays are taken of the spinal cord and/or nerve roots.

Myocardial infarction (MI) A condition caused by partial or complete occlusion of one or more of the coronary arteries, commonly known as a heart attack.

Myomectomy Surgical removal of a myoma (fibroid) from the uterus.

Nasogastric intubation The insertion of a flexible hollow tube into the stomach via the nose.

Nephroscope A nephroscope has a similar function to that of a cystoscope and is used for the direct visualization of the renal pelvis and calyces.

Nephrotic syndrome Abnormal condition of the kidney featuring proteinuria, hypoalbuminaemia and oedema.

Neurofibrillary tangles Tiny fibrils that extend and tangle in the brain.

Neurological observations Observations of mental state, best verbal response, best motor response, pupil reaction, respiration, pulse, blood pressure and painful stimuli.

Neurovascular observations   Observations of the colour, warmth and sensation of a limb.

Obesity   An abnormal amount of fat covering the body.

Oedema   An excessive amount of tissue fluid that occurs when the rate of formation of tissue fluid is greater than the rate of absorption.

Oophorectomy   Surgical removal of one or both ovaries.

Ophthalmic surgeon   A doctor with additional ophthalmic qualifications who is a fellow of the Royal College of Surgeons (FRCS).

Opioid   A narcotic drug containing opium or its derivatives, or with opium-like activity.

Optometrist   An optician who can test vision and dispense glasses or contact lenses.

Orthoptist   A professional, rather like an ocular physiotherapist, who is mainly involved with the diagnosis and treatment of patients with defective binocular vision or abnormal eye movement, in which the muscles of the eye are unbalanced.

Oscopy   Inspection of an organ or cavity.

Osteomalacia   A disease marked by increasing softness of the bones, which become flexible and brittle, thus causing deformities.

Osteoporosis   A reduction in the mass of bone per unit volume caused by the loss of both mineral and protein.

Osteotomy   Surgical division of a bone.

Ostomy   An opening or outlet.

Otomy   Incision or cutting of.

Pancreatojejunostomy   A surgical procedure to join the pancreatic ducts to the jejnum.

Papilloma   A benign tumour of the epithelium.

Paraesthesia   Disordered sensation.

Paralysis   Loss of motor function/power.

Paralytic ileus   The reduction or absence of intestinal peristalsis.

Paraplegia   Paralysis of the lower limbs and trunk.

Parenteral   Denoting any medical feeding route other than directly into the alimentary canal.

Patency   The condition of being open and unblocked.

Patient-controlled analgesia (PCA)   A drug delivery system dispensing a pre-set intravenous dose of a narcotic analgesic into the patient when he or she pushes a switch on an electric cord.

Percutaneous   Through the skin. In the case of percutaneous nephroscopy, a tract is made through the skin into which the nephroscope is inserted.

Percutaneous balloon mitral valvuloplasty   Insertion of a balloon catheter through the mitral valve. The balloon is then inflated to stretch the mitral valve to relieve mitral stenosis.

Percutaneous transluminal angioplasty (PTA)   A catheter is introduced into an artery through the skin and advanced towards an atherosclerotic or stenotic plaque. It is then compressed by inflating and deflating a small balloon at the tip of the catheter, which is then withdrawn. Also known as percutaneous transluminal balloon angioplasty (PTBA). The technique may be laser assisted.

Perfusion   The passing of fluid through spaces.

Peri-articular cartilage   Cartilage situated around a joint.

Pericardial effusion   A collection of fluid within the pericardial sac.

Pericardiocentesis   Needle aspiration of pericardial fluid under echocardiography guidance or close observation of the ECG.

Peripheral nervous system   The spinal and cranial nerves.

Peristalsis   A progressive wave-like movement occurring involuntarily in hollow tubes of the body, especially the alimentary canal.

Perthe's disease   Malformation of the femoral head resulting from congenital abnormality of the collateral circulation.

Phacoemulsification   Ultrasound is used to break up lens fibres prior to removal.

Photophobia   Abnormal sensitivity of the eyes to light.

Plethysmography   Measurement of finger blood flow.

Pneumonia   Inflammation of the lungs, caused primarily by bacteria, viruses and chemical irritants.

Polycythaemia rubra vera   An abnormal increase in the number of red blood cells.

Polyp   A small tumour-like growth projecting from a mucous membrane surface.

Polysomnography   Analysis of sleep pattern.

Positive end-expiratory pressure (PEEP)   Positive pressure that prevents complete alveolar closure on expiration. It helps to improve oxygenation and prevent alveolar collapse and atelectasis.

Post-cholecystectomy syndrome   A persistence or recurrence of symptoms which are indistinguishable from those for which the cholecystectomy was performed.

Pre-load   Left ventricular end-diastolic volume. A measurement of the force of myocardial contractility.

Proprioception   Joint position sense relayed by sensory receptors in muscles, tendons and joints which are stimulated by changes in tension.

Proximal   Nearer to the trunk of the body.

Pulmonary embolism   Obstruction of the pulmonary artery or one of its branches by an embolus from thrombosis in the lower extremities.

Pyloroplasty   Enlargement of the pylorus of the stomach.

Quadrantectomy   Removal of the quadrant of the breast containing the malignant mass.

Quinsy   A collection of pus in the tissues around the tonsillar capsule. Also known as peritonsillar abscess.

Raynaud's syndrome   Autoimmune disease often causing longstanding peripheral vasoconstriction, which may result in ulceration of the digits.

Regurgitation   A backward flowing, as in the return of solids or fluids to the mouth from the stomach, or the backward flow of blood through a defective heart valve.

Rehabilitation   The process of treatment and education that leads a disabled individual to attainment of maximum function, a sense of well-being and a personally satisfying level of independence.

Renogram   Procedure serving a similar purpose to an intravenous urogram in that it will reveal any abnormalities of the kidney. However, it has the added advantage that it will also give an indication of renal function.

Retrograde   Working backwards/against the flow.

Rheumatoid arthritis   A form of arthritis with inflammation of the joints, stiffness, swelling and pain.

Right atrial pressure   A reading of pressure in the right atrium, usually measured via central venous cannulation, can help to assess intracardiac pathology and haemodynamic abnormality.

Scleritis   Inflammation of the sclera.

Serology   The study of serum, originally for the presence of antibodies.

Slipped upper femoral epiphysis (SUFE)   A condition most commonly seen in adolescence, in which the upper femoral epiphysis becomes displaced by a fracture or through weakness of the growth plate.

Stasis   Impeded or halted flow through a blood vessel.

Steatorrhoea   State in which there is greater than normal amount of fat in the faeces characterized by frothy, foul-smelling faecal matter that floats.

Stenosis   Abnormal narrowing in, for example, an artery or arterial graft.

Stent   A device used to keep vessel patent by forming an expandable wire-mesh skeleton to oppose the elastic recoil of vascular stenosis.

Stomatitis   Inflammation of the mouth.

Stridor   Noisy breathing on inspiration owing to obstruction in the larynx.

Stroke volume   The volume of blood expelled from the ventricle in one contraction or systole.

Subarachnoid haemorrhage   Bleeding into the space between the arachnoid and pia mater.

Subchondral Osteoporosis   *See* Osteoporosis.

Subcutaneous mastectomy   Removal of breast tissue, preserving the skin, areola and nipple to allow for reconstruction.

Tamoxifen   A synthetic anti-oestrogen that may be given for at least 2–5 years following surgery for carcinoma of the breast.

Temporalis fascia   A fibrous tissue taken from the temporal region and used for grafting.

Thrombocytopenia   A deficiency of circulating thrombocytes (platelets).

Thromboembolism Condition in which a blood vessel is blocked by an embolism carried in the bloodstream from the site of clot formation for example, the deep veins of the legs to the lungs.

Thrombolysis Dissolution of arterial clot using an antifibrinolytic agent such as streptokinase or alteplase (rt-PA) via an arterial catheter.

Thrombosis The formation, development or existence of a blood clot or thrombus within the vascular system.

Thrombus A blood clot within the heart or a blood vessel.

Transfemoral An approach via the femoral artery.

Transient ischaemic attack (TIA) Condition resulting from temporary interference with the blood supply to the brain.

Translumbar An approach through the lumbar region used to inject dye into the aorta for aortography.

Transluminal Via the lumen of the vessel.

Tunica adventitia The outer layer of the wall of a blood vessel, composed mostly of elastic and collagen fibres.

Tunica intima The inner layer of the wall of a blood vessel, composed of a lining of endothelium (simple squamous epithelium), basement membrane and elastic lamina.

Tunica media The middle layer of the wall of a blood vessel, comprising smooth muscle and elastic fibres.

Turgor The resistance of the skin to deformation, especially from being grasped by the fingers.

Ultrasound imagining The use of inaudible high-frequency sound waves (20 000 intrations per second) directed in a beam into the body, the information provided by the echoes enabling an image of body structures to be built up. No radiation is involved.

Unstable angina Prolonged and severe episodes of angina occurring without increased oxygen demands.

Urinary flow rate measurement Common investigation used in outflow obstruction such as prostatic hypertrophy. The patient passes urine into a jug that rests on a transducer, which measures millilitres over time. This procedure can then be used as a post-operative baseline comparison to indicate that surgery has improved urinary flow rate.

Uterus The hollow, pear-shaped internal female organ of reproduction. It has three layers: the endometrium, myometrium and parametrium, or peritoneum.

Vagotomy Isolating and dividing the vagus nerve.

Varicose Dilated and tortuous, as of veins.

Vasculitis Inflammation of the blood vessels.

Vasodilatation Relaxation of the smooth muscle in the wall of a blood vessel, thus increasing the size of its lumen.

Ventilation Process enabling oxygenation of the blood.

Ventriculo-atrial/peritoneal shunt CSF is drained away from the ventricles of the brain into either the atrium of the heart or into the peritoneal cavity.

Ventrosuspension Surgically cutting and realigning the ligaments that hold the uterus in place, to correct its position.

Videocystogram A procedure similar to a cystogram that can demonstrate such abnormalities as outflow obstruction or ureteric reflux and therefore be used for diagnostic purposes. In this instance, however, a radio-opaque medium is used to fill the bladder and information is additionally stored on videotape. It has the added advantage that the bladder and urethra are observed on filling and voiding.

Vital signs observations Observations of pulse rate, respiration, blood pressure and, usually intermittently, temperature.

Vitreous Clear jelly-like substance in the cavity inside the eyeball and behind the lens.

Wedge resection Wide local excision with removal of the tumour together with a margin of microscopically normal tissue.

Whipple's procedure A surgical procedure involving resection of the head of the pancreas, the duodenum and the antrum of the stomach. Gastrojejunostomy, choledojejunostomy and pancreatojejunostomy reconstruction are carried out.

Index